HEALTH CARE
WITHOUT
MEDICARE

HEALTH CARE WITHOUT MEDICARE

A New Practice Manual for Community-Based Care Management

Joseph A. Jackson
LICSW, CCM

FOR

Nurses, Social Workers & Therapists
Long-Term Care Managers
Elder Law Attorneys & Finance Specialists
Physicians
Students & Family Caregivers

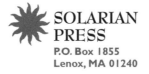

SOLARIAN
PRESS
P.O. Box 1855
Lenox, MA 01240

Solarian Press
P.O. Box 1855
Lenox, MA 01240

Library of Congress Card Number: 00-191374

Jackson, Joseph A.
    Health care without medicare: a new practice manual
for community-based care management/Joseph A. Jackson.

ISBN 0-9702208-0-4

    1. Community Health Services–United States.   2. Health
Self-Care–United States   3. Social Services–United States.
I. Title

Typesetting and Design by Dianne Cooper Bridges
Cover Design by Octavo Designs and Dianne Cooper Bridges

Printed in the United States of America

For my wife, Megan, and my girls, Eliza and Emma.

Table of Contents

xi

Acknowledgements

On January 16, 1999, two doctors, two nurses, a lawyer, two social workers, a financial planner, and a long-term care specialist gathered at my
home to spend a day in retreat to help me write this book. I would like
to extend my thanks to all of the book's contributors, whose willingness
to take a chance, and a long drive to the Berkshires on a winter's day,
made it all possible.

A special thanks to Heather Lorance for her transcription effort,
her patience and her reliability. Thanks to the editors, Janet Benton
and Amy Radbill of Benton Editorial, for their consistency and for
making me look like a writer. And thanks to Eric Bruun for editing that
last chapter. I also wish to acknowledge Fred Swan and Mimi Lewis
and the staff at Springfield Southwest Community Health Center, and
to express my appreciation for their support.

Above all, my thanks to the many home care patients, nursing
home residents, mental health and care-planning clients I have had the
honor to serve over the last two decades. Your faith in me, your
courage, and the risks you took taught me all I know about Community
LifeCare Planning.

Joseph A. Jackson, LICSW, CCM
September, 2000

To The Reader

This book can be used as a reference (buffet-style if you like) or it can be read straight through. Explore as you see fit. The conclusion summarizes the big picture nicely, and may be beneficial to read early. (I actually toyed with putting it in the beginning.) The appendices offer case examples that demonstrate the concepts described in the text. You may wish to use them in workbook fashion to further your learning.

Writing this book has been a rich experience for me personally. I would like to make it the most useful training guide possible and am very interested in your feedback and suggestions for improvement. Please feel free to share them with me.

My email is eldercare@earthlink.net or write to:

Joseph A. Jackson, President
ElderCare Advisors, Inc.
PO Box 1855
Lenox, MA 01240

No longer will older Americans be denied the healing miracle of modern medicine. No longer will illness crush and destroy the savings they have so carefully put away over a lifetime so that they might enjoy dignity in their later years. No longer will young families see their own incomes, and their own hopes, eaten away simply because they are carrying out their deep moral obligations.

– President Lyndon Baines Johnson
1965 Signing Ceremony for
Medicare Legislation

Introduction

Science has enabled all of us to live longer, healthier lives. By any measure, its success has been dramatic. Death by infectious disease is slowly disappearing from the medical landscape. In our trauma centers we are resurrected from injuries, illnesses and conditions that once would have been fatal. Average life expectancy is one and a half times longer today than it was just a century ago. We have all become marvels of modern science.

But our success has its price. As more of us live longer, we are more likely to develop chronic health problems. People with chronic illnesses and accompanying physical impairments, most of whom are over age 65, consume more health care. In the United States in 1999, the measurable cost of direct medical treatment—70 percent of which is given to chronically ill or disabled people—was nearly $1.2 trillion. This equaled approximately 13.5 percent of the U.S. Gross Domestic Product, nearly triple its percentage forty years ago.

It is clear that we can no longer afford the amount and kind of medical treatment on which we have grown so dependent. Our current health care approach is too expensive. And it does not meet the needs of the bulk of health care consumers. Ours is an acute-care system. It was not designed to treat illnesses that do not go away. Yet most consumers of health care services have chronic conditions. Today, we bend the needs of the chronically ill to meet the needs of the system, not the reverse.

Chronic illness requires chronic care. For several reasons, chronic care is not a health care system priority. It is neither high-tech nor high-profit. It isn't emphasized in medical schools, and it doesn't draw a lot of venture capital. But chronic care is the most important and the most overlooked issue in health care today. Unless we figure out how to provide adequate amounts of it, the health care and long-term care systems we have built over the last forty years will fail, because the less chronic care we provide, the more high-tech, high-cost, acute care we are going to need. And the more high-tech care we provide, the less we can afford. A health care system focused solely on acute care is on a one-way, dead end street. If ever a paradigm needed shifting, this is it.

The challenge we face in caring for our frail-elderly, chronically-ill, and disabled citizens will soon become the central political, economic, and ethical dilemma of our time. Many professional caregivers know the crisis is already upon us. It is less a crisis in health care itself than it is a crisis in consciousness. Outdated definitions of both health care and the health care professional's role are greatly to blame for our predicament. The problems can be solved, but first we need to change how we think about health care, prevention, and health care responsibility.

So where do we begin? How do we meet the growing needs of the most vulnerable among us and at the same time pay for the other infrastructures we need to thrive as a society? How do we resolve the conflict that is building between our human-service imperatives and our other societal needs?

As George Orwell wrote in his landmark novel 1984, "If there's hope, it lies in the proles." Our modified health care motto might become, "If there's hope, it lies in the patients." For years we have taught patients and their families a lot about compliance and precious little about self-reliance. Their dependency, the life-blood of our acute-care system, is untenable. It must now be transformed from dependency to interdependency. Patients now need to help their caregivers care for them, not just the reverse.

This book is not about changing our health care system. It is about changing our basic health care approach. It offers a model that empowers caregivers and patients to manage chronic illness and disability and to prevent illness exacerbation and injury outside the boundaries of system-based health care. Unlike system-fix approaches, this book argues for people-based health care that emphasizes the patient-caregiver partnership. It argues, too, that a people-based, preventive mode of care will never develop inside the current system of government programs and private, managed-care arrangements. The system is intractably fixed in a medical treatment paradigm that requires third-party reimbursement. And it appears to be incapable of change.

Chronically-ill and disabled individuals and their caregivers will need guidance if they are to move from system supports (third-party insurance, government subsidies, and so on) to self-supports. This book trains the professionals who will offer this guidance. It advances the premise that through education, counseling, and planning, chronic-care patients and their families can effectively manage most chronic conditions in community rather than medical settings. Better self-care management, coupled with supportive care planning, can prevent the worsening of illness or injury and the costly institutionalization that results. It can lower health care costs for our society, foster continued independence for the chronically ill, and reduce stress and inconvenience for caregivers.

This book is about two distinctly different tasks, care planning and care management. Care planning is to care management what architecture is to construction. They are interdependent and complementary enterprises; most health care and mental health professionals who do both rarely differentiate between the two.

Today, most care planners and care managers provide these services after completing specialized training in one or more health care subspecialties. But while a single, core discipline gives them a good foundation, it only provides the foundation. To become effective, most nurses, social workers, physical therapists, and others will need advanced training in the other lifecare disciplines including estate planning, financial management, insurance, and so on. At the present time, most do not pursue such training; such training hardly exists because few recognize its potential value. This lack of awareness stems primarily from today's restrictive and simplistic definition of health care as medical treatment only.

The knowledge base for long-term care planning comes in relatively equal parts from medical treatment, social work, legal services, financial planning, insurance, and the counseling professions. It also requires knowledge of housing alternatives, architectural modification, and the fast-moving field of supportive technology. The knowledge base for ongoing care management is more heavily weighted toward the clinical skills of medicine, counseling, and medical social work. Indeed, care management is often virtually synonymous with home health care.

In this writing, our aim is to dispel confusion, not to contribute to it. We have chosen to do this by using two terms throughout the book that we believe make sense. **Community LifeCare Planning** refers to the knowledge and skills that care planners and care managers must master if they are to help their chronically ill, impaired, or disabled clients achieve their most often-stated goals. Invariably these goals are to preserve independence (translated as the prevention of hospitalization and nursing-home placements), to preserve assets, and to maintain as comfortable a lifestyle as possible. We use the term **care manager** to refer to the practitioners of Community LifeCare Planning. While we differentiate between care-planning and care-management tasks, it is simply too cumbersome to consistently hyphenate these two references throughout the book.

In choosing the term care manager, we achieve three things. First, throughout the text we are able to distinguish practitioners of CLCP from the lawyers, physicians, accountants, financial planners, long-term care and health care practitioners with whom they collaborate. Second, we avoid the titling game all together and, we hope, offend fewer people in the process. Third, by following the K.I.S.S. rule (Keep It Simple, Stupid), the book is made shorter and easier to read.

Thus, we distinguish the practitioners from the knowledge and skills they need to practice. In so doing, we hope to create legitimacy and an identity for the care-management profession itself. Other theories and approaches will doubtless emerge over the coming years, just as different schools of psychotherapy have. We should welcome this evolution, this development of better ways of achieving good care plans and good care-management outcomes. But while many different types of professionals practice psychotherapy, they often share a core expertise and methodology, regardless of their credentials. Their orientation serves as a base for individual expression. We seek to create a similar foundation for a similarly adaptable profession.

As mentioned above, many professionals practice some variation of Community LifeCare Planning. They include social workers, nurses and physical therapists, as well as non-medical professionals such as paralegals and insurance advocates. When any of these professionals decide to become care managers, they face challenges similar to those faced by the one-event athlete who has decided to become a decathlete. They encounter a new scoring system and a new set of rules. To "win" as care managers, they must develop additional skills and broader capabilities. Community LifeCare Planning is their new field of training.

Community LifeCare Planning (CLCP) is the effort to help frail elders, the chronically ill, and the physically disabled to live in the least restrictive community setting of their choice through the strategic use of personal, family, and community resources. CLCP is always best provided through teamwork, usually by clusters of lifecare professionals. Practicing CLCP involves communication, advocacy, clinical services, education, planning, and advice. The care manager's greatest skill may not be in providing the services themselves, but in connecting clients with the specialists who are best able to help. Community LifeCare Planning is an all-encompassing term. "Community" connotes the broadest venue of practice as well as a sense of social connection and social responsibility. It also implies an all-inclusive approach that combines the ethics and purpose of each profession contributing to it rather than being driven exclusively by medical, psychosocial, legal, insurance, or financial considerations. And combining "community" with the terms "life" and "care" engenders a deeper sense of mission. Most people want to live and be cared for in their communities; today, CLCP is essential to achieving this desire.

This book serves many purposes. It is a training manual for care managers, a primer for a new profession. It fills a training void for those who wish to serve the Community LifeCare Planning effort. But by describing the strategies and skills of CLCP in depth, it also familiarizes the other members of the care planning team—health care, legal, and financial planning professionals—with the team care planning approach. A care manager's goal is most often to help the specialists—the physicians, the lawyers, the financial managers—achieve their goals of maintaining their patient/client's health and independence, while preserving assets and preserving choice. In our view, it is as important for care managers to learn CLCP as it is for all lifecare professionals to understand how they can work together more effectively. And last, but certainly not least, lay caregivers will also benefit greatly from reading this book, as gaining care-management information will help them to help their loved ones.

In preparing this comprehensive guide to CLCP, we have sought contributions from several professionals. Each of these players was set the task of formulating what he or she thinks a good care manager should know about his or her profession. As such, this book is a collaborative effort, just like CLCP itself. It grew out of the cumulative experience of its contributors, leaders in their respective fields who recognize the value of Community LifeCare Planning, and are eager to move the care-management profession from infancy to maturity as quickly as possible.

CLCP clears the way for health care change by challenging notions underlying current care models. It challenges the myth that patients and caregivers are impotent in the face of debilitating illness and a health care system teetering on the brink of collapse. It rethinks the standards of need for institutional care. It puts health care back into the hands of caregivers, patients, and families. And it regards the patient as the true care manager, because people support what they help create.

Ultimately, any health care system is partly an arbitrary arrangement. Our current system is a work in progress; it did not exist a hundred years ago, nor will it exist in its present form a hundred years from now. But the essence of health care is now and will always remain the expression of compassion between one human being and another. Human compassion is at once the foundation of healing and the most common thread of our evolution. Its expression provides all the quality improvement we need. Without it, there is no health care "system;" there is no care.

CHAPTER I

The Fundamentals of Community LifeCare Planning

Community LifeCare Planning (CLCP) is the strategic use of personal, familial, and community resources to prevent long-term institutional placement among the chronically ill. A basic tenet of CLCP is that the medical stability of many individuals with chronic health problems is as much determined by their behavior, knowledge of their condition, sense of self-efficacy, and chronic-care resources as it is by the severity of their illness. CLCP is a form of "lifecare" that includes medical treatment and non-medical care planning as equally critical to the short-term recovery, ongoing support, and long-term wellness of the chronically ill.

Whether we are well or ill, we all make decisions that determine the state of our health. Our psychology, emotions, and behavior drive the decisions we make. The lifecare decisions made by those with chronic illness and disability can determine whether they recover or decline, whether they live comfortably or uncomfortably, and whether they remain independent or become institutionalized.

For example, a stroke patient who is unable or unwilling to acknowledge his sudden disability may refuse short-term personal care from a home health aide. He may refuse to apply for long-term help from a community support program or to install a handrail in his shower or bathtub. This attitude can have medical consequences; might put him at risk for a hip fracture (due to the increased risk of a fall), an infection (due to increased risk of developing a bedsore), or to medication toxicity (due to the increased likelihood of inaccurate compliance), and so on. Whatever the outcome, difficulty adjusting to the sudden loss of independence creates significant obstacles to recovery from illness and maintaining medical stability.

In such a circumstance, non-medical interventions may lead to more favorable medical outcomes. Counseling, for example, may help this person acknowledge his disability and increase receptivity to support. He may accede to some home modifications, and may even accept some help with personal care. Advice from an elder law attorney may relieve his worry that he will automatically lose his home (or his children's bequest) if he enrolls in a state-subsidized, long-term care program. Financial planning may lead to the more efficient use of resources to support his stability and progress at home.

Time and time again we see that health care is not all medical. Community LifeCare Planning addresses both medical and non-medical lifecare interventions. CLCP is at once a service, a profession, a skill, and a body of knowledge. It completes our understanding of what supports wellness by acknowledging the influence of social systems on healing. These influential factors include finance, law, insurance, and housing, as well as those professions more traditionally associated with health care, namely medicine, counseling and social services.

WHY CLCP NOW?

Community-based, long-term care is more complicated today than it used to be. Not so long ago, most people with chronic illnesses, physical disabilities, and life-limiting conditions lived with their families until they died. People took care of themselves. When illness progressed to the level of incapacity, physicians would often say, "There is nothing more that we can do." In the not-too-distant past, chronic conditions progressed to complications and death far more rapidly than they do today.

Many, perhaps even most people who are advanced in age and/or have disabilities now live alone and far from their families. Unlike in times past, however, when they become so frail they can no longer fend for themselves, more often than not they hear from their physicians, "There's plenty more we can do!" We have made incredible progress in the delivery of health care and long-term care services. Double knee and hip replacement surgeries, coronary artery bypass surgeries, sophisticated combinations of chemotherapy, radiation therapy, and surgeries for the most virulent of cancers—all are commonplace. Housing options for those unable to be self-sustaining abound. For many, they compensate for the fact that family caregiving arrangements are less common than in the past. Aside from nursing homes, there are assisted living facilities, independent living facilities, continuing-care retirement communities, congregate care homes, intermediate care facilities, senior care homes, board and care homes—you name it. Today, there *is* plenty more we can do.

In the last few generations, health care and lifecare options for the elderly and the disabled have been subsidized from one main revenue source—taxes. Tax revenues have been channeled through three main social programs—Social Security, Medicare, and Medicaid. Through income supports, Social Security has provided some financial resources to those most at risk for needing chronic care—those over age 65 and those with disabling chronic conditions. Medicare and Medicaid have given nearly carte blanche medical treatment options to retirees, the physically disabled, and the poor. The result has been a near miraculous increase in longevity and quality of life for those with chronic health problems.

Yet nowhere in our health care or social service systems have we developed adequate decision-making supports to help people manage the complexities of modern-day, long-term care planning. Nor do we adequately teach people with chronic conditions how to better manage their illnesses so they can stay out of the medical treatment system. Hospitals, nursing homes, rehabilitation facilities, and home care agencies are paid to take care of people while they are sick; they don't help them plan how to stay well.

And a form of institutional codependency subverts the health care system's mission. Hospitals, physicians' offices, nursing homes, and home care agencies will usually provide only what their pay sources will oblige. Health care payers, namely for-profit managed care companies and public, not-for-profit programs (Medicare/Medicaid) remain steeped in their medical treatment focus. For 35 years it's been a relatively neat arrangement, but it is beginning to fail.

Both health care providers and health care payers acknowledge the importance of illness and injury prevention, but they provide very little education or prevention planning services. Case management as provided by health care payers is less a long-term care planning service than an effort to reduce exposure to claims. Insurance company case managers, most of whom are former bedside nurses, work to analyze and contain costs through utilization review. On the provider side, especially in hospitals, ever-shorter lengths of stay give hospital-based case managers and discharge planners very little time to do much planning at all. Subsequently, when the patient leaves the hospital, he or she is referred to a home care agency and/or the social service system. But home care is cutting back dramatically under the managed care approach recently imposed through the Medicare benefit, and nurses have very little time to do more than bring the patient back to a stable condition before they discharge. Long-term care planning and medical social work figures into the home care effort only at the margins. Outside the medical treatment system, community social services, mostly provided by state-sponsored elder and/or disability services case managers, don't so much offer planning as eligibility determination. And social service workers are asked to help people meet their medical care needs with little or no training in medical management. In short, we are left with an outmoded medical treatment/reimbursement system, onerous long-term care caseloads, and confusion about professional roles in both the health care and the social service systems. Nowhere do we offer adequately the time-consuming personal attention that chronically-ill individuals living in communities need to plan for wellness.

Where do people turn when they need lifecare assistance? Lawyers serve capably as estate planners; financial planners help with investment; physicians treat illness when it arises; but where can chronically-ill or disabled people turn if they wish to pull all the pieces together?

Increasingly, they are calling upon independent care managers. Care managers who practice CLCP offer an effective response to the growing need for guidance and decision-making assistance among the chronically ill, the physically disabled, and their families. They reconcile the growing discrepancy between what the health care system can provide (and what it needs to offer to remain solvent) and what chronically ill individuals need (and need to do) to stay well. Care managers serve as a bridge from the third party reimbursement model for acute care to a health care system/patient partnership that emphasizes self-reliance, self-care management and chronic-care planning.

CLCP addresses the broadest spectrum of influences on long-term care planning and medical stability for those most at risk for illness and injury. These considerations fall into the following general categories: Medical, Personal (which includes psychological, behavioral, emotional, and spiritual considerations), Socio-interactive (which includes family systems, legal advocacy, and community support services), Financial (which includes financial planning and management, insurance, and family financial support) and Environmental (which includes home modification, caregiving arrangements, and assistive devices).

A care manager must be an experienced specialist in at least one of these broad categories. He or she must also be well versed in all of the remaining categories. Yet CLCP is an interdisciplinary approach. Nurses cannot supply all its services by themselves, nor can lawyers, financial planners, CPAs, or medical social workers. Effective care planning and management requires a team effort.

THE KNOWLEDGE AND SKILLS OF CLCP

Maintaining medical stability for those with chronic health problems is as much a matter of acquiring and using resources as it is a clinical challenge. It makes sense, therefore, that someone should serve to link resource professionals with the treatment professionals. Care managers familiar with the lifecare planning professions serve as effective coordinators and communicators within the lifecare team.

Aside from the resource planning professionals—estate-planning attorney, financial advisor, insurance agent, accountant, and perhaps a trust officer—the care-planning team almost always includes a client's family members along with an array of medical treatment professionals and counselors. CLCP weaves these services together. It is also broadly applicable across the socioeconomic spectrum. It is useful to those with considerable financial means as well as to those who cannot afford the more expensive advice of attorneys and accountants. For low- to middle-income clients, a care manager can approximate some of the services of an estate planner, an insurance consultant, a financial planner, and more, while introducing clients to the possible need for focused services from these specialists. A care manager thereby increases the effectiveness of limited resources by educating clients of lesser means less expensively, then bringing in specialists for more defined purposes.

Let's take a look now at the categories of consideration listed above to see how CLCP promotes recovery and expedites caregiving for those that need it most.

MEDICAL SERVICES

Fundamental to the practice of CLCP is its focus on facilitating recovery for those who are sick, and on preventing illness and injury for those most at risk. Familiarity with medical treatment is the *sine qua non* of CLCP. Care managers serve as both client advocates and members of the caregiving team.

Frail elderly, chronically ill, and physically disabled people are vulnerable to all manner of ailment and injury. Skin tears, bedsores, fractures, infections, chronic, progressive system failures, and many other medical difficulties present a myriad of risks for those with a tenuous hold on health. Care managers must be knowledgeable about medical treatment systems in all venues—MD offices, hospitals, rehabilitation facilities, home health care agencies and nursing homes—if they are to be effective at prevention. They must be comfortable interacting with both specialized and generalist health care professionals. They must be familiar with health care regulations, public and private reimbursement systems, and the general criteria by which health care organizations determine both eligibility for and cessation of treatment.

Having served as medical social workers, nurses, and physical therapists, most care managers are already familiar with medical treatment systems and medical-surgical care planning. They have good firsthand knowledge of how the health care system does and doesn't work. Indeed, it is as important for care managers to understand how things go wrong in our health care system as it is for them to know how they are supposed to go right—an academic understanding of health care is not sufficient.

Care managers' experience leads them to approach the health care system with a healthy mix of respect and alertness. Care managers must recognize that, despite all of the highly credentialed professionals and bells and whistles of modern medicine, things don't always turn out the way they should. Hard working, competent, compassionate health care professionals can make mistakes. Patients can suffer as a result. While most hospital and nursing home stays are warranted by people's existing conditions, care managers believe that many, perhaps most hospitalizations and nursing home placements among those with chronic conditions are preventable. And once someone is in the health care system, a care manager can offer support for the patient and the health care professionals alike through education, counseling, and advocacy to come up with creative discharge planning options needed to help that person return home safely.

The simple truth is that today, health care professionals do not have the time to cover all of the bases their patients need covered. Because of this, many people are either discharged too soon or are sent to more restrictive settings than might otherwise have been possible. Care managers work as advocates for patients, whether by expediting a discharge from a hospital, a nursing home, or a rehabilitation facility or by advocating *against* discharge until a sufficient discharge plan is in place. In part, then, the benefit of a care manager's assistance turns on his or her ability to maneuver within the system during crisis periods.

There are four main CLCP objectives that make medical treatment and health care system knowledge instrumental to its practice: enhancing a client's sense of empowerment, client advocacy, efficient care planning, and accurate care planning.

Client Empowerment

Decision-making is hard enough when we actually understand what is happening and when the consequences of our decisions are somewhat predictable. Yet for most patients and their families, the health care system presents a bewildering array of circumstances that serve only to confuse, not clarify the decision-making process. For most people, even the language of medicine, let alone the rationale by which treatment is authorized or denied is gobbledygook. Care managers fulfill the role of interpreter for families and patients who need the in-depth information that health care providers have so little time to give. In the midst of a major medical treatment episode, families and patients are full of questions. What opportunities for recovery are available in a home care setting as opposed to a rehabilitation hospital? What preparations should be made before discharge to a home care setting, to assisted living, or to a nursing home? Will an estate-planning attorney's help be able to protect life savings from the exorbitant cost of nursing home care. What, they ask, are we to do?

Such questions challenge patients and their families. Suddenly, what was once the *possible* need for long-term care becomes an immediate need. Through teaching and guidance, care managers work to empower clients and their families to make good decisions. They work to reduce clients' anxiety and to decode the language and culture of the health care system. They seek to help clients learn to shape the long-term care process rather than having the process shape them.

Client Advocacy

In many instances, the health care machine works against a client's best interests. There are several reasons for this. Many health care professionals are less familiar with care planning in community settings than in institutional settings. Too often their best advice, although offered out of true concern for their patient's welfare, may not include the custodial-care options that can be created through CLCP, which can include strategic estate planning and financial planning. They may not recommend or even be aware of options such as privately paid live-in services, Medicaid waivers, community-based home care supports, and so on. Many fundamental skills of CLCP are simply outside the scope of their practice.

Time is also a problem. Health care professionals—in all venues and all disciplines—are under constant pressure to provide more care in less time. For many physicians, physician assistants, and nurse practitioners, nursing home placement is the quickest, least risky, least labor-intensive way to solve a complicated care-planning challenge.

Finally, and most unfortunately, nursing homes have no financial incentive for discharging residents into creative, community lifecare circumstances. Nursing home staff are focused on two things—providing care and maintaining census. Nursing homes go out of business if too many beds are unoccupied. And their incentive to discharge residents who are privately paying for nursing home care (at higher per diem rates than those who are publicly subsidized) is especially low. Ironically, these residents have the richest selection of community lifecare opportunities because of their more abundant resources.

Advocating for the least restrictive lifecare options requires that the care manager have a sophisticated understanding of both the capabilities and the limitations of today's health care system. The care manager must understand how a health care professional's perspective colors his or her decision-making. This enables the care manager to more effectively build support among medical treatment professionals for alternatives that might not otherwise have been considered.

As a client advocate, the care manager consults, negotiates, and serves alongside health care professionals. Without the care manager's understanding of the language of health care, communication between the patient, his or her family, the health care providers and the care manager is impaired and advocacy is less effective. If health care professionals perceive the care manager as a member of the treatment team who is working in support of the team's goals, they will be more receptive to his or her input. Here again, familiarity with medical treatment, with the language of medicine, and with the machinations of the health care system is the care manager's stock-in-trade.

Care Planning Efficiency

Efficiency is defined by the amount of energy expended in achieving a goal. The efficiency with which a care manager moves a client through the care-planning process can make or break a plan. Care managers must be able to help clients understand the risks associated with chronic conditions, the care-planning options, and the probability of success associated with each option. And they must be able to do so quickly. A good care manager, then, is an effective, low-cost communicator. The care manager's ability to ensure that all members of the life-care planning team are "on the same page" can expedite decision making and greatly improve a care plan's effectiveness.

Coordination is the key to care planning efficiency. Coordinated care planning promotes holism—the effect is greater than the sum of each team member's contributions. Without care plan coordination, time and money is wasted as care plan team members pull the client in different directions. For example, an attorney unfamiliar with a community-based, long-term care Medicaid waiver may draft an estate plan that actually undermines a client's eligibility. The care manager can help the attorney see that without the resources this program offers, a family's and physician's concerns about client safety in the community cannot be allayed. A different estate plan, developed through care planning coordination, permits eventual community program eligibility enabling the physician to postpone an otherwise avoidable nursing home placement.

A care manager must master the art of the two-minute consultation. High-priced professionals measure their time with the secondhand on their stopwatch. To facilitate care planning efficiency, the care manager must be able to communicate quickly, effectively, and in a manner that assures physicians, lawyers, financial planners, and so on, that time spent talking with the care manager was time well spent. They must be left with a clear understanding of the value-added benefit that CLCP has for both their client/patient and themselves.

Care Planning Accuracy

The care planning effort regularly brings several people together to accomplish a complicated task. Imagine how difficult it would be to plan if each of them spoke a different language. Without an interpreter what would be the chances of success? How could everyone have an accurate understanding of the physician's and nurse's treatment goals, the estate plan, the financial objectives, and the client's hopes and fears?

It is the care manager's job to facilitate this understanding, to serve as a kind of multi-lingual interpreter ensuring continuity of effort within the care planning team. The care manager helps the physician understand the family dynamics, helps the lawyer understand likely medical treatment outcomes, helps the financial planner understand the costs associated with future care needs, and guides the family and client toward understanding the likely benefits of better resource management and community program eligibility. Ultimately, the care manager helps everyone understand how the client's rehabilitation potential is affected by *all* of these concerns. Clarity of understanding within the care plan team creates synergy, a unified purpose, efficiency of effort, and increases the likelihood of success.

PERSONAL ISSUES

Today, the broadening focus on wellness and prevention is the most potent force for change in health care. But wellness maintenance and prevention for those with chronic conditions requires that patients learn to manage their own care better. Those who seek to help chronically ill individuals live a healthier life despite their disabilities must therefore understand the *person*. They must understand how emotions, behavior, spirituality, and social context influence a person's life.

For years the effort to incorporate psychosocial influences into medical treatment has been the purview of medical social work. Medical social work is a subspecialty of the social work profession that combines social work and medical treatment skills in support of wellness. Medical social workers have served as the glue that bonds the "community"–local, state, federal, and private support programs–to the person in recovery. They have also woven psychotherapy, supportive counseling, bereavement counseling, and so on into the fabric of medical treatment and palliative care.

Clearly this work is crucial. Yet, with the advent of managed care, medical social work has become marginalized. As managed care arrangements authorize less and less treatment, people find themselves more anxious and more depressed. Consequently, they are more at risk and more in need of counseling support and community connection.

CLCP provides these personal dimensions of health care. And, as no care-planning or care-management effort succeeds without the involvement and support of the beneficiary, CLCP develops a plan *with* clients, not *for* them. It is essential, therefore, that a care manager is highly skilled in interpersonal communication and that he or she can motivate and enable intrapersonal change. A care manager must have a mature awareness of the developmental milestones that govern the client's sense-of-self and his or her behaviors and motivations, as well as of the impact of one's spiritual life on decision-making. Without this awareness, the care manager will not succeed in engaging clients in the difficult emotional and psychological work that anyone challenged by chronic illness or disability must face. A care manager's perception of the client and definition of the client's problems is shaped by his or her ability to see clients as people, as well as patients.

SOCIO-INTERACTIVE CONCERNS

Human beings are socio-interactive. We interact with one another, and with groups of others, within a social context. At the same time, we create the social context within which we interact. Society affects each of us, and each of us affects society.

All of us live within a set of social boundaries, some clear, some not so clear. Laws, mores, social expectations, and personal expectations circumscribe our lives, affecting us physically, emotionally, and spiritually.

People want to feel secure, for themselves and for their children, especially when illness or disability strikes. How they feel affects the course of illness as significantly as any consideration. A client's fear that his or her last will and testament may not be carried out, for instance, affects his or her physical and emotional well being. Too much anxiety about financial security disturbs sleep, appetite, and metabolism as immediately as noncompliance with a medication regimen does. There is no mind-body split. Likewise, there is no mind-body-society split. Therefore, a care manager must take the client's social circumstances into account in developing the best possible care plan.

Care managers need to know how to guide individuals through social systems. This requires knowledge of a broad array of laws and regulations governing access to social supports. It requires an understanding of how society is set up to care for us when we become sick, and to manage our estates after we die.

Legal Advocacy

In every phase of our lives, laws proscribe our opportunities and our behavior. We impose our collective will on ourselves by statute. The laws that enable or restrict an individual's long-term care opportunities focus primarily on either the use or collection of personal and social resources. Care managers advising someone about how to obtain community support for chronic care must be familiar with both community support programs and the estate planning strategies that can enable access to them. This is the realm of what is now called elder law.

Elder law attorneys serve primarily as advocates for the elderly, but because of their knowledge of long-term care systems, they also serve people with chronic illnesses or disabilities. A significant amount of their work has consisted of providing estate-planning services to protect their clients' assets and to help clients qualify for Medicaid benefits. Elder law has become in many ways a long-term care service. The growing number of elders, coupled with their steadily diminishing health care benefits, ensures that more and more people will turn their attentions to estate planning as they reach their golden years.

Indeed, most CLCP clients will be elderly—over age 65, if not over 75. Most will be either currently or imminently disabled; most will be apprehensive about their futures and anxious to prevent their life savings from being consumed by the costs of long-term care. Most of these clients wish to remain free and independent and to leave a legacy for their children and their children's children. Estate planning with an elder law attorney helps to secure these most fervently held wishes, and a care manager must understand how the elder law attorney goes about doing so. He or she must also be able to interpret the immediate impact that estate planning can have on the client's short- and long-term medical stability—for attorney and client alike.

Once the preserve of the wealthy, estate planning is fast becoming a service for the middle class as well. A ranch house and $50,000 may not be millions, but it is well worth protecting. For those who have assets to protect but are unaccustomed to paying $175 per hour for anything, a care manager can interpret the value of such focused legal services and do the groundwork to expedite the process.

But estate-planning considerations may be irrelevant for many in need of chronic-care planning. What good is an estate plan if you have no estate? For those with average or below average incomes and few assets, CLCP practitioners offer an affordable long-term care planning option. Care managers can serve as a lower-cost connection to community support services that provide care to those who can't pay for their continuing-care needs. The care manager should therefore be capable of providing medical social services, whether directly or by referring the client to a community-based, medical social work professional.

Community Support Services

Medicare and Medicaid cutbacks are reducing home health care and rehabilitation services significantly. In this formula, medical social work services are minimized, if they are provided at all. Medical social workers, adept at connecting people to the community support services that help maintain wellness, have less opportunity to ply their trade. And, even when they are utilized by health care organizations, they increasingly find that the community resources they are so adept at connecting people to are disappearing as well.

Social work is a kind of brokerage service for community largesse. As budgets tighten, states will be less able to provide the services, let alone the service brokers. But our communities have not entirely abandoned the needy, and community support services, while less liberally furnished than in the recent past, will continue to exist for low- and average-income citizens. Care managers practicing CLCP will fill this service-access niche for many middle-income people willing to pay for the services once liberally subsidized by state and federal programs, Medicare, and Medicaid.

CLCP can be affordable for most people who fit the profile of the average Social Security beneficiary—someone with $800 per month in Social Security income and less than $50,000 in assets. Here again, we confront the question of value. A social services case manager, overwhelmed by an often unmanageable caseload, may not be able to find the time to develop a thorough long-term care plan for his or her community-dwelling, elderly/disabled client. The client might do well to hire someone who can. If a private care manager can find a way to help someone preserve his or her independence for even a few months longer, would this not be as valuable as so many services for which we pay without much hesitation, such as a car tune-up, home modification, or a lawyer-drafted power of attorney? Where the system cannot help us, we do well to help ourselves. Among the chronically ill, illness exacerbation and injuries occur as much from lack of resources and information as from illness itself.

FINANCIAL PLANNING

A care manager must alert his or her client to the possibility that different financial arrangements may create more favorable long-term care options. A care manager should be able to recognize when and how a client's investment portfolio could use some help. More fundamentally, he or she must understand how a client's financial resources can be spent most effectively to meet the client's needs. But it is not enough to assess current and future needs. Without some financial-planning acumen, a care manager will not understand the most effective way for available resources to satisfy unmet need. And the care manager could simply create more anxiety if he or she cannot help the client immediately understand his or her resource limitations or opportunities.

This is not meant to imply that a care manager must become a certified financial planner. The care manager passes the baton to the financial planner, bringing him or her a more receptive, better-educated client. Understanding and recognizing investment options is one way the care manager develops long-term care options.

Investment strategies, asset transfers, tax considerations, and so on, play into the long-term care planning process for most of the Medicare beneficiaries who own their homes or have savings. In general, these concerns have not typically fallen within the purview of case management (offered by health insurers), discharge planning (provided by health care facilities), or community resource linkage services (offered by medical social workers). Nurses and social workers offering these services have inquired into a person's financial situation only to determine eligibility for social programs and Medicaid waivers. Moreover, they have done so mostly in an era of liberal health care benefits paid for by Medicare.

As the ratio of working taxpayers to those in need of chronic care shrinks, the community support programs and public insurance benefits that help them will also shrink. Discharge planners in health care (primarily nurses and medical social workers), skilled at linking patients with community resources will find these skills less and less relevant to the task of helping patients meet their continuing-care needs in community settings. They will need to be further trained in Community LifeCare Planning to help their clients utilize their own resources effectively. Their ability to understand financial planning options as they impact long-term care will become indispensable to the work of preventing hospitalizations and nursing home placements.

Insurance

In our current system, groups—not individuals—pay for health care. At the time of this writing, Medicare serves nearly 45 million people, but an even larger group, comprised of both the beneficiaries themselves and the nation's wage earners (some 145 million people) funds it. Care managers must understand group-supported financial resources such as public and private health insurance, long-term care insurance, life insurance and viatical settlements. Insurance advocacy and guidance is the flip side of developing an effective personal financial strategy.

Insurance is a financial resource managed by a complex system of eligibility determination and utilization review, designed mostly to restrict the disbursement of limited funds. Care managers must be capable advocates for clients who need help submitting insurance claims and getting them paid when they are entitled to benefits. A care manager's effectiveness depends on the depth of his or her understanding of a beneficiary's health care or long-term care coverage. With the advent of long-term care insurance, the definition of health care will broaden to include chronic care.

Familial Support

When people plan long-term care they often overlook a third category of financial resources that was once the first line of defense—direct cash outlays and co-housing arrangements provided by friends or family. The care manager must regard these caregivers as invaluable sources of both emotional *and* financial support.

The day is fast approaching when more and more adult children will hear a line that has become almost taboo: "You may need to consider bringing Mom or Dad into your home." Long-term care has stood firmly on two pillars for years. The first, Medicare-subsidized home health and rehabilitative care, has recently been drastically reduced. For decades Medicare recipients have received liberal amounts of personal care assistance for their chronic-care needs at home. But home health care agencies can no longer provide these levels of care despite their patients' continued eligibility and need. Caps on the amount of care they can bill to Medicare have recently been imposed forcing them to cut services to their most needy chronically-ill patients. Once-commonplace weekly levels of care—20-plus hours of home health aide assistance, 3-plus hours of nursing, 3-plus hours of physical therapy, and 1-plus hours of medical social work, in some cases provided for a period of years—have all but disappeared. And similar cuts have hit the rehabilitation hospitals and sub-acute-care facilities. Federal belt-tightening has eliminated Medicare-subsidized custodial care in both homes and rehabilitation facilities from the long-term care formula.

The second pillar of long-term care, Medicaid-subsidized nursing home care, will soon crumble as well. Medicaid, which is administered and partially funded by state governments, will inevitably cut nursing home benefits as the demand for nursing home payments outstrips the supply of tax dollars. Unlike the federal government, states cannot fund anything on a deficit. They are constitutionally bound to balance their budgets, cannot pay on credit, and cannot print money.

What will we do as the pay source for custodial care in the home *and* the institution dries up? We will do what many did before Medicare and Medicaid existed: take our sick relatives home with us. As Medicare and Medicaid are whittled away, familial resources will become even more central to the long-term care equation. Adult children of chronically-ill parents, and the spouses and family members of those with disabilities will confront the possibility that there is no "room at the inn" for their loved ones.

Care managers can help families confront caregiving challenges when parental assets have been liquidated, when the Medicare home care budget has been exhausted, when there is no admitting diagnosis for the hospital, and when there is a waiting list for the state's long-term care Medicaid program. They guide families to long-term care solutions that utilize their own resources, not the state's or the federal government's. Care managers help by combining skills in resource planning and counseling. They offer clients an opportunity to adjust to and plan for challenges they never expected to face.

ENVIRONMENTAL RESOURCES

Most people with chronic health problems consider the home the venue of choice for long-term care. Yet for someone whose mobility is compromised and whose sight and hearing may be impaired, the home can be a help or a hindrance. The architecture of chronic care brings new meaning to the famed Chicago architect Louis Sullivan's dictum that "form follows function."

The safety and comfort of those with chronic, debilitating conditions often depends on environmental adaptation. A care manager should conceive of a client's living environment as dynamic, not static. Disability is usually progressive, and just as the required level of personal care tends to change over time, so should the home of a chronically ill individual.

The chronic-care environment must therefore be intelligent and responsive. It must accommodate the assistive devices and durable medical equipment that serve the disabled, chronically-ill, or injured person. The care manager must recognize the opportunity to create supportive environments for chronically ill persons and to find professionals to design and construct these modifications. The physics and mechanics of disability, then, are central to Community LifeCare Planning.

Knowing how to adapt an environment to meet the needs of a disabled individual requires both knowledge of the latest advances in assistive technology as well as good old-fashioned, hardware-store know-how. The care manager must be as familiar with the advantages of telemedicine, computerized pharmaceutical dispensers, home care monitoring devices, and sophisticated disability-support machines as he or she is with wheelchair ramps, hallway handrails, and shower stall grab bars. Care managers must also be skilled at acquiring the necessary adaptive equipment and arranging for home modification through either insurance, personal, or community resources. The right piece of equipment, communication device, or architectural modification can make the difference between independence and institutionalization.

SYNOPSIS

Ideally, community lifecare plans are developed in teams. A single professional cannot write the estate plan; manage the investments; write the prescriptions; provide the counseling, nursing, and personal care services; and so on. Neither is any physician, lawyer, financial planner, nurse, psychotherapist, nor social worker appropriately qualified to help his or her client/patient weigh every one of these long-term care considerations. And it is unlikely that the higher-priced professionals in this lifecare group—lawyers, physicians, and accountants—will cross train to become lower-cost care-planning professionals who are as familiar with community resources and adjustment-to-loss counseling as they are with law, medicine, or tax calculations.

Making decisions that provide for the long-term care needs of a chronically-ill individual requires specialized information. More often than not, clients and their family members must be eased into the process. This preliminary orientation/education phase of long-term care planning—often a time-consuming phase—is best provided by a sophisticated foot soldier. The care manager is familiar with each major system that affects a person with a chronic illness or disability who is struggling to maintain community-life options. As such, the care manager's perspective is unique in a world of specialized professionals. The care manager's goal is to avoid tunnel vision–to avoid the misperceptions of the proverbial blind men, each of whom describes the elephant as either trunk, leg, tusk, or ear, depending upon which part each is touching.

The art of Community LifeCare Planning develops from the care manager's broad, unprejudiced perception and understanding of life's many stressors. The following chapters clarify the building blocks of this perception.

CHAPTER 2

The Health Care System

The health care crisis we currently face is analogous to the phenomenon of global warming. One of the predicted symptoms of global warming is a rise in sea level as the ice sheets melt. Algorithmic calculations show how much the sea level is expected to rise in response to projected rises in the average global temperature. This temperature rise, and the heightened sea level it creates, first will manifest in weather pattern changes that will make extraordinary storms both more commonplace and far more damaging. Storm surges will cause more significant flooding and the inundation of low-lying, often densely populated land. We don't realize how much trouble we're in until the storm is upon us.

The crisis in health care is building in a similar fashion. In global warming terms, health care's "sea level" is measured by the prevalence of chronic illness in the population—the higher the incidence of chronic illness, the greater the need for health care. Sixty percent of disability and chronic illness in the U.S. population exists in those above age 65. While those over age 65 currently comprise 13 percent of the population, the population of some rural American counties has already reached 25 percent over the age of 65—the anticipated national average by 2050. Many other regions are well above average. For example, in Berkshire County, Massachusetts, 18 percent of the population is over the age of 65, which is expected to be the national average by the year 2025.

The consequence of this growth in chronic illness within the population hits the health care system in a fashion similar to the extraordinary storms mentioned above. Consider the flu epidemic of 1999, which hit New England especially hard. At the flu epidemic's height, the acuity level of the patients in one Massachusetts hospital was so high that a veteran ICU nurse triaged the same bed four times in one night—meaning that someone sicker came in to the hospital, or someone already in the hospital became sicker than the patient just received into ICU. At the same time, there was a five-hour wait in the emergency room for a chest X-ray. Already filled with a high "sea level" of chronic illness, the flu epidemic washed into this hospital like a Tsunami. It couldn't handle the sudden inundation of acute illness because it was filled to capacity beforehand.

The number of people with chronic illnesses and physical disabilities is growing very quickly. Today, nearly 5 percent of the U. S. population is unable to perform one or more Activities of Daily Living (ADLs). Over thirteen million U. S. citizens are unable to do one or more basic activities alone, such as walking, bathing, eating, dressing, or using the toilet. The health care system is struggling with the intractable problem of caring for them.

But our health care system is not set up to provide chronic care. Nor is it designed to prevent the exacerbation of chronic illness. It is set up only to care for those who become ill enough to need "treatment." But as more and more of us need chronic care (the health care equivalent of the sea level rise described above), hospitals will become bottlenecks through which fewer and fewer will comfortably pass.

Several system "fixes" are currently well underway. They are supported by extensive data collection and outcome measurements, system analyses informing Medicare and Medicaid revisions and managed care arrangements, and a panoply of well-reasoned reforms. These will make a dent in the problem, but most are focused only on the acute care we actually provide in hospitals, rehabilitation facilities, home care agencies and physicians' offices. Acute care is a piece of the action, but not all of it.

Our health care system is itself in ICU. Thus we should not minimize the importance of health care system fixes. We need a thriving, effective health care system. But to achieve this we must rethink how those most likely to consume health care—our infirm, disabled, and chronically ill citizens—access the chronic-care services they need. The delivery of acute care will become less costly and more manageable if we not only fix the system that provides this type of care, but also change the behavior of those receiving most of the health care treatment in the United States. A consciousness shift toward prevention-minded self-care management among those who consume the most expensive medical treatment will deliver the greatest results for our efforts. Chronically-ill patients and their professional and informal caregivers need a bridge to better self-care management and a new kind of patient/caregiver partnership.

In the words of Fritz Perls, founder of Gestalt therapy, "Awareness is curative." We begin building our awareness of the changes needed in how we provide health care by examining our health care system, a system whose greatest imperative must now be the successful prevention of illness and injury among the chronically ill and disabled.

THE HEALTH CARE SYSTEM

Today's health care system is a care-continuum that begins with the physician's office and progresses from hospital, to rehabilitation facility, to home health care, to nursing home. At last count, we were able to identify thirty-six levels of care currently available in this country:

1) Acute Care
2) Observation Unit Care
3) Swing Beds
4) Emergency Department Care
5) Ambulatory Care
6) Short Stay Unit Care
7) Same Day Surgery
8) Outpatient Surgery
9) Hospital Clinic
10) Free Standing Clinic
11) Urgent Care
12) Inpatient Rehabilitation
13) Acute Rehabilitation
14) Outpatient Rehabilitation
15) Ambulatory Infusion Clinic (AIC)
16) Occupational Health Care
17) School Health Care
18) Home Health Care
19) Home Infusion Care
20) Hospice Care
21) Respite Care
22) Adult Day Care
23) Physician Office Care
24) Partial Hospitalization
25) Day Hospital Care
26) Nurse Based Clinic
27) Correctional Facility Clinic
28) Skilled Nursing Facility Care
29) Intermediate Care Facility Services
30) Pharmacy Benefits Management
31) Women's Health Center Care
32) Medical Foster Care
33) Self-Care
34) Family Care
35) Subacute Care
36) Transitional Care

This list shows how complex our health care delivery system has become. In the years prior to 1983, when the hospital acute-care setting was the center of health care delivery, the options for entry into the health care system were somewhat limited. Continuing health care services were more or less restricted to a nursing home or to home health care where the care was focused more on custodial care rather than interventional services.

A BRIEF HISTORY OF HEALTH CARE

The recent history of health care is the history of government-administered health insurance. In 1965, Medicare and Medicaid were signed into law. The impact of these two programs on the development of our current health care system cannot be overemphasized. Many medical treatments considered commonplace today either didn't exist or existed only for the extremely wealthy prior to 1965. When Title XVIII (the statute that authorized the Medicare program) and Title XIX (the statute authorizing Medicaid) were enacted into law, the average life expectancy of an American man was 65 years of age. Today the average life expectancy of an American man is 74; an American woman can expect to live to age 79. It is probably safe to say that no single development in health care is more responsible for our incredible success at prolonging life than the Medicare and Medicaid programs.

Medicare and Medicaid were enacted as titles; all Americans eligible for these programs became *en*titled. The significance of this is important to appreciate: A government program to which all eligible citizens are entitled has no spending caps. So, for over thirty years no significant cost controls were imposed on a health care system that rapidly grew to depend on reimbursement under the Medicare and Medicaid programs. Not only did the system come to rely on public subsidy, but our population also grew to expect it. A population entitled became a population justified in demanding all manner of treatments and surgical procedures.

Following the creation of Medicare and Medicaid, the story of health care became the story of how these programs were modified. In 1974, a significant development occurred in health care with the passage of the Employee Retirement Income Security Act (ERISA). ERISA marked the beginning of medical management, utilization review and outcomes monitoring. Then, in 1980, the Omnibus Budget Reconciliation Act (OBRA) repealed the three-day prior hospitalization required to establish home care eligibility for Medicare beneficiaries. In 1982 the Tax Equity and Fiscal Responsibility Act (TEFRA) was enacted, establishing Diagnostic Related Groups commonly referred to as DRGs. Through TEFRA, and nearly twenty years after the inception of Medicare, the federal government began to review and control the length of hospital stays. The message to the Medicare patient was clear: Medicare is cutting back.

Shortened hospital stays dramatically changed the delivery of health care leading to the birth of a burgeoning alternative-care market that especially addressed the long-term care sector. Functional assessment tools, notably those developed by Katz in his work titled

"Assessing Self-maintenance: Activities of Daily Living, Mobility, and Instrumental Activities of Daily Living" (1983) were being developed. Functional assessments targeted the growing field of long-term care in the community.

In 1983, there were two primary types of alternate or long-term care: home health care and nursing home care. As highlighted in the list above, today there are several dozen alternatives for health and long-term care services. Needless to say, it has become difficult for physicians, case managers, medical social workers, and discharge planners to sort out the differences between many of these levels of care, and even more difficult for them to determine what is best for their soon-to-be-discharged patients.

By 1986, Aetna Health Insurance began providing individual case management for each of their hospitalized patients. Aetna rightly concluded that if frail-elderly patients enrolled in Medicare could be discharged from hospitals fairly quickly, the same might be achievable in even less time with the more able-bodied, privately insured population. They focused on the high-cost/high-volume cases, much to the consternation of the hospitals that counted on those cases to ensure solvency and profitability. "Managed care" would soon become a household phrase.

In 1988, an attempt was made in the Catastrophic Care Act to remove the three-day hospital stay required for Medicare payment for rehabilitation in a skilled nursing facility or rehabilitation hospital. Unfortunately this act was repealed in 1989 when a very active group of seniors rebelled at another provision in the bill that would have resulted in their paying a higher premium for some Medicare services. They felt that there would be erosion of their entitled services and this very important change fell with the other changes in Medicare.

By 1990, the hospital re-engineering effort among insurers was in full swing. The delivery of care became scrutinized with no holds barred. The ratio of registered nurses to patients began to drop. Nonprofessional, non-licensed technicians and aides began providing more and more care. Ambulatory care found favor among insurers and health care administrators. Observation beds and ambulatory surgeries became fixtures of both hospital-based and non-hospital-based care. Advances in technology supported this movement from the "acute" care bed to a more ambulatory level of care. The cost of health care had become public enemy number one.

In 1993, we witnessed the great health care reform that failed. The Clinton Administration's Health Care Advisory Board, run by Ira Magaziner and Hillary Clinton, analyzed health care reform in detail, but produced little substantive change. Perhaps their fatal misstep was the failure to include a physician on the board. Politicians, lawyers, and policy makers don't provide much in the way of health care in this system; physicians do. But despite the failures of health care reform in the early '90s, the essence of the Health Care Advisory Board's recommendations has come to fruition. This essence is what we call "managed care." Like it or not, managed care has come to Medicare and Medicaid.

In 1993, we also saw a considerable harvest of outcome studies that measured the efficacy (or lack thereof) of many medical and surgical treatments. "Efficacy" is a relative term, however. It can refer to cost effectiveness as well as quality of life. The latest in a string of buzzwords in outcome measurement is QALY (Quality Adjusted Life Years), indicating that adding to the quality of life is a valid reason to recommend a costly treatment. Insurance companies were taken aback when studies revealed that more women who received hysterectomies reported statistically significant improvement in the quality of their lives after the surgery than did women who were treated medically. Such a finding had obvious negative consequences for the insurance industry's bottom line. Clearly we face a considerable political, economic, and social challenge as we weigh financial considerations against quality of life concerns.

In 1996, Congress passed the Health Insurance Portability and Accountability Act (HIPAA). This act made health insurance portable for America's workers, so long as they could afford the payments for eighteen months after losing their jobs. It required significant protections of confidentiality in health care records, especially those transmitted electronically. It also made long-term care insurance tax deductible and authorized the expenditure of significant federal government resources to ferret out fraud and abuse among health care providers, insurers, and providers of durable medical equipment.

These provisions have had both intended and unintended consequences for the quality of health care in this country. Unscrupulous health care providers notwithstanding, who can measure the consequences of the defensiveness among health care professionals that our fraud and abuse investigations have spawned? It is conceivable that the cost-effectiveness of so much fraud investigation is at best minimized and at worst negated when, for example, long-term care facilities must hire one nurse to provide the care and another to explain it, document it, and argue that it's necessary. And how effective can a paranoid physician or nurse be? Yet how can providers be anything but paranoid when they see their colleagues sanctioned on technicalities and when they hear, whether rumor or fact, that the FBI is training its agents to pose as home health aides to hunt down fraud and abuse in the home care industry? As legitimate as the effort is to find and prosecute fraud and abuse, we cannot avoid the unfortunate consequence that many creative solutions will not be tried because of it.

Legislative action has continued to change health care in other ways as well, always seeking to control costs. The Balanced Budget Act of 1997 (BBA) was perhaps the most sweeping revision of the Medicare Program since its inception. Most of its provisions are designed to achieve one overarching goal: to protect the Medicare-A Trust Fund by slowing the rate of growth in expenditure. BBA has brought us a new Medicare component—Medicare-C or Medicare+Choice. And through a new Prospective Payment System (PPS) it has imposed maximum reimbursement amounts for home health care services and for rehabilitation services provided in both subacute and nursing home facilities.

PPS in home care and rehabilitation services means that the Medicare dollar is going to be scrutinized and managed, and no longer offered to the health care system without limitation. These two initiatives are an effort to change our "entitlement" mentality to a "management-of-resources" mentality. Health care professionals and health care consumers need to move from the idea that there is no limit on health care services to accepting that money is a precious resource and that there are limits on what can be spent.

Among the many other provisions of the BBA is the Transfer DRG Law. In this provision, ten Diagnostic Related Groups (DRGs) have been identified as using more post-hospital services than any other diagnoses. Under this law, hospitals will be financially penalized for discharging patients with these ten conditions before they have stayed their so-called "geometric length of stay." The geometric length of stay is a number used to calculate the (roughly) per diem equivalent of a fixed amount of compensation for a particular DRG, regardless of the number of days a patient stays in the hospital. The Transfer DRG Law means that hospitals can no longer count on making money under the so-called DRG flat rate, which paid a fixed amount of compensation no matter how long (or briefly) the patient stayed in the hospital.

The geometric length of stay is based on data collected by the Health Care Finance Administration (HCFA) for specific DRGs for the previous year. For example, in DRG 14 (Stroke) the geometric length of stay is 6 days. If the hospital discharges the patient at 4 days to a post-acute provider for related services, the flat rate DRG payment is divided by 6 and the hospital is paid a per-day fee rather than the full DRG. Essentially, hospitals are now penalized for discharging patients early where once they did so with immunity from rate reduction. Under the old system the hospital was reimbursed the same amount for the patient who came in for the same treatment and stayed 6 days as for the one who stayed for 4.

Under the Transfer DRG law, the ways Medicare calculates the appropriate length of stay, which it uses to pay hospitals, have also been made more complicated by the establishment of two levels of reporting for patients. One level is for patients who stay either to or beyond the geometric length of stay and the other for those discharged before the geometric length of stay. Two patients with the same exact DRG, but who have different lengths of stay will need two different types of bills. The geometric length of stay is used to calculate the formula for payment to hospitals for patients who stay beyond their expected length of stay and who still require care.

As a result, the hospital is now given the incentive to keep the patient until the geometric length of stay is completed and then to discharge, so to avoid regulatory scrutiny. However, any changes to patient care patterns based solely on a financial incentive draw scrutiny regarding quality of care issues. The irony here is that hospitals that worked to be efficient in their care delivery and were successful in decreasing the length of stay while maintaining quality are now being penalized for that efficiency. While the Transfer DRG Law may prove to be a good idea, for the time being, it gives providers a difficult message.

Hospitals must now relearn how to take care of patients for *longer* periods, providing, for instance, a total-hip replacement patient with physical therapy and a regular diet for a five-day post-operative period, instead of fewer days under the previous system. This development probably signals the end of the prospective payment system for inpatient care (DRGs). Over the last fifteen years, hospitals have adjusted to it *and* learned to make money under it, but their ability to profit under it will soon be eliminated. It would appear that HCFA, the budgeting and financing arm of the federal government that controls Medicare and Medicaid, now sees that further savings can be realized at the hospitals' expense.

The following list illustrates the DRGs included in the Transfer DRG Law.

TOP 10 DRGS / USERS OF POST-ACUTE CARE

DRG 014   Stroke (50 percent discharged from hospitals to either a skilled nursing facility or a home health care agency)

DRG 113   Amputation for circulatory system disorders

DRG 209   Total hip and total knee replacements without complications (77 percent of these patients receive post-hospital care, mostly in short-term, inpatient rehabilitation facilities)

DRG 210   Other hip and femur procedures without complications

DRG 211   Other hip and femur procedures with complications

DRG 236   Fractures of hip and pelvis

DRG 263   Skin graft without complications

DRG 264   Skin graft with complications

DRG 429   Organic disturbances and mental retardation

DRG 483   Tracheotomies

Soon other diagnoses and procedures may be added to this list. They include cardiovascular surgeries and pneumonia.

Other BBA provisions have had significant effects. By early 1999, the Interim Payment System (IPS) in home health care, a BBA provision in effect since late 1997, had resulted in both significant cost savings to the Medicare program and the closure of thousands of home care agencies nationwide. In early 1999, the Prospective Payment System (PPS) was imposed on rehabilitation services for Medicare beneficiaries. We have yet to see its full impact. And PPS was imposed on home health care in the October 2000. The 1999 Balanced Budget Refinement Act has produced some relief for post-acute providers, but the overall approach to managing costs will not change.

On the political front, the federal government has indicated its support for the long-term care insurance industry and family caregiving, proposing tax breaks for both of these arrangements. Universal access to health care seems to be a theme gaining the most attention, but the reality of the cost of an "unmanaged" health care delivery system is also at the forefront of public debate. The receivership of Harvard Pilgrim HMO and the liquidation of the Tufts Health Plan of New Hampshire (during the last month of the last century and leaking into the first month of the next) has shocked many providers and sent patients into a tailspin lack of confidence in managed care. Managed care may not be the answer, but the policy question of the day is—"What is better?"

These and other soon-to-arrive changes mark the beginning of a new era in health care. One of the hallmarks of this new era is that the hospital is no longer at the center of the health care delivery system. The health care system is being consolidated and re-engineered out of the inpatient treatment model. Community LifeCare Planning is an increasingly critical service for a health care system in transition.

HEALTH CARE IN THE PRESENT: FOUR AREAS TO WATCH

The Medicare Home Health Care Benefit

Two factors have contributed greatly to the loss of home health care options and the high rate of hospitalization and nursing home placement among the elderly and disabled: public confusion over what Medicare provides, and a general reluctance among Medicare beneficiaries to anticipate and plan for functional decline and personal care dependency. The system's response to these problems has been woefully inadequate. First, we look at what Medicare can and can't do for those with home health care needs.

Medicare beneficiaries cannot rely on their home health care benefit to do more than help them regain medical stability after an illness or injury. Medicare does not pay for long-term health maintenance or custodial care services in the home no matter how much they may be needed. It covers short-term, intermittent care only. Medicare pays for home care only when all of these circumstances coexist: the services of a registered nurse (RN), a physical therapist (PT), an occupational therapist (OT), or a speech therapist (ST) are medically necessary for recovery from an illness or injury; a physician orders these skilled services; and the patient is homebound in the sense that his or her illness or impairment significantly restricts mobility. (The operational interpretation of "homebound" differs among regional Medicare intermediaries.)

Aside from the services of the above-cited professionals, Medicare home care patients can receive personal care assistance from a home health aide, as well as supportive counseling, long-term care planning, and community resource linkage services from a medical social worker. Personal care assistance and medical social work are not stand-alone services under the home health care benefit, however. "Skilled" services (RN, PT, OT, ST) must be both medically necessary and currently provided in order for aides and social workers to provide services billable to Medicare. This means that once the patient has recovered to the extent that skilled services are no longer justified, *all* services are discharged. Further, the number of hours of care patients can receive in a week are limited. Nurses and therapists treat the illness; aides provide scheduled personal care (such as dressing, bathing, and mobility assistance) for brief increments of time; and medical social workers provide counseling and planning help when social or emotional problems impede recovery from the primary diagnosis.

Under the auspices of Medicare, then, recipients of home health care services, most of whom are chronically ill and elderly, are helped back to a baseline of wellness. They must then rely on themselves, their families and community supports. Although the services that helped them recover may be continuously needed to prevent a relapse, and while Medicare still does authorize provision of medical management services when relapse is likely, reimbursement caps have made the provision of ongoing services all but impossible for most home care agencies to offer. Essentially, Medicare will not pay for services after recovery has been achieved despite the probability that relapses will occur (chronic conditions aren't cured, they're managed) or the likelihood that subsequent hospital and rehabilitative treatment will cost more than preventive measures would have.

For years, the terms "homebound," "short-term," "intermittent," and "medically necessary" have been liberally interpreted by home health care agencies. Under a fee-for-service reimbursement system, the home care industry grew throughout the country. Recently, however, home health care has been tarred with a reputation for fraud. While many of the accusations may be unfounded, those that weren't drew the attention of the Health Care Finance Administration (HCFA). The entire industry came under scrutiny in an effort to reduce actual fraud and to save some Medicare dollars in the process. Increased oversight, combined with the imposition of per-patient reimbursement limits, has forced home health care and visiting nurse agencies nationwide to trim the amount of care they provide under the Medicare home health care benefit.

HCFA's wish to reduce both Medicare fraud and Medicare cost will likely be realized. But what of the unintended consequences? Consider this: in the mid-1970s there were more people over the age of 85 in nursing homes than there are today, *despite the fact that as a percentage of the population, they were half as numerous!* It is reasonable to assume that this lessening of the most elderly population in nursing homes has been made possible by the Medicare home health care benefit. It is also reasonable to assume that home care cuts will continue, despite the fact that most chronically-ill and disabled individuals need medical management services in their homes to avoid illness exacerbation and injury. The federal government clearly intends to make chronic care the primary responsibility of the individuals (and their families) that need it most. It is why Community LifeCare Planning is so vital a health care service today.

Case Management
Another trend in health care likely to have far reaching consequences is the care-planning role that hands-on caregivers will continue to fill under the managed care approach to disease management. Both health care providers and insurers have been hiring clinical medical staff, most of whom are nurses, away from the bedside and into case management. Perhaps the most unfortunate consequence of this exodus is the growing shortage of experienced nurses throughout the health care continuum, especially in hospitals. Many go eagerly to case management to get away from the increasingly stressful demands on bedside caregivers in today's hospital environment. What they often find, however, is a different kind of stress. Their new roles require new skills and make demands upon them for which many are unprepared.

Many hospital- or insurance-based case managers may be unfamiliar with community-delivered chronic-care services. For the most part, case managers hired by insurance companies and hospitals are pulled from the ranks of the in-patient workforce. Many have never worked in ambulatory care, nor did the nursing schools in which they trained offer extensive community-based experience. While they understand very well the nature of acute exacerbations of chronic illness, the impact of comorbidity of chronic conditions during non-acute phases has not usually been a part of their experience or training. Many have spent little time in patients' homes. And their nursing experience providing chronic care for the elderly has probably been limited as well; those with such experience have likely learned it in a nursing home, the current venue of choice for teaching nurses primary care skills such as bathing and toileting.

Today's case manager, therefore, is generally an experienced, inpatient, bedside nurse who is now working in an office, making treatment and planning decisions about patient care rather than providing the care itself. These case managers must now depend on other health professionals for information on which to base decisions. Insurance company case managers call a hospital for utilization review and get a clinical snapshot of a patient that may or may not take into consideration the patient's medical or psychosocial complexity. Hospital case managers have very little time to help their patients, usually no more than a few days. What these case managers need is a video, not a snapshot, but they rarely have the time to get a true, full picture of the clinical and personal circumstances affecting the patient's recovery.

Care managers practicing CLCP must learn to work effectively with system-based case managers. Care managers also depend on others for patient assessment information and must be fluent in "clinical-speak," the language of health care in the clinical setting. They must quickly become familiar with their CLCP clients' medical histories, medications, and disease processes. They must remember that the usual purpose of communicating with case managers is to gain some understanding and agreement on a plan of care from the third-party payer. Case managers' receptivity to suggestions from a privately-hired care manager (whose payer is the patient!) will be based on their respect for the care manager's understanding of the case manager's world, not the reverse. Once trust has been built, then the care manager may find opportunities to address psychological, social, legal, and/or financial considerations and their impact on the client's long-term prospects. When working with case managers, these considerations should be couched in concrete terms, however. Case managers need information that is measurable and that can be usefully incorporated by physicians and administrators.

Insurance- and hospital-sponsored case managers have three missions: to ensure quality of care, to reduce hospital length of stay and to reduce the cost of care within the length of stay. Hospital-based and insurance company-employed case managers are usually charged with getting patients out of the hospital as the hospital remains the insurance company's major cost center. Some insurers have even placed their own case managers in hospitals, where they assume discharge-planning responsibilities alongside hospital staff. But regardless of their employer, case managers will continue to play a critical role in the provision of health care and long-term care services. Care managers must be able to work with them and help them bridge the gap between what the system can provide for patients and what patients will need to provide for themselves.

The Decline of Discharge Planning

True discharge planning requires time. Unfortunately, hospital discharge planners, whether medical social workers, nurse case managers or both, have very little time to plan their patients' discharges. What they are doing is more akin to crisis intervention. In 1983, the average length of stay in a hospital was somewhere between eleven and twelve days; today it is a little less than four. These averages include occupants of ICUs and maternity units. How much planning can take place in these time frames when the discharge planner may spend no more than a few hours with the patient and his or her family during the patient's hospital stay?

In 1990, a survey was conducted to measure the need for discharge planning services among those admitted for inpatient hospital stays. Unfortunately, this study coincided with the hospital re-engineering initiative that began in 1982 with TEFRA and the imposition of DRGs, as well as the growing managed care movement, so the results were not well publicized. The results indicated that approximately 17 percent of those admitted at that time needed some help developing a plan that would enable them to be discharged safely. In other words, over 80 percent of those admitted to hospitals in 1990 had little or no need for help with discharge planning.

These figures would likely be reversed today. With the advent of ambulatory care, many of the 80 percent who didn't need discharge planning help in 1990 are no longer admitted to hospitals at all. Today, cataract surgeries, hernia repairs, breast biopsies, even gallbladder surgeries are commonplace in the "day-stay" unit; we are admitting only the most acutely ill to our hospitals, most of whom have one or more chronic illnesses, are elderly, and need extensive discharge plan-

ning assistance if they are to remain independent in a community setting following discharge. Yet even so, the new discharge-planning rule
appears to be "Out of the coma and into the cab."

We must be careful to differentiate between a short hospital stay, on
the one hand, and a short hospital stay *without planning* on the other. A
shortened length of stay in a hospital can be a good thing, even an *excellent* thing. However, for those most vulnerable to a fall, or to skin
breakdown secondary to incontinence, or to the exacerbation of a
chronic illness, discharge back into the home care setting without planning and follow-through nearly guarantees re-hospitalization.

Discharge planning is required by law, but discharge-planning services are in a shambles largely because of the re-engineering of hospitals. A primary nurse on a unit finds it very difficult to forge a good plan
for the patient who is ready for discharge. He or she often has twelve or
more patients to care for, seven of whom are likely to be unstable, requiring frequent vital sign checks, PRN (as needed) medications, and
sophisticated diagnostic services. At least two others have probably just
returned from surgery. And, if possible, each nurse working under these
circumstances must somehow limit the patient's length of stay to less
than three or four days. Here, then, is the sum and substance of discharge planning today: The patient who is stable is discharged!

Thus, as system-based discharge planning continues to decline, patients will be forced to do their planning themselves. Community-based
care managers will find an expanded role as care-planning advocates
during the transition from acute care to home care.

Disease Management

Linked to case management and discharge planning, a relatively new
concept called disease management is changing how chronic care in
America is being delivered. Disease management is an attempt to control the cost of care for chronic conditions, especially for those diseases
that take a toll on quality of life. Providers and private insurers share
the risk and the responsibility when chronic illness results in higher
costs of care. And Medicare may subsidize disease management efforts
as when a Medicare beneficiary enrolls in a Managed Care/Medicare
plan under the Medicare+Choice program.

Disease management protocols specify a program of care for a specific chronic illness or combination of chronic illnesses. Comprehensive services are provided with the goal of wellness maintenance.

Insurance companies have authorized disease management programs for asthma, diabetes, congestive heart failure, and chronic obstructive pulmonary disease. Problems arise when patients have more than one chronic illness (comorbidity). Case managers may have difficulty determining which slot to fit the patient into.

While such programs are a positive development, they are very difficult to maintain. Many HMOs covering the Medicare beneficiaries most likely to need disease management are not overanxious to offer these programs. The reason is not immediately apparent. Consider, however, that Medicare beneficiaries enjoy nearly unbridled freedom of movement; they are able to change health insurance plans with relatively little advance notice. Therefore, managed care companies covering Medicare beneficiaries under Managed Care/Medicare Plans may take a dim view of long-term care planning. They hesitate to invest in prevention (and who can blame them?) when the investment they make may yield dividends to one of their competitors if the Medicare beneficiary changes plans.

DISCUSSION: THE CARE MANAGER'S FIT

It is difficult to imagine a crueler irony than that of discharge planning falling to the cost-cutters scalpel. Take the case of the patient with mild dementia who visits an emergency room for a burn that occurred while she was cooking. She is admitted to the hospital through the ER for observation. She is subsequently discharged to the home care agency, which can assess her wound and treat her inpatient-diagnosed cellulitis, but cannot touch her biggest problem—*she lives alone!* In short, we treat the least of her problems in the most expensive way. No planning is provided to ensure a safer circumstance after her discharge from the most expensive, acute-care setting, and all because we can't afford it!

We cannot fault the health care professionals for these often-tragic twists of priority. No one in the acute-care system is truly assessing preventive needs, primarily because they have neither the time nor the authority. Many also lack the skills, for the focus of their training is almost entirely acute care. Our current payment system is set up so that if they do engage in non-medical care planning activities, their employers (the hospital, rehabilitation facility, or home care agency) risk reimbursement denials. The concept of need, so narrowly defined by "medical necessity," forces health care providers to ignore chronic-care needs and to treat only symptoms. A wound is a wound is a wound whether on the hand of an 86-year-old widow with early-stage Alzheimer's Disease who lives alone, or on the arm of a 65-year-old man whose spouse and two adult children live with him.

This is not an argument for giving health care professionals more latitude to address a broader definition of need. Most health care professionals are not trained to meet the resource-management needs of someone with a chronic illness who lives alone in the community. They are not trained as family-care coordinators, financial managers, or home care resource professionals. Nor is it likely that the system will figure non-medical planning and support into the medical treatment equation any time soon. Indeed, there is a legitimate question as to whether it should. How can we expect our physicians, nurses, surgeons, and therapists to competently handle the growing number of acute-care problems we place at their doorsteps and at the same time to forge creative long-term care options with families, lawyers, courts and financial managers? They have their job and community-based care managers have theirs. And in a very real sense, the care manager's job is to protect the health care system (from landing in bankruptcy?) and its caregivers from getting burned out and overwhelmed.

Community LifeCare Planning can promote safer discharges by providing the system and the patient with care-planning and caregiving strategies that most effectively blend system and patient resources. Advocating for his or her clients' needs is part of the ever-expanding role of the private or community agency-based care manager. This advocacy is often complicated by a certain amount of understandable defensiveness in the hospital, rehabilitation facility, nursing home, and home health care staff; a defensiveness that stems primarily from their belief that the care manager's service is redundant. Health care professionals care deeply about their patients and want to serve them comprehensively, and some may view the care manager's involvement as a threat to their opportunity to do so. Others may be concerned that a care manager's intervention may have a negative effect on their patients' outcomes.

In addressing these attitudes, it is important to remember that the privately hired health care advocate is a new kid on the block. The care manager must take the lion's share of responsibility for helping system-employed health care professionals grow comfortable with this new relationship. Without question, acceptance and trust can only be built if the caregivers on the system side of the equation experience the care manager as appreciative of their efforts, empathetic with their plight, and, above all, dedicated to client benefit.

In sum, no one begs more for better-coordinated, interdisciplinary caregiving than the individual dwelling in the community who is frail, elderly, chronically ill, and physically disabled. Yet no piece of the formal health care system provides this service adequately. Indeed, a health care system set up to treat illness and injury may be structurally incapable of promoting the kind of prevention planning and patient behavioral changes that prevent treatment from becoming necessary in the first place. After all, the primary goals of all institutions and bureaucracies (and health care is one of the largest institutions in the country) is self-sustenance and survival. Like all "healthy" bureaucracies, the health care system will have difficulty accommodating any effort that reduces the need for the services it must provide to survive.

Let's look now at the knowledge and skills base for the new professional who will fill this void in preventive care planning and care management.

Suggested Readings

Boland, P. *Making Managed Healthcare Work.* Aspen Publishers, 1993.

Fries, J. and C. E. Koop, et al. "Reducing Health Care Costs by Reducing the Need and Demand for Medical Services." *New England Journal of Medicine* 329:321-325 (July 29, 1993).

Grosel, Charles, Melinda Hamilton, Julie Koyano, and Susan Eastwood. *Health & Health Care 2010: The Forecast, the Challenge.* Prepared by The Institute for the Future. San Francisco, CA: Jossey-Bass, Publishers, 2000.

Hoffman, C., Rice D., et al. *Chronic Care in America: A 21st Century Challenge.* San Francisco, CA: The Institute for Health and Aging. Princeton: The Robert Wood Johnson Foundation. August 1996.

CHAPTER 3

The Assessment

In the initial planning phase, the care manager must quickly learn a great deal about the client. Armed with the knowledge of CLCP and having engaged the client and his or her family in the long-term care planning process, the care manager's first task is to complete the continuing-care needs assessment. The goals of the care needs assessment are to define unmet needs and to determine how best to meet them given the resources at the client's disposal.

The care manager's ability to acquire the right information turns as much on establishing trust with the client as it does on knowing what questions to ask. In order to achieve this trust, the care manager must express respect for the client's dignity and autonomy while also showing competence as a guide and advisor. Compassion and empathy are as much the tools of the care manager's trade as estate planning acumen, health-care system knowledge, medical treatment and counseling skills.

The assessment, then, must be completed with accuracy, sensitivity, and diligence. The following steps are meant to serve as a guide to completing a thorough care needs assessment.

STEP I — CLARIFY YOUR ROLE AND VALUE

No care-planning client should answer a question without understanding why it is in his or her interest to do so. A continuing-care needs assessment will not succeed unless the care manager can clearly describe his or her role and confirm that the client clearly understands it. Without exception, a care manager must begin every assessment by building client receptivity to the care-planning process, ensuring that he or she understands its purpose, and clarifying each player's role in the process.

A Sample Introduction

Imagine that you have been contacted by a family caregiver seeking help for her 84-year-old mother. Even before you meet this mother and daughter and learn about the mother's situation, you can bet on one thing: Neither knows what you do! As the care manager, then, your first job is to educate your prospective clients about your profession, your CLCP approach, and your value—quickly and thoroughly.

What follows is an illustration of how to accomplish this task. In practice, details will differ to suit each care manager's background and personal style.

The care manager arrives at the client's home. Introductions are made. The mother, the daughter, and the care manager are seated in the living room—the room in which the mother feels most comfortable. The mother is nervous. The daughter is hopeful. The care manager initiates the meeting with an overview:

"I always like to begin these meetings by describing what I do. I find people are more comfortable when they understand exactly what my role is and why I ask some of the questions I ask.

"My background is in health care. I've worked for years as a medical social worker, primarily in home health care, but also in hospitals and long-term care facilities. So I know about the health care system, and what it can and can't do. And over the years I've learned that many people wind up in hospitals for a lot of otherwise preventable reasons. And I believe the key to prevention is planning, but that not all of the planning we need to do is about our medical treatment. Good planning requires input from many different "lifecare professions" as I call them. And these include medicine and social services, but also law, and finance, and insurance, and counseling, and even architecture.

"So now I call myself a care manager. My training as a medical social worker has helped me understand how the community can support long-term care. That's what medical social work is. But health insurance and community supports aren't the only resources we have to help us meet our long-term care needs. I've also had to learn a lot about the professions that help people develop their own resources. Resources are key in my work. Long-term health and security have come to depend as much on our resources as on medical treatment.

"So I usually start by looking at my client's resources much as an estate planning-attorney, a financial planner, or an insurance agent might. I then combine my knowledge of health care and social services with these other professions to help you use your own resources better or to acquire a community-based service to promote long-term health and security.

"I don't represent myself as an estate-planning attorney or a financial planner, however. But I can usually recognize when one of these professionals might be useful. And I can also help you understand how to make use of their skills.

"In addition, I can help you and your advisors—whether they include a lawyer, a doctor, a financial planner, a relative, or anyone else—to see how they might help one another. For example, I can help health care professionals under-

stand how an estate plan or some available financial resources might provide you with options that they didn't think were possible. Many times I've been able to stave off a nursing home placement or a hospitalization simply by letting the physician know that something else could be done. Care planning, then, is a resource challenge. In my opinion, six resources are critical in developing long-term care and asset protection plans.

"First is health insurance. You're (the planner nods at the mother) covered by Medicare, I assume. And Medicare pays for a lot of the care that you might need if you get sick. You may also have a supplemental policy to pay for what Medicare won't cover. So health insurance is of obvious importance to your long-term security. Lately, another insurance is becoming very popular. It's called long-term care insurance. I'm seeing more and more people buy this type of insurance. Both health insurance and long-term care insurance are resources that pay for much of the care that most of us couldn't afford otherwise.

"The second resource is our own money—whether it's money from income, such as Social Security and pensions; or money from investments, such as annuities, stocks, and CD's; or home equity; or life insurance policies with cash value.

"Third are the community resources that include local programs here in town, as well as state programs, federal programs, churches, charities, volunteer groups, and so on. I view the community as a primary long-term care resource.

"The fourth resource is the home. And it can be a good resource or a not-so-good resource. For instance, if someone is unable to climb stairs and the bathroom in his or her home is upstairs, then the home isn't yet the best resource it could be for that person. Sometimes people need to make their homes more accessible, whether with a ramp, handrails, or other assistive devices. The point is that changes may enable the home to help keep someone independent longer.

"The fifth resource is more personal: family, friends, and neighbors. People who have relationships with us tend to do things for us. In fact, if you think about it, family, friends, and neighbors provide most of the health care in this country. The help they provide, such as the ride to the pharmacy or the doctor's office, or the help with shopping, cleaning, and laundry, is very important. A person's family, friends, and neighbors are caregiving resources, no different than one's insurance or income might be. You might say that our family and friends are a form of equity. Or as my uncle used to say, 'I have friends I haven't even used yet!'

"The sixth and probably most important resource is the person for whom the plan is being developed. Individuals are able to contribute to their own care and care planning to varying degrees. Perhaps someone can remember when to take medications and thus doesn't need prompting, but does need assistance with get-

ting out of bed or getting dressed. Almost everyone is a self-care resource to some degree, and each person's plan should always build upon his or her capabilities.

"So, you might say that I'm a resource management professional. I begin by asking a lot of questions to try to get a full understanding of your circumstances, your resources, hopes, and goals. I want to know what you want to do, and then I help figure out how you can do it. If I can begin by asking you (the mother) some questions, I can determine how I might be able to help you. Or, if someone else might be more helpful, I can tell you who that someone might be."

And so the assessment begins. I have given this speech a thousand times and each time I make good eye contact and convey a sincerity of purpose. Within a few minutes, both mother and daughter understand why I will begin to ask so many seemingly disparate, incongruous questions about family circumstances, home ownership, advance directives, past and current medical status, community agency involvement, income and assets, health insurance, and so on.

It is also useful to continue reminding clients throughout the initial interview that there is a purpose to the questioning. In the above example, the mother may wonder why the care manager wants to know how many children and grandchildren she has, where they live, and what their ages are. She may need a gentle reintroduction to the concept of family members as caregiving resources and decision-makers.

The point of this introduction is to engage the client in the process. Understanding begets compliance. Since a care manager is most often paid hourly by the client, his or her value is measured partly by the amount of time it takes to complete the assessment. A well-educated client, confident of the care manager's ability, tends to stay on task and to provide thorough, informative responses, expediting the assessment.

STEP II — INFORMATION GATHERING

Information gathering begins ahead of the first meeting. The client or a family caregiver can prepare the way for the care manager by completing a questionnaire ahead of the care manager's first visit. A sample questionnaire, the Initial Consultation Checklist, is included in Appendix A. This questionnaire is similar to an attorney's or tax accountant's estate inventory. If it is provided to the client in advance of the first meeting, much if not all of it can be completed prior to that meeting.

Also in Appendix A is the Initial Interview Form, a one page, at-a-glance assessment tool that helps remind the care manager of what information must be obtained. Many clients who have received the Initial Consultation Checklist ahead of the first meeting will not have completed it. They may find it too difficult, or they may be unable to find the relevant information, or they may simply choose not to complete it. If the checklist has been completed, the care manager may find it useful to transfer some information onto the Initial Interview Form to create a one-page reference for future discussions with the client. If the checklist has not been completed, the Initial Interview Form will prove useful because it condenses all areas on the checklist into boxes, all on one page. This ensures that the care manager, despite interruptions and distractions, will ask all relevant questions. The care manager's goal should be to complete this interview form as fully as possible; it is essential that each box be filled in.

During the first meeting, all roads lead to the bottom box on the Initial Interview Form, "Service Needs/Referrals." The care manager uses the Initial Consultation Checklist and the Initial Interview Form to establish a profile of the client's needs, both met and unmet, as well as his or her resources, both currently available and unavailable. In short, the assessment is the job estimate. It defines the client's problems and determines what services and resources are needed to address them. The assessment process engages the client and his or her family and friends in the care-planning partnership, and it establishes the care manager as a trustworthy guide.

STEP III — EVALUATING THE RESOURCES

Long-term care resources might be thought of as the equivalent of the assets of a military campaign. They are the troops, the ordnance, and the hardware with which clients fight the battle for their independence, wellness, and control. Let's take a closer look at the six long-term care-planning resources that we listed in the introductory speech above.

Resource I — Health Insurance

Health insurance, in all its forms, is both a long-term care planning resource and a first line of defense against the high cost of health care. In the United States, there are now four general categories of health insurance. They are Medicare, Medicaid, private health insurance, and long-term care insurance. These four insurance vehicles pay for the lion's share of medical/surgical treatment and long-term caregiving in all venues.

Care managers must appreciate that these insurances support a client's long-term care security in two ways. First, they pay for the medical treatment that the client probably cannot afford otherwise. They spread the financial risk among the many and minimize the financial risks of catastrophic illness for the individual. In paying for intensive, high-cost, acute-care services, they preserve individual assets and, thus, also reserve private paid continuing-care options. Second, they protect not only an individual's solvency, but that of the medical treatment system as well.

It is well beyond the scope of this book to describe the minute details of insurance. Some general concepts are clarified below.

Medicare

Medicare is without question the most abundant pay source for health care for the elderly and physically disabled in this country. Indeed, Medicare drives the health care system. A comprehensive understanding of how Medicare pays for services is critical to the practice of Community LifeCare Planning.

As noted earlier, Medicare is also running out of money. Medicare cannot continue to subsidize acute-care services in anything like the manner to which we have grown accustomed. Indeed, both current and imminent Medicare spending cuts are primarily responsible for the increasing need for Community LifeCare Planning.

It is important to understand what Medicare will pay for and what it won't. Medicare is medical *treatment* insurance. It does not pay for prevention, except in the case of certain diagnostic tests, such as bone density scans (which look for evidence of osteoporosis) and cancer-screening tools, including mammograms and colonoscopies. The good news is that Medicare beneficiaries can find out if they are developing chronic illnesses that will threaten their life or their independence; the bad news is that Medicare will not pay for the chronic-care services that may be needed after the illnesses develop.

As described in chapter 2, recent political developments have changed Medicare forever. It is less and less a fee-for-service, indemnity-style insurance coverage than it is a managed care-type plan. But managed care may not be the shining white knight that will save Medicare, as its proponents so vigorously represent it. Disturbing questions are being raised about the quality of care the Medicare population receives under managed-care arrangements. In 1996, the *Journal of the American Medical Association* published "The Difference in 4-Year Health Outcomes for Elderly and Poor, Chronically Ill Patients Treated in HMO and Fee-For-Service Systems." The author noted that, while mental health outcomes for this population were better under managed-care arrangements, the physical health of the Medicare-risk patients (or managed-care Medicare patients) in this study group deteriorated twice as much as the health of those in the traditional fee-for-service Medicare plan.

And the cost savings of managed-care coverage for Medicare recipients do not appear sustainable. Recently we have seen an HMO exodus from the Medicare market. One reason is that per-capita marketing costs—associated with the effort to persuade seniors into HMO's—increase significantly in regions where Medicare-Risk plans have been marketed for some time. This also makes the inevitable disenrollments more costly for the insurer. On the whole, it appears that the managed care approach of policing health care, with gatekeeper case managers overseeing utilization, may be ill suited to a population that needs close monitoring and regular access to care.

Economic realities will continue to force policymakers to reduce the services covered by Medicare, but social and political realities will continue to make it more difficult for them to do so. The viability of a health care system addicted to Medicare dollars will remain in question until the continuum of physicians' offices, hospitals, rehabilitation facilities, home care agencies, and nursing homes receives help from its most abundant resource—its patients. CLCP aims to enable patients to provide that help by making it possible for them to utilize their own resources more effectively in managing their chronic conditions and expanding their long-term care options.

Medicaid

Medicaid is health insurance with a twist. Aside from paying for primary care in the doctor's office, in-patient care in the hospital, and medications, it also pays for custodial care for chronically-ill and physically disabled individuals in nursing homes and community settings. Medicaid is a means-tested health care and long-term care insurance available to those who fall within certain income and asset limitations. Many states also allow middle-income citizens to acquire Medicaid in community settings under so-called "Medicaid Waiver" programs. And considerable marital assets can be disregarded for some Medicaid applicants if they are necessary to provide income for the well spouse who is living at home.

But Medicaid, too, is running out of money. Since it is half funded by state governments and almost wholly administered by them, it operates under limitations that federal programs do not. As mentioned above, the most important distinction is that all states must annually balance their budgets. They lack the deficit funding option. So while Medicare may be headed for a bridge of questionable structural integrity, Medicaid is headed for a brick wall. States are seeking ways to reduce Medicaid expenditures to lessen the impact of the collision. But how do you cut an entitlement program?

You don't. You simply change the eligibility rules. States have begun restricting eligibility for institutional Medicaid by changing the formula for the reimbursement of nursing homes. In Massachusetts, nursing homes are reimbursed at varying per diem rates that correspond to Medicaid beneficiaries' levels of disability. Each beneficiary's level of disability is determined by the nursing home's clinical staff, which completes a "Managed Minutes Questionnaire" or MMQ. The MMQ determines a resident's need for personal care, socialization, and emotional support throughout the course of a day. The resident's MMQ score translates into a reimbursement category that is subsequently assigned a letter from H to T. If a resident earns an H, the lowest score, he or she has the lowest level of need that the state will pay for. The nursing home is reimbursed at the lowest per diem rate. If he or she is assigned a T, the nursing home is reimbursed at the highest per diem rate. This is but one example of a host of modifications that states will have to try to slow the growth of their Medicaid budgets.

Such developments make expectations of Medicaid coverage in long-term care planning far less predictable, and their consequences will be significant soon. Many residents of assisted living facilities are currently "spending down" their assets, anticipating that once the money is gone, they will select a nursing home that will be paid for by Medicaid. But what will happen if these individuals can no longer afford to live at the assisted living facility, but do not meet the required level of disability to qualify for long-term care Medicaid? Not long ago, the daughter of a woman planning to move to an assisted living facility posed this very question to me. The only answer I could give was that either the assisted living facility would help the resident find an affordable housing option, probably by referring the resident to local social services, or that the daughter would receive a phone call to come and collect her mother.

The viability of community-based Medicaid is similarly unpredictable. In most states, community Medicaid Waivers allow higher income eligibility limits for special community-dwelling applicants including the elderly, people with AIDS, disabled children, and so on. They provide additional chronic-care services for eligible individuals living in their homes. But they also operate within limited budgets. During annual budgeting sessions, states find themselves walking a budget-balancing tightrope as they seek to fund community-based services adequately, but not excessively. Waiting lists for enrollment develop regularly when legislators do not authorize program support increases in time. Both the beneficiaries and the states lose when the underfunding of community-based, long-term care services leads to higher rates of nursing home placement. This eliminates the cost savings that the community-based waivers were supposed to help states realize.

The budgetary constraints on all forms of public insurance are forcing everyone to utilize their own resources more effectively. Care managers working in concert with estate-planning attorneys, financial planners, and insurance specialists have become the private sector's health care finance administration.

Private Health Insurance

Most CLCP clients have health insurance either through Medicare or Medicaid. They may also be covered by a supplementary policy through a private, for-profit or not-for profit company. The supplement may pay the health care costs not covered by Medicare. Private insurers, including HMOs, PPOs, and so on, may also be "primary" (the payer of first resort) for those Medicare beneficiaries who have elected coverage under the Medicare+Choice program. This has come to be known as "Managed-Care Medicare." For example, Medicare beneficiaries can enroll in a participating HMO and have the Federal government pay most of the HMO's annual premium. The HMO becomes the Medicare beneficiary's health insurer, the same as it is for other privately enrolled, non-Medicare beneficiaries. Many Medicare beneficiaries elect this Medicare+Choice option to access benefits that are otherwise not provided under Medicare, such as pharmaceutical assistance, for example. Under the Medicare+Choice option, a beneficiary's monthly premium co-pay for full coverage of hospital, outpatient, and pharmaceutical costs is usually affordable–averaging approximately $125 per month at the time of this writing. The supplementary cost is less than a standard Medigap policy (see below), but the beneficiary is subject to the constraints on choice inherent in the managed care model.

Medicare beneficiaries may also have private insurance policies that are "secondary" or supplementary to Medicare. Such policies may be offered as part of a pension benefit package or they may be paid privately by the beneficiary him or herself directly to the insurance company. These "Medigap" or "Medex" policies will usually pay the portion of a Medicare beneficiary's health care bill that is not otherwise paid by Medicare. Medigap policies are available in three tiers–so called Bronze, Silver, and Gold policies. Bronze policies are the least expensive, Gold the most expensive. At the time of this writing, Medex Gold policies cost as much as $300 per month and offer full supplementary coverage including prescription assistance. Bronze policies cost one third as much, and offer no pharmaceutical coverage and less coverage for annual Medicare deductibles, hospital deductibles, and so on.

Private health insurance, just as Medicare itself, is *not* long-term care insurance. Care managers are not likely to find a pay source for CLCP services through private health insurance, nor will they interact with private health insurance company case managers to acquire chronic-care benefits. Whether managed-care or fee-for-service/indemnity plans, private health insurance policies subsidize *medical treatment*, whether given in MD offices, hospitals, rehabilitation facilities and home care. They pay for pharmaceutical assistance, durable medical equipment, and hospice care as well, but rarely do they subsidize home modification, personal care assistance, homemaking and so on. Care managers may advocate on behalf of their CLCP clients to dispute claim denials or they may assist when clients are deciding which supplementary policy to buy, as for Medicare beneficiaries deciding whether or not to enroll in Medicare+Choice.

Long Term Care Insurance

Long-term care insurance (LTCI) is the newest kid on the health insurance block. We have included LTCI as a health insurance resource since "health care" includes chronic-care services, such as ongoing personal care assistance, homemaking, and other CLCP supports. LTCI will continue to grow as a pay source for long-term care services, spreading risk across the growing pool of "covered lives". It will also become a pay source for Community LifeCare Planning as insurers with long-term care risk begin to perceive CLCP's value.

Home health care and rehabilitation agencies, staffed primarily by nurses and physical therapists, are currently vying for care coordination contracts with LTCI companies. However, the medical necessity model with which they are most familiar may not be sufficient for LTCI as it does not address the problem of developing alternate resources to pay for necessary chronic-care services. Nor does it adequately identify or provide time to address the problems of client engagement, family care coordination and planning. And its practitioners have rarely developed the skills needed to do so. These and other necessary Community LifeCare Planning tasks generally have not been assigned a primary position in the medical model's hierarchy for long-term caregiving. Disease management, as widely practiced by medical personnel working for long-term care facilities and managed care companies, also lacks the resource management and client engagement aspects of Community LifeCare Planning.

The best care coordination deal for both the LTCI company and the LTCI beneficiary will likely come from care-planning professionals who have not only medical treatment experience, but also skills in counseling, financial planning, estate planning, and community resource access. Family care coordination, client engagement, and resource management will minimize LTCI claims making CLCP attractive to insurers. LTC insurers are also interested in seeing beneficiaries opt for effective, low-cost home care services whenever possible, which CLCP also advocates. For the insured, these services will help ensure the strategic use of the finite LTCI benefit. Care managers working with LTCI insurers and insureds will need to anticipate continuing-care needs in 2 to 4 *year* time frames, not the 2 to 4 *month* time frames that current home care and rehabilitation facilities consider.

RESOURCE 2 — PERSONAL INCOME AND ASSETS

As public long-term care supports diminish, self-paid health care—including chronic care services in the home—will become much more common. How could it be otherwise? Consider the following statistics describing the demographics and economics of disability.

- A chronic illness or chronic condition disables one in four people over the age of 65.

- 5 percent of the U.S. population is currently physically disabled and unable to perform one or more activities of daily living. By the year 2050, that percentage will double.
- Medicare and Medicaid are primarily subsidized by working taxpayers. Social Security beneficiaries contribute only a small fraction of the annual cost of Medicare from their retirement benefits. Indeed, many Social Security beneficiaries have long since consumed their contributions to the Social Security system as well. [1]
- Currently there are slightly less than four taxpayers for every individual over the age of 65. By the year 2030, there will be two. In 1935, when the Social Security program started, there were forty.
- The median average net worth of individuals over the age of 65 is nearly $100,000.

It is clear that personal income and assets are the second long-term care resource. Nearly everyone with a disability wants to stay in his or her home and the numbers of people with disabilities is greatly increasing. At the same time the programs that once paid for significantly lower percentages of disabled people within our population are already diminishing. Thus, the net worth of disabled individuals, primarily those over the age of 65 and with the means to pay, will be spent more often to avoid nursing home placement.

Resource 3 — Community Resources
Communities are organized to care for their members. Whether the community is a family, a subsidized apartment building for seniors, a

---

[1] An average wage earner who retired in 1990 at the age of 65 contributed $40,787 in taxes to the Social Security system throughout the course of his or her working life. Adjusting for interest that these contributions might have earned, with an initial benefit of $720 per month, this Social Security retiree recovers his or her contribution within five and a half years. For those who retired earlier–those currently over age 75–the number of months to recover is incrementally less for each earlier year of retirement. For example, the average 1980 retiree recovered his or her contribution within two years. Source–Social Security Administration, Office of the Chief Actuary. May 6, 1999. Informational Memorandum–Social Security Retirement Benefit Amounts and Number of Months-to-Recover the Value of Past Social Security Taxes, Comprehensive Illustration, Table 3.

town, a city, a state, or a country, the people within it look out for one another. They do so voluntarily by contributing their time to community members in need, by providing financial support to community organizations, and by offering food, clothing, shelter, services, and money to those in need.

Extreme wealth is not a prerequisite to long-term care security. Community LifeCare Planning pays immediate attention to the community support option. Churches, charities, and civic groups, as well as local, state, and national government agencies, are all considered as potential sources of long-term care support. In fact, Community Lifecare Planning is often a brokerage service for community lifecare *giving*, as it connects individuals in need to the common wealth. Chapter 7 (Community Care Planning Resources) offers an in-depth exploration of community support services.

Resource 4 — The Home

Operating rooms are designed to maximize a surgeon's efficiency. They are well appointed to minimize the risk of infection and to maximize the management of surgical crises. The operating room itself is a resource for patient and caregiver.

A CLCP client's home and everything in it should be viewed as a long-term care operating room. The home itself can either help or hinder the caregiving effort. It should be as accessible as possible to caregiver and client alike. The accessories of long-term caregiving, which include bedside commodes, shower chairs, stair elevators, soon-to-arrive conveyor belt beds,[2] and the like, are deployed to improve the home's caregiving capability.

Identifying the necessary adaptations for disabled individuals is typically the province of physical therapists–health care's biomechanics experts. Physical therapists work to improve their patients' structural integrity in many ways. They also assess how modifying the environment, itself an extension of the patient's body, will promote physical rehabilitation, help maintain stability, and work to ensure patient safety.

---

[2] One of the latest innovations in caring for disabled individuals is the conveyor belt bed. The bed's six-inch mattress is a conveyor belt that can move a patient who cannot transfer independently off the foot of the bed into a specialized wheelchair, and vice versa.

Modifying the home and acquiring the necessary durable medical equipment and assistive devices makes the client's living environment a more effective caregiving resource. Thus, care managers need to understand how such processes can be put in motion. They should have a general knowledge of accessibility building codes, accessibility design, costs associated with building modifications and renovation, and so on. They should also understand that modifying and adapting the home is not simply a mechanical task. The *client* must adapt as well. For most of us, our homes are manifestations of ourselves. Many home care clients resist even minor changes, not because they don't make sense, but because of the personal change they require. A widened door or a wheelchair ramp is a symbol of disability. The client who needs a more accessible living environment experiences these adaptations not just as barrier modifications, but also as demands for *identity* modifications. Care managers must therefore understand that recommending home modifications, let alone actually arranging for the work to be done, may require a period of personal adjustment. The same is true for acquiring durable medical equipment or a residential rehabilitation loan or subsidy.

Resource 5 — Family, Friends, and Neighbors

Those who care for us because of long-standing relationships do things that we might otherwise have to pay for. You might say that friends and family have equity—relationships *are* resources. As indicated in the client introduction speech, my uncle understood this very well when he said, "I've got friends I haven't even used yet."

If health care is the expression of compassion between human beings, then the most abundant health care resource is the one from which the most compassion flows. Family, friends, and neighbors do more laundry, provide more transportation, prepare more meals, provide more hands-on personal care, and give more emotional support than all of the professionals in our health care and social service systems combined. Family, friends, and neighbors are the ways and means of long-term care. We have addressed the issue of family caregiving in depth as part of our discussion of housing alternatives in chapter 6.

Resource 6 — The Client

We describe people who can "take care of themselves" as resourceful. Chronic illness and/or physical disability does not entirely destroy that resourcefulness. Rarely is an individual so incapacitated that he or she cannot contribute in some way to his or her own care.

But it may be difficult for the care manager to differentiate between capacity and willingness. Can the client truly not remember when to take her medications, or is she feigning incapacity to retain her daughter's attention? Why does one CLCP client resist following a nurse practitioner's recommendations, risking dire complications, while another with the same capacity and similar conditions follows the practitioner's suggestions exactly?

Our acute-care model of healthcare makes patients into health care "consumers" and health care professionals into "providers." Yet no treatment succeeds without the patient's contribution. Healing happens *because* patients are good reporters of their experience. No health care is effectively provided until after professional or lay caregivers "consume" accurate information from the patient. Rarely are effective care plans developed, much less implemented, without client input and authority. A client's motivation, as well as his or her ability to act as a partner with his or her caregivers, determines the client's value as either a resource or a deficit to the care-planning and management effort. The client is in many ways the most important long-term care resource.

STEP IV — DETERMINING CONTINUING-CARE NEEDS

From the very first contact with a client, the care manager is evaluating the client's continuing-care needs. The care needs assessment is done concurrent with the resource assessment.

There is a difference between long-term care goals and needs. *Goals* are determined by one of two people. When the client is competent, the client describes his or her goals. When the client is incompetent, the authorized decision-maker defines the goals. Long-term care *needs* are not so much determined as they are identified. The care manager recognizes needs based on a functional assessment of the client, an evaluation of client safety issues, a review of the client's medical history and current medical status, and consideration of what the client or his or her decision-makers define as the goals. It is the care manager's job, in concert with the client's other professional advisors, to determine and recommend how to meet these needs best in order to achieve the client's goals.

Nearly every goal identified by a care-planning client falls into one of the following categories:

- Recovery from an illness or injury that is immediately affecting function
- Maintaining an acceptable level of functioning and medical stability
- Preserving assets
- Providing for the future of one or more family members
- Remaining independent/Preventing institutionalization
- Assuring continued comfort and dignity

The purpose of the continuing-care needs assessment is to determine what the client must do to increase the likelihood of achieving his or her goals. There are three categories of need: action, service, and resource. **Action needs** refer to those tasks the client and his or her social support system will engage in to overcome a resource deficiency, a clinical problem, or a safety risk. **Service needs** refer to those outside services necessary to recover from illness, to maintain the client's safety or medical stability, to acquire resources, and so on. **Resource needs** refer to resource deficiencies that must be overcome through resource acquisition or through the more efficient use of available resources. Throughout the initial interview and beyond, the care manager is searching for the answers to three questions that correspond to the three categories of need. These questions are:

- What does the client or his or her support person(s) need to do to achieve his or her goals?
- What services and/or referrals will enable the client to achieve his or her goals?
- What resources must the client acquire, modify, or develop to improve the likelihood of achieving his or her goals?

Needs cannot be identified until goals have been established, the resource snapshot has been taken, and the functional assessment is completed. The amount of personal care assistance (**service need**) required to maintain client safety and medical stability (**goal**) cannot be determined until the client's reporting accuracy (**self-as-resource**) has been evaluated. The care manager (**service need**) may not be able to develop a strategy for locating personal care assistance (**service need**) without meeting the client's family (**action need/resource**) and determining the client's ability to pay (**resource**). Acquiring durable medical equipment (**resource need**) will likely require a physical therapist's or a home care nurse's evaluation (**service need**) as well as the funds from either personal or insurance sources (**resource need**) to pay for the evaluation. If an electric wheelchair is recommended (**resource need**), but the client does not have the money to buy one, the care manager might assist the client or his or her family with an application (**service need/action need**) to a community resource, such as Medicaid (**resource need**), that will pay for one. Here we see that the care manager coordinates many layers of activity to meet needs and achieve goals.

The continuing-care needs assessment reveals how best to meet the client's needs ahead of a crisis *and* teaches us what we need to know to prevent further injury and illness whenever possible. A sample assessment form—the Continuing CareNeeds Assessment—is included in Appendix A. Completing the Continuing CareNeeds Assessment form requires clinical assessment skills, as well as input from the client, his or her family, and his or her medical treatment team. Its completion clarifies the caregiving challenge posed by the client's functional deficiencies and medical risk.

Every time a chronic illness worsens, or precipitates an injury, the care manager is presented with both a caregiving challenge *and* a learning opportunity. To learn from an illness exacerbation or injury, the care manager must conceive of even the commonest injuries and syndromes suffered by chronically ill, elderly, and physically disabled individuals as *accidental* rather than inevitable. In other words, a fractured hip must be seen as an accident that was not effectively prevented. A stroke, too, must be conceived of as a breakdown in the planning and services that might otherwise have decreased the client's blood pressure enough to prevent it. A care manager must train to think ahead of the problem.

After a chronic illness has exacerbated, the caregiving challenge is both to respond to the accident *and* to learn from it. Over time, we become able to identify and work to prevent the "accident-waiting-to-happen," whether for the same client or for another who presents a similar mix of circumstances at a later time. We must remember that, sooner or later, most chronically ill or physical disabled clients will not escape needing some medical treatment. A fall may be inevitable, but the care manager "fails less" when he or she incorporates the care-planning lesson that can be learned because of the fall.

A care manager must begin every assessment with the expectation that prevention planning works. The predictability of fractures among frail elders makes their prevention a legitimate focus of many lifecare plans. The most basic principle of Community LifeCare Planning is simply this: Planning is the prerequisite to the success of all human endeavor. Long-term care "success" is no exception. In this effort, assessment is everything. The assessment informs the plan, and often, an assessment will need to be done more than once. A recent care management "accident" that results in a hospitalization requires a new plan based on a new assessment. The old plan must be retrofitted, or perhaps discarded altogether, in light of new developments and new information. Time and time again, we see inadequate care planning result in rehospitalization and subsequent nursing home placement. To save time, discharge planners hope the old plan will work one more time. This is the Procrustes bed[3] syndrome in care planning, in which the patient is stretched or trimmed to fit the plan and not the reverse. The time required to do the new assessment is always time well spent.

We must remember, too, that just as the client's circumstances change, the client will change as well. And because people change, usually what appears to be impossible isn't. An individual desperate to avoid a nursing home placement may be willing to take risks, spend resources, or consider options that were formerly dismissed out of hand. The best policy by far is to keep as many options open as possible during the assessment process. What the client, the family, or the care manager thinks can't happen, can.

[3] Procrustes was a figure in Greek mythology who tricked passers-by into his Inn with the promise that all beds always fit perfectly. After check-in, patrons were stretched on the rack, or had their legs cut off if they were too short or too tall for his accommodations.

CHAPTER 4

Counseling For Care Managers

The need for CLCP invariably arises from either sudden-onset or gradual, progressive disability. Disability *is* loss. It is therefore essential for care managers to understand the psychosocial, emotional and developmental impact of loss.

Most long-term care plans succeed best when supported by the client. In most cases, without client support and engagement, plans never even get off the ground. Initiating a care plan for someone who has not yet acknowledged the need for it is a little like throwing a surprise party and failing to invite the guest of honor. Exuberant to make good things happen, we forget whose life it is we are planning for in the first place. As well-meaning caregivers—whether family members or professional care managers—we wind up "all dressed up with no place to go" unless the most important guest—*the client*—is invited to the CLCP "party."

In health care parlance, a client/patient's unwillingness to do what his or her more enlightened caregiver "knows best" is most often rubber-stamped as "non-compliance." This disconnect between the client's priorities and those of his or her professional or family caregivers may be the unrecognized leading cause of hospitalization and nursing home placement today. Far too many care plans fail for lack of client involvement in the plan's creation. In our view, this stems less from client resistance per se than from the difficulty many well-meaning caregivers have working with this resistance.

Anyone adjusting to loss must resist that adjustment. It is, as they say, human nature to do so. Indeed, we would interpret any prompt, immediate and uninterrupted adjustment to a major loss, such as the functional decline following a debilitating stroke or the loneliness following the death of a spouse, as abnormal. Far more frequently we see the normal reaction to loss as being denial, resistance, bargaining, anger, sadness, fear, guilt, apprehension, and so on—*practically everything but compliance!* Yet in case after case we see prevention opportunities missed because well-meaning caregivers are unable to perceive either the developmental nature or the value of the adjustment-to-loss process. They are untrained in the art of grief counseling.

Successful CLCP turns on client engagement. Successful client engagement turns on the care manager's understanding of loss and the purpose of grieving. It can be difficult for care managers to exercise patience with clients who are unwilling to adjust to loss. As care managers, we are often cursed with a vision of our clients' futures. We become frustrated as we see that, despite their need to work through their loss, our clients' long-term care choices must often be made quickly. How then do we shepherd them through denial, resistance, anger, depression and resignation, to the acknowledgement of loss and the need to plan to compensate for it?

HEALING AND ADJUSTMENT TO LOSS

Adjusting to loss is a pivotal challenge everyone faces in life. It affects us emotionally, psychologically, socially, spiritually, and physically. For those afflicted with chronic illness or disability, the struggle to cope with loss impacts medical recovery and complicates the ongoing, day-to-day challenge of living with a debilitating chronic condition. Care managers must therefore understand the meaning of loss and the care manager's role as the client works through the adjustment-to-loss process.

All of us react to loss through a series of adjustments that we express in a creative, emotional way. We call this process grieving. Grieving enables us to resume outward-focused living following loss. *But grieving is the solution to loss, not a problem to be resolved because of loss.* It is how we grow *because* of loss. And when we grieve, we all do the same thing. We grieve by spending a certain *necessary* amount of time refusing to believe we have to change; wishing we didn't have to; being depressed, remorseful, angry, and so on, when we know we have to; then, finally, we find the courage to reset our lives.

Why do we do this grief work? Is their a purpose or value we can understand given the universality of this experience?

Indeed, there is. Grieving and the emotional pain that follows significant loss results less from the actual loss of a loved one, an ability, a role, or cherished possession than from a fundamental shift in our experience of who we are. *The pain of loss results from the separation from ourselves.* Grief is how we experience and express this pain. It is the shock and disbelief, the sorrow and anger we feel when we realize that we can no longer be who we were when we had that person in our lives, that ability, or that important role.

Each of the emotions we express as we adjust to loss are critical to the primary task of grieving–letting go of our former self and clearing the way for a new self to emerge. We grieve when we permanently lose a relationship that was a critical part of our self-concept. The lost relationship may be with another person or with a capacity inherently vital to our life, such as the ability to walk, or to see, or to speak.

Grieving, therefore, is transition work. It is our journey of change to a reinvented self. We do not make this journey on foot. The river of emotion takes us there. On this journey, we must be careful not to strive too vigorously for progress and closure. Too often, our struggle to get through grief to "acceptance" turns our grieving into a pressure-filled exercise in self-judgement. As care managers, we may help our grieving clients find solace by de-emphasizing a goal-oriented, problem-solving approach in deference to one more responsive to the client's emotional experience, here and now. For those who are grieving, much self-imposed (and sometimes counselor-imposed) pressure dissipates when clients are free *not* to show progress in their grief work. Acknowledgement of loss and the freedom to express the feelings associated with that acknowledgement are often sufficient to enable the healing inherent in the grief process to unfold. Indeed, the harder we press to accept the loss and adjust to it, the longer and more difficult our grief journey becomes. Eventually, we will get there. For now, it is enough to say, "The loss is real, and I'm still here."

It is not possible for a care manager practicing Community LifeCare Planning with a frail elderly, chronically ill, or physically disabled client to succeed in developing a care plan without addressing the client's loss on some level. Care managers will find a counseling role with their clients who are adjusting to loss–or it will find them. Loss is always the primary psychosocial issue for those who have lost control of some aspect of their lives. It is central in the mind of an elderly man who resents the mere sight of his walker, let alone his need for it. It is the reason an elderly woman at risk for falls will refuse to take up her oriental scatter rugs. It is why we attend to the emotional well being of so many disabled and chronically-ill people.

So how are we as care managers to be with our clients as they move through loss toward closure and a new beginning? How can we be effective catalysts for the affirmations of grieving and the reawakening that follows?

The answer is full of paradoxes. When we grieve, appearances deceive. What look and feel like problems that must be resolved are often themselves solutions. The anger and depression we feel carry us beyond loss. Only through experience and expression can these "negative" emotions help us adjust. So, what looks in need of repair may actually be the *work of* repair. "Failure"–in the form of a deepening depression or intractable denial–may in fact be success. The deeper we *feel,* the sooner we exhaust the feeling. Recognizing these apparent inconsistencies, as care managers working with clients who are grieving, we must often refrain from trying to make something happen for our clients and, more effectively, "Don't just do something, stand there!"

The fundamental paradox of grieving is that short-term emotional pain (a few months to even a few years depending on the severity of the loss) is unavoidable, even necessary, if we are to ever feel "better" again. Reestablishing a stable sense of self following significant loss requires that we grieve. However, as care managers, most of us were trained to relieve pain in our healing work. It feels foreign to suspend our impulse to help our clients solve what appear to be deeply disturbing adjustment problems. We don't feel useful when, for those who are grieving, our role is usually and simply, to be aware with our clients; to listen only. We ask, often in frustration, "But isn't there something we should do or say–some way to 'help'?"

Indeed, there is, but what appears to be doing nothing, i.e. "active listening," is anything but. Active listening (listening to listen, not listening to respond), is inherently therapeutic. Active listening accomplishes two things. First, it creates the opportunity for the client to feel the pain of separation from self, deepening the awareness of loss and facilitating the transition of grieving. Second, it keeps us from satisfying our own need to be "helpful" (and from interrupting the client's grieving process in the bargain). Awareness *is* restorative. The more deeply aware of our loss we become through emotional experience, the more readily we can acknowledge our changed circumstance and adjust to the new circumstance we find ourselves facing. As counselors and care managers, our job is most often to stay out of the client's way rather than pushing them along at our pace, not theirs.

Care managers must remember that grieving is not pathology. We can help our clients and ourselves immeasurably by appreciating painful emotions (sadness, anger, remorse) as indispensable solution steps toward resolving the central problem and challenge of grieving–letting go of that part of ourselves that no longer works (or "fits") in light of the loss. To do otherwise is to attempt to fix the solution. When grieving is the issue, every time we interpret our task as "I must make this person 'feel' better"–we trap ourselves and our clients into viewing the solution (grieving) as a problem to be overcome. Thereafter, they and we are in quick sand. First, it is not likely we will "succeed" in enabling them to feel better. As counselors and caregivers, we then come away feeling we've failed. Second, if we do succeed in this, most likely we will have achieved only a temporary interruption of their grief work, consigning their necessary pain to the limbo of repressed emotion. While we say, "See what a good boy/girl am I–my client feels better already!", the client feels inadequate when the feelings of grief surface again, as inevitably they will. Thus, when faced with our client's uncomfortable emotions, we must guard against our impulse to "make it all better." All too often, albeit with the best of intentions, we only prolong our clients' grieving by trying to fix not only what is not ours to fix, but what really isn't broken to begin with.

Grief is the river we cannot push. Our job as care managers, as listeners, and as healers, is not to pull the oars for our clients, but to sit in the boat with them, holding a light. We seek to create an environment within which our clients can safely build awareness and express the difficult emotions of grief. We do this by practicing self-awareness first, so that we can be with those who are in pain and catch ourselves from rescuing them before they have healed.

In his insightful work *Transition Therapy: An Existential Approach to Facilitating Growth In the Light of Loss,* Ken Moses offers a valuable prescription for grief counseling. He combines some of the basic tenets of Client-Centered Therapy, as developed by Carl Rogers, and the Gestalt approach, primarily developed by Fritz Perls, to create a template for Transition Therapy and to set parameters for the counselor's use-of-self. He calls his process "ENUF." ENUF honors the dictum that grieving is the client's work, not the counselor's, and that it is for our clients to feel what they must, for as long as they must, in their own way, not ours, if they are to move through grief to closure.

The Process of ENUF

Reprinted here, is a part of Moses's work on the ENUF process.

"Grieving takes place only in the context of a relationship with a significant other who is willing, and able, to be authentically present for, and witness to, the journey of the bereaved. It is a relationship-based interactive process. It

is the quintessentially human phenomenon. The most profound experiences and psychosocial forces are felt, and must be shared with significant others, for the work to be fulfilled. Facilitating that process requires that helpers have a map for the journey and a map for the relationship-based process. Through a model called ENUF, Transition Therapy provides a map for the interactive process of relating to the bereaved.

"The practice of ENUF is defined as Empathizing, Nonjudgementally, Unconditionally, through Focusing on feeling. The practice of ENUF is an open-minded process. It is dynamic, fluid and changing, rather than a set of fixed responses, formulas, or recipes.

"ENUF is a set of attitudes about human interaction, rather than a technique of psychotherapy. Taken as a whole, this set of attitudes about the 'hows' and 'whys' governing the helper's responses creates an environment which provides the structures and boundaries essential to facilitating the work of grieving."

For care managers, ENUF offers a model to rely on when doubt comes to call. Care managers will inevitably encounter the issue of loss and the feeling states of grieving. They will need some confidence that they know how to be with clients who will weep about their loss, express anger about their loss, deny their loss, and so on.

ENUF is simple and effective in its emphasis on the experience of emotion as inherently valuable, and in setting up guideposts that ensure the care manager will not rush in and try to "fix" the emotions of grieving. When the care manager finds the client in grief, he or she should strive to convey empathy. Empathy is not "I know how you feel," but "I feel for you, and with you."

This attitude of empathy should be expressed without judgement, i.e. Nonjudgmentally. No one's genuine feelings of loss should be censured or labeled as "wrong." The client should feel the care manager's respect for his or her experience is unqualified and Unconditional. The client should feel not only approved of, but valued as well. These three concepts—Empathy, Nonjudgement, and Unconditional positive regard—offer guideposts that help the care manager "listen-to-listen" and not interfere with the grieving process. They set the stage for the real work of grieving—Feeling.

Ultimately, the process of ENUF creates room for the client to feel. This last, and perhaps most important feature of ENUF emphasizes the therapeutic value of the expression of emotion. Grieving is nothing if not feeling. Concentrating there keeps the care manager honest.

Our purpose here is not to authorize care managers as psychotherapists or grief counselors with the simple offering of a technique, but to make the issue of loss tangible and understood. In all aspects of Community LifeCare Planning—legal, medical, financial, architectural, and interpersonal—it is inappropriate for any single individual to try to perform every task. Aside from being impossible, it would be very confusing for the client. (Imagine the client's question "Are you my doctor today, or my lawyer?") If in the care manager's opinion a client's grief has become a primary obstacle to successful care planning and care management, the client should probably be referred to a competent Transition therapist or bereavement therapist. The care manager's familiarity with the grief counseling process is all-important in recognizing this service need.

DEPRESSION

The incidence of depression and suicide among Medicare beneficiaries is twice that of the general population. Depression is unquestionably the most prevalent psychological disturbance among CLCP clients. Depression is a mood disorder that may be precipitated by a variety of physiological changes or life experiences. For many elderly and physically disabled individuals, depression may be precipitated by loss, but it also may become sustained and arrest the grief process.

Depression is existential—those who are clinically depressed may experience their depression less as an illness or malady than as a state of being. Depression is defined by a sense of hopelessness, an absence of life-direction, an inability to experience pleasure (anhedonia), and the nagging expectation that hope, pleasure, and purpose will never return again.

As disabling as depression can become for able-bodied individuals, it is doubly so for the chronically ill and physically disabled. Those who have already lost function due to a medical problem may experience further decline because of their depressed mood. Depression wreaks havoc on all areas of functioning—sleep is disturbed, memory is impaired, thinking may become disorganized and confused, appetite is erratic, even mobility can be lost due to lack of motivation to do anything. And those already struggling with a chronic, disabling medical condition are far less likely to achieve their highest level of wellness or rehabilitation when their recovery is complicated by depression.

Depression is especially insidious for the elderly whose life expect-

ancy is relatively short. As described above, depression is characterized by a lack of purpose or direction. For many homebound elders, as
well as those who must live out their lives in nursing homes, it is very
difficult to reconnect to a sense of purpose or meaning, especially
when time is running out. For many elders consigned to a life of dependency in an environment over which they have little control, life is
as depressing as they are depressed.

Depression is treatable by counseling, pharmacologic intervention
and a host of therapies—from acupuncture to loco-therapy (manipulation
of the environment to affect mood). Different individuals respond to different types of therapy. There are also different types of depression.

Normal Depressed Mood and Grief

We have addressed the normal depressed mood that associates with
grieving in the adjustment-to-loss section above. But depression precipitated by the loss of a loved one or a loss in function, despite its nor-
malcy, is depression nonetheless.

All of the symptoms associated with a clinical depression may also
manifest in depression associated with grieving. These include insom-
nia, appetite disturbance, weight gain or loss, guilt, confusion, impaired memory, and so on. As suggested above, we "recover" from the
depression associated with grieving *by* grieving. However, if after a reasonable length of time following a loss an individual has not regained
a sense of equilibrium and adjustment, then the mood states of grieving, including depression, may be seen as psychological disturbances
per se. The individual may be unable to emerge from grief because the
loss has deepened a preexisting depression, or perhaps depression remains a defense against acknowledging loss. In either case, care managers may appropriately recommend mental health intervention from
a psychiatrist who may work in tandem with a psychologist or a clinical social worker. The psychiatrist may manage the antidepressant
medication regime, and the psychologist, social worker or mental
health counselor may provide psychotherapy services.

In addressing a normal depression, it may be difficult to determine
the boundary marker between what is a reasonable grief reaction and
what is a mood disorder. Care managers should consider the severity
of the loss and the impact it has had on the client's sense of self. We
may be depressed about a stock market loss for a few days or weeks,
but may remain depressed and anxious for a year after the loss of a

spouse. A client's depression may not call for immediate treatment if his or her sense of hopelessness is a reasonable response to a core-level loss or life challenge. Adjustment-to-loss counseling may be indicated.

Adjustment Disorder with Depressed Mood

Our moods are affected by our changing life-circumstances. "Life" forces us to adapt and alter our expectations of others and ourselves. Sometimes the difficulty we have coping with a life change manifests as depression. Such depression usually lifts when we regain our bearings and adjust to our changed life circumstances. As with grieving, the depression we feel when we have difficulty adjusting may grow out of proportion to the life change that precipitated it. Short-term counseling and/or pharmacologic intervention may be appropriate to help us regain our existential equilibrium.

Mild Depression (Dysthymia)

Dysthymia is a chronic, depressed mood that often associates with a poor sense of self-esteem. It may have no precipitating factor or event, and all of the symptoms associated with major depression may manifest, although to a lesser degree of severity. Dysthymia may already be an entrenched personality characteristic or it may emerge precipitously. This sudden change in personality can be confusing for the individual experiencing it and for his or her friends and family as well.

Major Depressive Disorder

Major depression is a profound mood disturbance that affects all areas of functioning. It can be incapacitating to the point where the individual in a major depression cannot work, sleep, have sex, feel pleasure, eat, or even get out of bed. Major depression is a total loss of interest in living coupled with the expectation that the thrill of life will never return again. Indeed, this all-pervasiveness is the feature that distinguishes a major depression from the other forms of depression. Individuals suffering a major depression may experience a severe loss or gain in weight; they may become anxious, easily irritated or agitated; they may lose the ability to sleep or may sleep excessively; and their hygiene may deteriorate as they become incapable of performing even the simplest routine personal care tasks.

Major depression can occur in a single episode or it can be chronic– differentiated in *The Diagnostic and Statistical Manual of Mental Disorders*

(DSM IV-R) as Major Depressive Disorder, Single Episode (Diagnostic Code-296.2x) or Major Depressive Disorder, Recurrent (296.3x). Major depression may or may not be triggered by an identifiable life event, crisis, or developmental milestone. Such a marked disturbance in mood with no apparent cause may become almost as difficult emotionally for the loved ones of the individual experiencing it as for the individual him or herself.

The DSM IV-R identifies a major depressive episode when ". . . Five or more of the following symptoms have been present during the same two-week period and represent a change from previous functioning; at least one of the symptoms is either 1) depressed mood or 2) loss of interest or pleasure." These symptoms are:

1) Observed or reported depressed mood most of the day, nearly every day
2) Markedly diminished interest or pleasure in almost all (or all) activities
3) Marked sleep disturbance (increase or decrease)
4) Marked appetite disturbance (increase or decrease) with weight gain or loss
5) Changes in psychomotor activity
6) Chronic fatigue or decreased energy
7) Feelings of worthlessness, hopelessness or severe guilt
8) Disturbed concentration and/or uncharacteristic indecisiveness
9) Suicidal ideation; suicidal gestures, planning or attempts; recurrent thoughts of death

The symptoms of a major depression may be present in several medical conditions. For example, depression may be confused with a sudden-onset dementia that may have been caused by a transient ischemic attack (TIA) or "mini" stroke. Differential diagnoses must account for an individual's medical status, age, and possible adverse drug-drug interactions (polypharmacy). Care managers should encourage clients to consult with a mental health clinician or their primary care physician when symptoms of major depression are observed.

Seasonal Affective Disorder (SAD)
By its name, Seasonal Affective Disorder (SAD) implies that one's

moods are affected by the seasons. SAD refers to the depression that many people experience during the winter months. The defining characteristic of winter—*the cold*—is caused by a reduction in the amount and intensity of sunlight that reaches the earth's surface. Therefore, SAD or the "winter blues" is a mood disorder that is precipitated by an absence of light.

SAD itself has varying degrees of severity. In its mildest form it may resemble "cabin fever"—the increased irritability, fatigue and malaise many people feel by the end of winter. In its moderate form, people feel more overt symptoms of depression throughout the winter. Functioning is impaired, sleep and appetite may be moderately disturbed, productivity is reduced, even a person's appearance changes due to an observable weight gain or loss. In its most severe form, Seasonal Affective Disorder leads to markedly impaired functioning equivalent to that observed in major depression.

As indicated above, the incidence of SAD is related to the reduction of light in the winter. SAD is therefore more prevalent further north or south of the equator. As with other forms of depression, SAD is more prevalent among women and the elderly, although it does occur in children as well as adults.

Because SAD is so closely associated with changes in light, scientists have investigated the biological changes that take place within our bodies, and especially our brains, resulting from our exposure to light. Research has focused on the pineal gland, which is stimulated by the optic nerve. As the light recedes in winter, the pineal gland receives less stimulation from the optic nerve and, as a result, secretes an increased amount of the hormone melatonin. As melatonin output increases, reproductive behavior decreases. Thus the birth cycle among many species is regulated to coincide with seasons during which food supply is more abundant. Human birth cycles also follow a similar pattern as a result of the melatonin response, verifying that human behavior is itself also directly regulated by the presence or absence of light. Scientists have found that many of the same metabolic changes that occur in the hibernating and the migrating animals and birds also occur in humans as the days grow shorter and light grows less intense. Indeed, SAD has been labeled as the "hibernation response."

Not surprisingly, phototherapy (prolonged exposure to full-spectrum light) has proven to be an effective treatment for SAD. SAD sufferers can take a vacation in the middle of winter to sunny climates or they can invest in a light box (a specialized lighting unit developed for those with SAD) and turn it on every morning during breakfast. SAD sufferers have achieved significant improvements in mood by adhering to light therapy treatments during the late fall and throughout the winter months.

Anxiety vs. Depression

Anxiety and depression share a similar set of symptoms. Both progress to the level of a "disorder" when they persist beyond a reasonable time frame relative to their precipitating circumstance.

Anxiety is the sense of urgency we feel when our current situation is unacceptable *and* we lack the confidence that we will be able to change it. The larger the gap between what we have and what we want, the greater our anxiety.

Anxiety can worsen the health problems of CLCP clients in an insidious cycle of events. For example, someone with chronic obstructive pulmonary disease is likely to become anxious because of the immediate association between shortness of breath and anxiety. As anxiety grows, heart rate increases and respiration shortens even further. As breathing becomes more shallow and labored, and heart rate quickens, the COPD is itself exacerbated. The COPD sufferer may additionally go into congestive heart failure. As the patient's illness exacerbates, the patient becomes more anxious, which, in turn, exacerbates the illness, and so on.

Both anxiety and depression can manifest in obsessive thinking, catastrophic expectations, physical and behavioral problems including sleep and appetite disturbance, irritable bowel syndrome, fatigue, and panic attacks. Those who experience anxiety and depression concurrently may also be at higher risk for suicide.

Treating Depression
Counseling

Care managers who have mental health training may recognize depression and understand the treatment options more readily than those with primarily medical treatment backgrounds. But this does not mean that care managers who are also trained in mental health services should automatically serve CLCP clients as either psychotherapists or bereavement counselors. As we have suggested, it may be too confusing for the client to sort out the care manager's role if the care manager is serving in both an administrative and a clinical capacity. Nor is the care manager always the best psychotherapist for his or her CLCP client.

Thus, in the same way that care managers should cultivate relationships with several "resource managers"—attorneys, financial planners and insurance brokers—they should also be able to call upon different mental health professionals when a psychotherapist's or a psychiatrist's services are indicated. For most CLCP clients it is also important that care managers find mental health practitioners willing to visit clients in their homes.

It is well outside the purview of this book to teach care managers all of the different approaches to psychotherapy, but it is appropriate for us to offer suggestions that will help care managers make appropriate mental health referrals. First, care managers must understand that a client's relationship with a psychotherapist is deeply personal. Indeed, the trust that develops between a psychotherapist and his or her client has been likened to that between an individual and his or her priest, rabbi, or minister. Psychotherapy is defined less by the *therapy* than by the *therapist*. Who the therapist is as a person, and the extent to which he or she is able to build trust and engage the client in the therapeutic process, is usually more important than his or her psychotherapeutic orientation. Therefore, the therapist-as-person is a significant concern in a care manager's decision to make a mental health referral.

Second, care managers should be no less selective when referring clients for mental health services than they are when referring to medical managers, lawyers, or financial planners. Not only are care managers invested in maintaining the quality of the services that their clients receive, but they must also remember that every referral reflects on the referent. Care managers should have confidence in and a personal connection with the mental health professional whom they lead their clients to.

Such confidence is built over time and through experience. Care managers face a unique challenge in developing this confidence. It may be difficult for them to understand how an individual psychotherapist works due to the personal nature of the counseling service. Mental health services explore the intricacies of our inner selves. They are less concrete than perhaps any of the other CLCP services. The clinical issues underlying depression, marital stress, or adjustment-to-loss can be arbitrary and unpredictable as compared to the sometimes more concrete challenges of developing an appropriate investment portfolio or writing advance directives. It may be easier for care managers to learn a financial planner's or a lawyer's competence in these areas than it is for them to develop the same level of familiarity with a mental health practitioner's style and ability.

Third, as mentioned above, many psychotherapists work in tandem with psychiatrists, especially in treating those with depression. It may even be that a mental health clinic will only treat a patient within their team. Team communication is no less critical in mental health services than it is in medical, surgical, or chronic care. Care managers must be familiar with how a psychotherapist, a psychiatrist and a social worker communicate as a mental health team if they are to keep the care planning service timely and relevant.

Care managers develop confidence in mental health practitioners no differently than they do with the other lifecare professionals— lawyers, doctors, insurance brokers, financial planners, and so on. They do so over time and through experience. And while a care manager must respect the intimacy and confidentiality of the psychotherapist-client relationship no less vigorously than for any of the other lifecare professions (perhaps, in some cases, even more), the mental health practitioner is clearly an integral part of the care-planning and care-management team. Here again, the care manager's communication skills become all-important to the success of the Community LifeCare Planning effort.

Antidepressant Medications

Antidepressant medications can be very effective in treating depression. They may take time to have effect, but most people suffering from depression will benefit from them. It is not unusual for patients to undergo a trial and error period to determine which antidepressant medication will have the most favorable effect. Many who suffer from depression are understandably hoping for relief and may find the time lag associated with this trial and error very disappointing. Their trial may be further complicated when they have difficulty tolerating a medication's side effects.

Antidepressant medications are not magic, nor is taking them always free of inconvenience or discomfort. They may be expensive for those without prescription coverage. But antidepressants are effective for as high as 60 to 80 percent of those who take them—*as prescribed.* Fortunately, most antidepressant medications are paid for through community support programs that offer pharmaceutical assistance to income-eligible seniors and physically disabled individuals.

Antidepressants affect the neurotransmitters in the brain. Neurotransmitters are the chemicals that allow electrical nerve impulses to jump the gaps (synapses) between nerve endings. The electrical impulse travels down a nerve and is "sent" across the synapse when the sending nerve releases the neurotransmitting chemical. Following the transmission, special enzymes clear away the neurotransmitting chemical from the synapse, enabling the next impulse to be transmitted.

Depression has been associated with extraordinarily low levels of neurotransmitters, including serotonin, epinephrine, and norepinephrine. Antidepressant medications slow the process of clearing neurotransmitters from the synapse following transmission of a nervous impulse by interfering with enzymes that eliminate them, a process known as "reuptake inhibition." Different antidepressants act on different neurotransmitters uniquely. Psychiatrists rely on subtle descriptions of symptoms from their patients to determine which enzyme inhibitor (or antidepressant) to prescribe.

MAO Inhibitors (Nardil, Parnate)

MAO inhibitors were the first antidepressants. They were discovered by accident when researchers found that they were ineffective against tuberculosis, but that they did make TB sufferers feel better emotionally. Over the years their use has declined due to an unfortunate side effect–patients can suffer dangerously high blood pressure when MAO inhibitors combine with tyramine, an amino acid that appears in fairly high concentrations in many popular foods.

As with all antidepressant medications, MAO inhibitors affect the brain's neurotransmitters. MAO inhibitors are so named by their mechanism of action–they interfere with monoamine oxidase, a naturally occurring enzyme, which helps clear serotonin, epinephrine, and norepinephrine from synapses in the brain.

Selective Serotonin Reuptake Inhibitors (Prozac, Zoloft, Paxil, Celexa)

Selective serotonin reuptake inhibitors (SSRIs) were developed during the '90s for treatment of depression, panic, obsessive-compulsive disorders, anorexia, and bulimia. SSRIs block the reuptake of the neurotransmitter serotonin from nerve synapses in the brain. SSRIs have become very popular and Prozac has become the most frequently prescribed antidepressant medication.

SSRIs have many of the "normal" side effects of antidepressant medications, including dizziness, drowsiness, nausea, diarrhea, tremor, weight decrease, and sunlight sensitivity. Nearly half of SSRI users report dysfunction in sexual arousal or performance. Many also complain of sleep disturbance in the form of short intervals of wakefulness in the night, contributing to fatigue during the day. While many SSRI users find substantial relief from the symptoms of depression, they sometimes pay the price in these potentially disturbing side effects.

The Tricyclics (Elavil, Pamelor, Tofranil, and Others)

Tricyclic antidepressants are so named due to the three-ringed chemical structure of the molecule. They inhibit the reuptake of the neurotransmitters serotonin and norepinephrine. They also affect the metabolism of amine compounds in the central nervous system. Tricyclics are nearly as old as the MAO inhibitors. Users may experience a variety of side effects including dry mouth, blurred vision, nausea, vomiting, dizziness, anxiety, sexual function changes, confusion, constipation, urinary retention, tremors, GI distress, headache, fatigue, agitation, and rashes. As with all antidepressants medications, tricyclics must be monitored for efficacy and side effects. These and all antidepressant medications must be taken as prescribed for physicians and psychiatrists to accurately manage their use.

Suicide and Depression

One in one thousand Americans attempts suicide every year—one in ten thousand succeeds. Indeed, the signs of depression are also the signs of suicidality. Care managers should be able to perform a suicide risk assessment for all CLCP clients suffering from depression. Those CLCP clients believed to be at high risk for suicide must be referred to a physician, a psychiatrist or a mental health practitioner with whom the client is familiar, or to a mental health outreach/crisis intervention service.

Care managers practicing as licensed nurses or social workers are "mandated reporters"—they must report *suspected* abuse, exploitation, abandonment, neglect, self-neglect, and danger to self or others, to the appropriate authorities. Filing a report of suspected abuse or danger to self might be one of the most difficult and at the same time most important tasks a care manager may perform. Not only is the client's life at stake, but a care manager's report of a client's suicide risk to either a physician or adult protective services' worker may destroy the trust the care manager has so assiduously worked to establish. The care manager may lose a client as a result, but there is far more to lose if he or she fails to report and something goes horribly wrong.

The operative word in most mandated reporter rules is "suspect." The reporter does not need to *know* that his or her client will actually attempt suicide. Reasonable suspicion is the rationale for reporting a client's danger to him or herself, just as it is for reporting when an incapacitated client is at risk for being abused by someone else. In those rare cases when a client's safety is at extreme risk, care managers are wise to file a report and let the psychiatrists and physicians assume the responsibility that is rightfully theirs.

Most people suffering from a depression so severe that they are considering suicide want to be helped. Most often, they are less interested in dying than in feeling better, but lack the confidence that they can change their suffering. Persuading a suicidal client to seek appropriate help immediately is the care manager's first course of action. Usually it will work. A mandatory report may be precluded by escorting the client to the hospital, or by a verbal or written contract following the client's voluntary contact with a doctor or psychiatrist. But the bottom line should always be that all threats of suicide are taken seriously and must be addressed by an assessment performed by an appropriate clinician. A sample Checklist of Suicide Risk Factors is included in Appendix B.

CLIENT INVOLVEMENT:
THE KEY TO CARE PLANNING SUCCESS

Client support and involvement is critical to the success of any care-planning effort. Successful engagement with clients can only develop in a relationship characterized by trust. Trust between the client and the care manager, established through genuine empathy and contact, is the cornerstone of effective care planning.

For the care manager, earning the client's confidence and securing his or her involvement can be a daunting task. Time may not be on the care manager's side. The care manager must often work quickly to engage with an anxious client, as well as with overwhelmed family caregivers, given the pressures of a progressive illness. Relationship building has a small window of opportunity.

The planning tasks themselves are equally imposing. It is no small feat to persuade someone (whose vigorous independence has enabled long life) to embrace a lifestyle of even partial dependency. Resistance builds as clients are asked to consider initiating life changes they feel no immediate need to make, changes that may be totally inconsistent with long-standing attitudes of self-reliance and independence. How does the care manager engage the resistant client in acknowledging that problems exist, let alone in disclosing personal information about finances, family, and personal problems? How is the client then motivated to reallocate resources, or change his or her lifestyle, based on abstract notions of injury prevention? How are we to persuade clients to spend money on problems they often don't think they have!?

The care manager overcomes resistance by convincing the client that planning is in his or her best interest. The client must first believe that the care manager is honest and has the client's best interests at heart. The client must then believe the care manager is competent. This perception of competence enables the all-important client concession that "the care manager knows more about where I'm headed than I do."

The care manager must establish these conditions without threatening the client's autonomy. This may be difficult for a care manager who is often a generation (or two) younger than the client. It can be even more difficult for a close relative with a well-developed role history. Yet, no care plan succeeds without some measure of client surrender. By following certain "rules of the road" a care manager has a much better chance of developing the trust necessary to overcome client resistance to the often-difficult care planning tasks.

Rule 1: Always meet the client where they are, not where you or they think they should be.

When we serve as care managers, we are agents of change in the lives of our clients. Naturally, we hope to help clients make favorable change, but it doesn't always work out that way. Clients won't always follow our good advice. We may even increase resistance when clients experience our efforts to facilitate change as an affront to their dignity and a threat to their autonomy. If we persist despite this resistance, our own urgency and frustration builds and we may wind up more invested in solving clients' problems than the clients are.

Care managers must curb an overactive desire to be helpful in the face of client resistance. Trying to persuade resistant clients who are also in denial to do what is "best" for them can be a Sisyphean task. We roll the stone up the hill all day long, only to find it at the bottom of the hill the next day. To guard against this disconnect between the client's goals and our goals as care managers (or as loving family members) we must continuously ask ourselves, "Whose life is this, anyway?" In *all* cases where the client is oriented, capable and competent, we must recognize our frustration with client noncompliance as an indicator that we are not attending to our client's needs, but to our own. We are probably trying to fulfill our own need to be a "successful caregiver" at the expense of client autonomy and *the client's right to make bad decisions!*

Allowing someone to make a "bad" decision is not the same as supporting that decision, however. We can suspend our frustration while we encourage a different, more therapeutic course of action. It is our frustration that gets us into trouble, not our interest in healing, increasing client safety or bringing comfort. The key is not to interpret our inability to persuade clients to safer choices as a sign of *our* inadequacy. The minute we do this we begin to obsess on what is the matter with us and we lose awareness of our client's actual needs. We have violated this first rule. We are neither recognizing nor validating the client's experience.

We can help our clients and ourselves greatly by appreciating the value of resistance and denial. Our chronically ill or recently disabled clients (and their caregivers) most frequently employ denial as a defense against what is too painful or too threatening to acknowledge. Care planning cannot be based on the perspective of a client or caregiver in denial, but neither should the care manager pose client denial as a "problem" to be overcome before care planning can be initiated. Denial must run its course, giving the client and his or her family time to mobilize themselves for psychological and emotional change.

Denial is a blown fuse that protects our circuitry from overload in the face of too much stress. It is a necessary and valuable defense—an indispensable self-preservation mechanism. Realistic care planning cannot begin when denial is active, but clients cannot adjust to loss without expressing some measure of disbelief. The care planning process may serve as a vehicle for the client to work through his or her denial. However, instituting a care plan before this transition occurs almost always results in the plan being sabotaged by the very person it is intended to help.

Rule 2: Don't make promises that you can't keep, and—Don't take no for an answer!

Care managers eager to be effective must not allow their own desire for change to instill unreasonable expectations in the client. As a care manager, never suggest you'll deliver what you know you cannot. It is better to deal with difficult limitations straight on than to diffuse a client's painful emotions momentarily by giving them false hope.

On the other hand, it is often equally important to persevere in creating opportunity where no opportunity appears to exist. Any care manager willing to accede to limitations will be given plenty of opportunity to do so. Many care-planning limitations are more perceptual than actual. The money *may* be available from somewhere, but you may have to dig. The housing alternative *may* be there; it just might not be where you or the client would prefer. The community support program *may* exist, just not in *this* state. Finding solutions where there appear to be none may require that the care manager pose difficult, even presumptuous questions. "Is relocating to alternative housing a possibility?" "Have you considered living with your adult-children, or they with you?" "Is there a friend or relative who can pay for your care, or from whom you can borrow the money you need to install a ramp or accessible bath?"

As care managers, we must learn not to take no for an answer. Very few problems are impossible to solve. If the care manager does not believe this, he or she will operate with the diminished effectiveness of a "can't do" attitude. Care managers are not in the pacification business. They are in the advocacy business. Proceeding with the attitude that "we can find the solution," while communicating no guarantees other than perseverance, makes the care manager the client's ally.

Rule 3: Learn about the resources that enable client choice and control.

Good care planning can reestablish your client's sense of power, choice and control. Anyone dealing with illness or disability has two challenges for the price of one. First, and most obvious, is the day to day challenge of summoning the courage to deal with the medical treatment regime, the pain, and all the major and minor inconveniences of being sick. Less obvious is the identity crisis we must face when suddenly, after years of independence, we cannot take care of ourselves. When we suffer a stroke, for example, we may not be able to make a phone call, take a walk, drive a car, perform on the job, or offer wisdom to our children. We feel humiliated as we lose control of our environment and ourselves. We feel we've lost our membership in the human race. We say, "I'm no longer a person," or "I'm only a burden to those I love." The unspoken conclusion is, "and I will never be who I was again."

Paradoxically, one of the most important steps in our recovery is reconnecting to a sense of control. In this, CLCP becomes a part of the treatment. A client feels empowered after a favorable experience with a care manager. The care manager employs adjustment-to-loss counseling skills, shares knowledge of community resources, and shares personal experiences to pull the client from a sense of hopelessness into a sense of possibility. The care manager's job is to bring a fresh perspective. Successful CLCP should reinvigorate the client with regained self-respect. This enables the client to risk believing that what once seemed impossible might be possible, that what he or she believed couldn't happen can. The scale is often tipped by acquisition of seemingly marginal resources. A ride to the doctor's office or an hour of companionship can make all the difference.

Rule 4: Engage the client in a contactful, trust-building relationship in every meeting.

Expertise is one thing; contact is quite another. It is far more important for a client to feel genuinely cared for by a real person than it is for him or her to receive instruction and information on program eligibility and application processes. The care manager is a resource *and* a person. Community LifeCare Planning should lead to the resolution of practical problems *and* the reduction of anxiety, apprehension, frustration, or fear. Emotional change is accomplished through emotional contact; the relationship between client and care manager may be as important as the plan itself. We find it easier to risk change in the context of a therapeutic, supportive, contactful relationship. We listen to those we trust.

CONCLUSION

The best efforts of any care manager will evaporate in the absence of trust. Three fundamental qualities must exist for CLCP to succeed. First, clients must believe the care manager's eagerness to serve, which means that they must feel they are cared for *personally*. Second, they must feel confident that the care manager is well informed and competent. Third, clients must appreciate the care manager's willingness to communicate what they, the clients, may not want to hear. The care manager's depth of concern, tempered by objectivity, keeps the care plan on a realistic course. Practice the four rules of the road:

1) "Be here now," with your clients and yourselves;
2) Promise tenacity at least, favorable results at best;
3) Know where the resources are that enhance choice for your clients; and
4) Build trust—*intentionally!*

By doing so, care managers can successfully engage clients in their own planning and self-care management. Clients are empowered to meet the challenges they face in illness, infirmity or disability, supporting what they help to create.

Suggested Readings

Duffy, Michael. *Handbook of Counseling and Psychotherapy with Older Adults.* New York, NY: John Wiley & Sons, Inc., Publishers, 1999.

Diagnostic and Statistical Manual of Mental Disorders, 4th ed. Washington, D.C.: American Psychiatric Association, Publishers, 1994.

Moses, Ken, and Robert Kearney. *Transition Therapy: An Existential Approach to Facilitating Growth in the Light of Loss.* Evanston, IL: Resource Networks, Inc., 1995.

CHAPTER 5

Medicine For Care Managers

Community LifeCare Planning supports medical treatment and chronic-care management. Indeed, helping the medical team achieve its treatment goals is often the care manager's primary focus. And since he or she who helps the physician also helps the physician's patient, the care manager directly impacts medical management outcomes.

Most CLCP clients want to remain independent, living in their homes for as long as possible. Helping them do so is a fundamental tenet of Community LifeCare Planning. In service of this goal, care managers must understand how health care services are delivered for chronically ill people in their homes. Here we focus on two areas of community-based care management—primary care in the home and end-of-life care. And since most CLCP clients have one or more chronic illnesses, we have included descriptions of several chronic conditions and their basic medical-management protocols.

PRIMARY CARE IN THE HOME

Anonymity is one of the greatest barriers to delivering health care to frail elders and physically disabled individuals who live alone. Too often, they come to the attention of the health care system through a hospital emergency room, and by then it may be too late to prevent costly institutional care. These individuals do not access regular medical treatment for many reasons. The cost of transportation to and from a physician's office may be prohibitive on a fixed income or they may simply be disinclined to visit a medical practitioner or facility of any kind. Whatever their reason for not getting care, they frequently fall into a cycle in which they move from anonymity, to crisis, to hospitalization, to discharge, and back to anonymity.

Home-delivered health care is often the answer for the sickest, most vulnerable, and socially isolated of our citizens. The expansion of Medicare's home health care benefit in the mid-1980s and the development of Medicaid waivers that provide less expensive chronic-care services have increased the use of home care within the formal health care system. The home health care industry has been built on the visiting nurse or visiting therapist model. When deciding whether to order continued nursing, therapy, home health aide, or medical social work services in the home, physicians have traditionally relied on a nurse's or therapist's treatment report and assessment of a patient's needs. But this approach is changing.

Although Medicare remains the primary paysource for home health care, looming fiscal insolvency has forced cutbacks in all services. Due to the recent imposition of reimbursement caps under Medicare, home health care agencies are no longer able to sustain ongoing medical-management services for their patients. In 1998, over two thousand home health care providers nationwide closed their doors following the 1997 imposition of Medicare's Interim Payment System (IPS) for home health benefits. IPS ended unrestricted fee-for-service billing in home care. It forced home care providers to calculate average service costs per patient per year, and to stay within assigned limits. For example, if a home care agency served only two patients in a year, one of whom received $500 worth of care, the other $10,000, the average annual per-patient cost was $5250. If the agency's assigned limit was $4500 per patient, the agency was not reimbursed the per-patient billing overage—in this example, $1500 for that year (or $750 per unduplicated patient). Since over 95 percent of home care patients are chronically ill and in need of ongoing care to stave off health crises, home care advocates argue that these service cutbacks will cost Medicare more money in the long run because they are likely to result in higher rates of hospitalization.

While Medicare home care services have been cut back significantly, the rate of pay for doctors willing to make home visits has recently increased. Physicians, physician's assistants, and nurse practitioners are leaving their offices to oversee directly the care provided to patients in their homes. Since one out of every twenty persons on Medicare is homebound, increased physician participation ensures that the trend toward home-delivered health care is likely to expand despite home care agency cutbacks.

There are pressing economic incentives for home care. As the numbers of people with chronic conditions grows, hospitals will strain beyond their limits to care for them. Hospitals will be forced to discharge patients sooner with higher levels of acuity than ever before. Many chronically-ill hospital patients are discharged to nursing homes. But nursing home care is becoming increasingly unaffordable, and state budgets are lurching toward insolvency under their mounting fiscal burden. Nearly all of these patients will want to return home, and many will be willing to pay privately for their care to avoid long-term nursing home placement. Thus, post-acute care provided in a home care setting will need to be overseen by more highly skilled practitioners. Our physicians will once again need to carry black bags.

As physicians become providers of home health care services, there will be more emphasis on primary care than there is in the current visiting nurse system. Home-delivered primary care is defined as *comprehensive, coordinated, continuous, preventive, medical assessment and management of chronic health conditions in the home care setting.* It is an old model for the delivery of health maintenance and medical treatment services that is likely to become the new model once again. The primary consumers in this new system will be the frail elderly and people with disabilities and chronic illnesses.

The home-based primary care practitioner assesses the patient's needs in terms of prevention, acute care, chronic care, and palliative care. The medical assessment is the primary focus of service, but the impact of other areas of the patient's life on his or her medical stability must be considered. Primary care in the home must be holistic. It must also assess the context of care, which is as important as the client's medical treatment and personal care needs. The home is devoid of institutional caregiving supports, so methods of support must be created within the home care setting. Additionally, the patient is in control of and is most familiar with the caregiving environment. This impacts the patient-caregiver relationship significantly. In the home, the professional caregiver most often accommodates the patient's needs, rather than the reverse.

The medical professional offering home-based treatment initiates care in a fashion similar to office-based care. Socio-demographic considerations, end-of-life directives, treatment preferences, past medical history, family history, and physical examination all inform the continuing-care needs assessment. A functional assessment determines the patient's capabilities, both physical and cognitive, as well as his or her homebound status. Further valuable information is routinely determined through laboratory studies, including EKGs (electrocardiograms) and chest X-rays. Nutritional status is an area of primary concern.

But the home care practitioner has additional assessment opportunities *because* he or she is practicing in the home. For example, the "pantry biopsy" can reveal whether a canned diet has made the patient hypertensive and increased the risk of congestive heart failure. In many ways, this closet-inspection approach is a metaphor for home health care. Peoples' homes reveal their values, their history, their habits, their eccentricities, and, as revealed in a pantry full of high sodium canned foods, even their physiology. The home health care practitioner's diagnosis and prognosis turn not just on an analysis of a patient's internal physical, emotional, or psychological reality, but also on an analysis of the environment they create. The design of the home or apartment is a critical factor in this analysis. The home care practitioner evaluates the way in which the patient interacts with the home and how the home itself supports or impedes the patient's recovery and stability.

Home care physicians should be knowledgeable about chronic care and geriatric care, since the majority of patients who are unable to get to a doctor's office are frail elderly individuals or younger people with disabilities. For instance, dementia is a common complication among the homebound geriatric population. Physicians must be aware that dementia may be either reversible or irreversible, and they must be able to identify the possible underlying causes of reversible dementia, including hypothyroidism, polypharmacy, depression, and malnutrition. Falls are another common problem for homebound elderly people, and those who fall are at the highest risk for hospitalization and nursing home placement. In fact, fractures are the leading cause of nursing home placement in the United States, and the death rate among elders who have sustained injury from a fall is twice as high as for those who have not.

Preventing falls among the elderly often requires home renovation and barrier modification, as well as physical and occupational therapy with the acquisition of specific assistive devices and durable medical equipment. It always requires that both the patient and the caregiver acknowledge that falling presents an immediate risk. It may require personal care assistance, or even some form of restraint. All of these prevention strategies may be experienced as an assault on an individual's independence. As discussed in chapter 4, the care manager's ability to engage clients in the care-planning process can overcome a client's resistance to perceived threats to his or her autonomy. Familiarity with adjustment-to-loss counseling strategies can help clients deal with change and increase their safety.

Depression and anxiety are common geriatric syndromes. The incidence of depression and the rate of suicide are twice as high among the elderly as in the general population. And nearly 20 percent of all Medicare beneficiaries experience symptoms of major depression. The negative effects of depression on an individual's health are well documented, including the fact that depressed patients are five times less likely than non-depressed patients to recover their highest level of functioning following a major surgery, an injury, or a hospitalization due to illness. Depressed patients are also less likely to survive strokes and heart attacks.

Social isolation is a primary cause of depression among the elderly. Nearly 40 percent of people over the age of seventy-five live alone. Loss of functioning, loss of independence, loss of spouse and friends—*loss* in general—makes depression a primary syndrome in this population. Sensory impairments such as loss of eyesight or hearing often complicate the treatment and medical management of homebound elderly people, and may precipitate depression. Given that 95 percent of the information our brains process is visual, adjusting to the loss of eyesight can be especially difficult. Deafness or severe impairment to hearing can also impose a feeling of social isolation.

Iatrogenesis, or illness or pathology that is induced inadvertently by a physician, must be included in the constellation of syndromes that complicate treatment among the elderly, the chronically ill, and the physically disabled. Since this is the population receiving the lion's share of medical treatment, it is logical that they will also receive the lion's share of medical *mis*treatment. In a study published in the *Journal of the American Medical Association* it was shown that nearly 8 percent of hospital admissions among the elderly are caused by adverse drug reactions. Frequently these reactions are due to interactions between prescription drugs.

Polypharmacy and its iatrogenic effects can result from a combination of factors. Medical practitioners tend to rely on drug cures. This can sometimes worsen, not cure a patient's condition, especially when combined with a patient's belief that drugs will relieve a medical problem quickly and easily. Patients who are dissatisfied with one physician's treatment often switch physicians and fail to disclose their medication regimen. In some cases the new physician may learn of the former physician's prescription, but may decide that it is unwise to have the patient discontinue taking it immediately. The medical consequences of withdrawal become a primary concern. It may be that the patient also resists discontinuing the drug. Under pressure to *prescribe*, whether to fulfill the patient's expectation of a cure or to feel effective in helping bring relief, the new physician may prescribe new drugs even when they may be unnecessary. The cycle can continue as the medications grow both in number and complexity of interaction.

Ironically, once patients have become reliant on their medication mix it may take a great deal of the physician's time and monitoring to wean them. This is formidable task, and often impossible for a physician whose time is no longer billable. Fixed reimbursement rates are a condition of participation in most HMOs, and the physician is likely to be too anxious about the patients sitting in the waiting room to spend a great deal of time on treatment of one chronically-ill patient. High rates of hospitalization for drug interactions may also be taken as evidence that the managed care system does not meet the needs of those with chronic conditions. People with chronic medical conditions require regular monitoring, thorough evaluation, and regular access to care, and these things cannot be delivered in ten or fifteen minute office visits.

Under the current system, a physician may order medications for a homebound patient without having seen the patient in many months, possibly not since the patient initially became ill. At the time of this writing, Medicare does not require a rigorous schedule of regular contact between physicians and their home care patients. Eager to be responsive, a physician or mid-level practitioner will make medication changes by relying on a report from either the home care nurse or the patient. But the primary physician may not know, for example, that the patient was recently treated by an orthopedist who prescribed a muscle relaxant. The drug he or she prescribes without this knowledge can interact with the muscle relaxant to cause symptoms that confuse the third physician—the one who sees the patient in the emergency room and thinks he or she has an accurate picture of the medication regime from the primary MD.

Even when drugs are prescribed at the correct dosages, our susceptibility to drug side effects greatly increases as we age. Dosage standards often differ significantly for frail elders, primarily due to the slowed rate at which they metabolize and excrete medications. There are also many new medications that are constantly being introduced to the market, and their effects have not been tested over time and for all populations. Most drug testing is done on people under age sixty-five. Therefore, we know relatively little about the general effect of many modern medications on today's population of elders.

Medical treatment providers may not be aware of the impact of certain drugs on their elderly patients. Valium has a half-life of twenty-four to thirty-six hours for a thirty-year-old. One day after a dose is taken, half of it remains in the body. By the age of eighty, that half-life increases to ninety-six hours. For an eighty-year-old, half the Valium taken on Monday is still in the body on Friday, nearly four times as long as for the young adult! To further complicate matters, Valium may relieve a patient's anxiety, but also greatly increase the risk of falling. The cumulative effect of an even slightly too high dosage of Valium, combined with a little drowsiness and disequilibrium, could spell disaster for a frail elderly woman with osteoporosis. Her Valium-induced fall could land her in the nursing home for the rest of her life.

Digoxin is another example of a drug that is metabolized differently by younger and older patients. It is primarily filtered out of the body by the kidneys, and kidney function declines over a person's lifetime. The kidneys of a seventy-year-old may function half as effectively as the kidneys of a thirty-year-old. Digoxin toxicity can cause dementia, poor appetite, or even anorexia.

The expectation and acceptance of death might also be seen as a normal syndrome of aging. Those who have lived a long life are aware that their time is coming to an end. Many elderly people feel that death is imminent, whether or not they have been chronically ill or have been given a terminal diagnosis. It is not unusual for those who feel they are nearing death to want only to be made comfortable for as long as they will live. They have acknowledged the closeness of death and want only assurance that the transition from life to death in their final days will be smooth. They are perfectly prepared, even content, to die.

This lack of resistance to dying is too often labeled pathological and viewed as a sign that a patient is depressed and suicidal. But receptivity to death among the elderly may be less a pathology of the elder than a manifestation of the personal values of the caregivers. We must exercise caution before imposing our own "never-say-die" values upon the extremely old, when it may be appropriate and meaningful for them to embrace the inevitability of death. Managing end-of-life issues is the ultimate eldercare challenge.

Physicians and other mid-level clinicians cannot provide all the home care services that their clients require. As we have seen, home-delivered primary care for patients with chronic illnesses and physical disabilities must address non-medical concerns as well as medical treatment. The patient's resources and the home environment determine treatment and medical-management options. On a hospital floor one needn't be so concerned with care giving resources and environmental obstacles—the hospital is designed for caregiver access and patient support. But ignoring these factors in the home is to overlook some of the most important factors impacting recovery. The plan of treatment cannot be determined without an assessment of the context in which that treatment will be administered.

Physicians do not have the time, or in many cases the skills, to perform a full resource assessment or to help chronic-care patients and their families administer day-to-day care. While primary care practitioners are now being compensated more adequately for medical home visits, families, friends, and neighbors will be the ones to meet most of the needs of home care patients. These people will need professional guidance from those who are capable of linking them to the support services they need at a price they can afford, and care managers can offer this link at the lowest cost. It takes a lot of time and knowledge to find home care aides, teach patients about household employer and workers' compensation issues, give appropriate advice on barrier modifications, determine a patient's eligibility for community support programs and then help the patient apply for such programs, and coordinate family members to provide home care resources that are no longer subsidized by the government. These resource-management and care planning tasks often must be addressed if those with chronic illness are to remain safe in their homes at affordable costs. The role of the care manager will become increasingly important in sustaining continuity of care for home care patients.

Privately paid care managers and privately hired personal care attendants may not be affordable to the poor, but CLCP can be provided through public programs to assist lower income individuals in accessing community resources (see chapter 7 for a complete discussion of how CLCP helps clients access community support services). CLCP as practiced by independent care managers will provide some measure of relief to the Medicare program itself as well. CLCP clients who use their own resources to meet their chronic-care needs reduce their risk for illness and injury, thus reducing their health care costs. And when they do become sick, as inevitably they will, care managers can help intervene to expedite recovery. Society also benefits when middle- or upper-income individuals successfully plan for and manage their own long-term care. After all, Medicare *is* a social welfare program. It provides health insurance to the rich and poor alike. Thus, CLCP is a social service to the extent it can reduce Medicare expenditures through successful care planning and prevention for its beneficiaries.

END-OF-LIFE CARE

End-of-life care may also be known as palliative care, terminal care, or hospice care. End-of-life care has a unique set of treatment goals and is defined by its focus on quality of life. Quality of life for a dying patient is achieved through a caregiving partnership that includes the medical treatment team, the dying patient, and his or her family.

Although it has gained considerable attention in the United States in the past ten or fifteen years, end-of-life care has not yet become a major training concentration for medical students. Indeed, at the time of this writing, it is emphasized more in nursing education than physician training. But in the coming years, eldercare will replace childcare as the number one dependent-care service in the country and end-of-life care will inevitably become a more widely practiced medical specialty.

End-of-life caregiving is a multifaceted, multidisciplinary service, and CLCP can be as critical to hospice care as it is to medical treatment and long-term, chronic care. Decision-making assistance is a key feature of end-of-life care, and patients frequently need help making sense of the legal documents they must sign regarding end-of-life treatment preferences, resuscitation status, designation of surrogate decision makers, health insurance issues, and so forth. The severity of the decision to elect hospice care makes education, emotional support, and help with setting priorities a central focus. Patients and their caregivers must be keenly aware of the consequences and limitations of the hospice approach if they are to make a well-informed decision. Care managers who are knowledgeable of the medical, legal, and personal issues affecting hospice patients and their families can offer valuable guidance and support.

The success of the palliative care effort is measured in quality of life, not quantity. Palliative care is defined as ". . . the active, total care of patients whose disease is not responsive to curative treatment. Control of pain, of other symptoms, and of psychological, social and spiritual problems is paramount. The goal of palliative care is achievement of the best possible quality of life for patients and their families."

("Cancer Pain Relief and Palliative Care," World Health Organization, Geneva, 1990). The goal of palliative care is to promote quality of life by controlling pain, managing symptoms, and helping the patient maintain his or her dignity. Psychological, social, and spiritual issues must be given the same priority as issues of medical management. But these goals tend to be antithetical to the philosophy instilled in physicians and medical students. Most health care practitioners learn from the beginning of their medical education that their goal is to cure illness. They are not taught how to talk about the process of dying, much less how to facilitate a comfortable death. Death is defined negatively–as evidence that treatment or surgery has failed–rather than as the natural, inevitable conclusion of life. And comfort care is not emphasized as satisfying a physician's mission to heal and *save* life.

The result is that the skills required to provide end-of-life care often go undeveloped in our physicians. And these skills are not just technical, but interpersonal as well. Achieving hospice care goals is determined as much by the medical treatment provider's knowledge of pain and disease management as it is by his or her ability to communicate with the patient and their family members about the dying process. The quality of a dying person's life is enriched if the medical team is able to communicate directly about death. Many people who are dying want to talk about it. Honest communication about their imminent death may enable patients to work more closely with the treatment team in managing their care. Unfortunately, medical clinicians untrained in end-of-life care may avoid or even hide issues surrounding a patient's imminent death, not because the patient does not want to address them, but because the clinicians themselves are uncomfortable doing so.

Pain management is the primary challenge of end-of-life care. Many people believe that pain is inevitable at the end of life, but this need not be true. Unfortunately, the fear of pain can exacerbate it and preclude good pain management. Pain management is contingent on the reporting skills of the patient or his or her primary caregiver, and if they are afraid and confused it is difficult for the medical professional to get an accurate picture of the patient's pain. Pain is therefore one of the most under-treated and/or inaccurately treated symptoms in medicine. The skillful use of opiate and adjuvant medications, nerve blocks, advanced medication delivery systems (e.g. intraspinal morphine, the transdermal duragesic patch, and so on), and non-medicinal interventions such as relaxation techniques and acupuncture are effective methods of pain management, but such management depends on effective communication.

Nausea, vomiting, anorexia, and anxiety are examples of other symptoms that may be ignored or inadequately treated at the end of life. Many times patients or caregivers do not alert treatment professionals to these symptoms. They may be unable to differentiate between symptoms that indicate the worsening of a condition and those that are temporary. They may also choose not to call attention to symptoms out of denial or for fear that their catastrophic expectations will be confirmed. Because depression is considered a reasonable condition in a dying patient it may be ignored. Many times, however, depression results from inadequate control of other symptoms, especially chronic pain. Treatment of other symptoms can result in the improvement of depression. But depression may also be the cause of pain or somatic complaints, and it should be vigorously treated when it is diagnosed. As covered in chapter 4, we possess excellent antidepressant medications as well as methods for measuring a patient's depression and response to medication.

On the other hand, depression may also be one of the most *over* treated symptoms of terminal illness. Indeed, what is labeled as major depression in people with terminal illnesses is frequently the normal and necessary grieving process. The *Diagnostic and Statistics Manual of Mental Disorders, Fourth Edition (DSM IV-R),* which is used by psychiatrists, psychologists, and clinical social workers in diagnosing psychopathology, recognizes that bereavement in the face of recent or anticipated loss often masquerades as major depression. It suggests that major depression should be ruled out as a primary diagnosis when a client is dealing with the recent death of a loved one. Much of what is labeled as clinical depression among the dying and/or their loved ones is, more simply, sadness. While such sadness feels like and mimics clinical depression, it is necessary to the process of grieving, whether in anticipation of death (one's own or that of a loved one) or in reaction to the death of someone significant.

However well meaning it may be, much treatment for the denial, depression, guilt, and fear associated with grieving is often administered to relieve the caregiver's emotional discomfort rather than the patient's. Pain is not easy to witness, and many caregivers may seek to minimize their own discomfort in the face of their patient's or their loved one's inevitable emotional pain by trying to make the patient feel better emotionally as well as physically. If they cannot cure the disease, at least they can anesthetize the patient and themselves against the dark night of the soul. But our despair at the end of life is often purposeful and transitory. It is important for lay caregivers and professionals alike to recognize the purpose of grieving and to approach it not as a problem to be treated and eliminated, but as a vehicle for growth—even at the end of life.

End-of-life care requires sophisticated assessment methods and often-unorthodox treatment for physical symptoms. Emotional distress may exacerbate physical discomfort. If anxiety and panic are causing dyspnea, or severe shortness of breath, these symptoms may legitimately be treated with narcotics, which are most often used for purely physical pain. Palliative care practitioners often struggle against standard protocols limiting the administration of addictive substances. The social stigma against the use of narcotics and other controlled substances often inappropriately enters into palliative care protocols. For example, the controlled administration of narcotics to a person dying of cancer may provide comfort unavailable from other interventions.

End-of-life care is often complicated by the side effects of drugs used to control symptoms. Nausea or constipation is often the result of treatment for pain. The hospice care team must control these secondary symptoms if the patient's quality of life is not to become further compromised. Skillful use of laxatives and anti-nauseants provides the patient with important improvements in quality of life and these drugs are often given concurrent with narcotics.

At the time of this writing, hospice patients and their families receive relatively generous support from hospice services subsidized by Medicare and Medicaid. While these benefits provide substantial help, they are often insufficient to maintain the comfort of the dying person adequately in a non-institutional setting. Like most medical services today, end-of-life care is "managed." Visiting nurse agencies are given a per-diem budget for hospice care, and the patient is only eligible if a physician has "certified" that he or she will die in six months or less. These requirements present a significant obstacle to care management. By definition, hospice services are "back loaded," or provided in higher amounts toward the end of the patient's life. Hospice professionals face the challenge of providing as much help as necessary, but as little as possible in the beginning, knowing that the care will become far more expensive the nearer the patient is to death.

Because enrolling in a hospice benefit is a formal process requiring that patients state and sign their intention not to seek medical treatment for reasons other than comfort maintenance, it requires that the patient acknowledge that his or her illness is terminal. Thus patients tend not to sign on to the benefit until late in their illness. A delayed enrollment in the hospice benefit means that the hospice program may not be able to offset the higher, end-stage cost of care with the excess per-diem funds that might have been stored away if the patient had signed on earlier. This presents an ethical and financial dilemma to caregivers who often accurately anticipate that they will not be able to care adequately for their dying patient *and* remain solvent. Many hospice programs manage to remain viable from donations, fund-raising efforts and endowments.

Medical providers can help ease this resource dilemma through careful clinical assessment and aggressive symptom management. Families and friends must be educated early to anticipate increases in the need for support and assistance during the last weeks of life. If adequate supports cannot be provided at home, the patient may need to be admitted to a more supportive care environment such as a nursing home or an acute-care setting. Under the Medicare hospice benefit, these alternatives are to be used sparingly and only in the absence of alternative care at home.

Insufficient reimbursement often restricts professional caregivers from adequately supporting the families of hospice patients as well. The result is often caregiver burnout, which may lead to the need for more costly hospital and nursing home care. Care managers can play a critical role in the prevention of caregiver burnout by helping to find additional resources to support them. Third party reimbursement need not remain the only paysource for the provision of hospice care. As federal and state budgets strain against the rise in the costs of care and the growing numbers of those in need, care managers can offer affordable help for families developing hospice care strategies, just as they do for families developing chronic-care plans.

In truth, the difference between "hospice" care and "chronic" care is mostly semantic. Eventually, most chronic-care patients become likely candidates for hospice care. End-of-life care is the final part of the care continuum that includes acute, chronic, and palliative responses. It is a continuation of the care that has preceded it.

End-of-life planning, terminal care issues, and symptom management become the caregiver's focus in the face of a life-limiting illness. There are encouraging educational efforts under way to train clinicians in this work. In 1997 the John Hartford Foundation recognized the need for such training by authorizing a grant called the Expansion of Home Care into Academic Medicine. It is the first grant specifically intended to support the study of home health care and end-of-life care in American medical schools. The grant was provided to ten medical schools to allow them to develop curricula to teach students the art and science of home health care, the importance of the interdisciplinary team, the skills required by hospice and palliative care, and the role of the physician as a professional support for family caregivers. Students' reactions have been overwhelmingly favorable because of the emphasis on real human contact and not just pathophysiology. The development of these training programs has greatly increased the ability of physicians to be skilled managers of the palliative care effort.

The challenge of palliative care for physicians is the struggle between quality of life and quantity of life. Physicians are traditionally encouraged to embrace quantity of life as the most important patient care issue, but palliative care requires a shift in thinking. It requires that the treatment team moves from thinking, "Keep the patient alive at all costs," to "Let the patient die unimpeded and in comfort." It is essential for physicians who find themselves at the head of an end-of-life care team to re-evaluate their outlook on death if their training is inconsistent with this approach, or they may be left with an overriding sense of guilt and inadequacy.

The prevention of suffering is the essence of palliative care, and the goal of the care team is to ensure the comfort and the quality of life of their dying patient. The care manager's role is to help create a secure, supportive environment in which the care team can accomplish this goal. As resources dwindle from both the public and private insurance sectors, care managers fill an administrative and counseling support role for the team. They assist the team members in acquiring other funding and caregiving resources, as well as helping them to nurture themselves. As part of the hospice care team, the care manager's goal is to reduce the sense of urgency felt by caregivers, families, and patients when resources are strained. The care manager seeks to keep the distractions of care administration to a minimum, so that the physician can focus on managing symptoms and keeping the patient and his or her family apprised of the progression of the illness.

No other type of medical care challenges professional caregivers like hospice work. The foundation of this end-of-life care is respect for a patient's right to die as he or she chooses, but this takes a tremendous amount of time and effort, and hospice relationships between caregivers, families, and patients simply are not nurtured within the standard HMO structure of fifteen minute office visits. In the coming years, the greatest challenge to hospice care will be maintaining adequate funding to provide care and support to dying patients and their families.

CHRONIC ILLNESS

The following chronic conditions are described in this chapter:

1) Congestive heart failure
2) Chronic obstructive pulmonary disease
3) Spinal cord injury
4) Multiple sclerosis
5) Diabetes
6) Hypertension
7) Myocardial infarction
8) Cancer
9) Cellulitis
10) Urinary incontinence
11) Urinary tract infections
12) Alzheimer's disease and the dementing illnesses
13) Fractures of the hip and knee
14) Osteoarthritis and rheumatoid arthritis
15) Cerebrovascular accidents (stroke)
16) Ocular disease
17) Osteoporosis
18) Parkinson's disease

These are the chronic conditions most likely to be encountered by care managers. The following synopsis will assist care managers in understanding the basics of medical management for these conditions. Care managers will likely run into many other chronic conditions in the course of their practice. We encourage readers to continue their education by exploring further in other sources and have supplied a more extensive list of additional readings at the end of this chapter.

Congestive Heart Failure (CHF)

Congestive heart failure occurs as a result of the heart's inability to pump blood effectively, resulting in blood backing up in the lungs or the rest of the body. If the right side of the heart is involved, blood backs up in the body and commonly causes swelling of the lower extremities. If the left side of the heart is involved, blood backs up in the lungs and causes pulmonary edema or fluid in the lungs. Congestive heart failure has many causes, but on the simplest level those causes can be classified either as a failure of the heart muscle itself (the myocardium) or of the valves. Heart muscle can fail because of an injury to the muscle or from pumping against too great a vascular resistance. Muscle injury results from ischemia (temporary deficiency of blood supply) due to narrowing or closure of the coronary arteries or various external agents such as viruses, bacteria, or direct trauma. The heart can also fail to pump if the heart rate increases or decreases too drastically.

When circulatory resistance in the lung capillaries increases to excessive levels, it produces a condition called pulmonary hypertension. The right side of the heart receives blood that is returning to the heart from the body, and it pumps blood to the lungs. Pulmonary hypertension can cause hypertrophy (enlargement) of the muscle of right side heart chambers (atrium and ventricle). This enlargement occurs because of the increased load placed on the muscle of the right side of the heart. Ultimately, the cardiac muscle may not be able to tolerate pumping against such increased resistance, and when the right side of the heart fails, blood cannot be effectively pumped to the lungs. Backward pressure causes blood to pool in the rest of the body and produces edema (swelling) of the legs. Oxygen, usually administered continually by nasal prongs, is the treatment of choice for pulmonary hypertension, because it causes the capillaries in the lungs to open and reduces the resistance against which the heart must pump.

The left side of the heart can fail due to problems similar to those that cause right-sided heart failure. Increased resistance in capillaries other than those in the lungs causes an increased amount of work for the left side of the heart. Since the left side of the heart receives oxygenated blood returning from the lungs and pumps this blood to the rest of the body, if the load on the left side becomes too great and it fails to pump efficiently, blood will back up in the lungs, producing pulmonary edema (fluid leakage into the small airsacs of the lung).

Treatment of left-sided heart failure is focused on reducing the workload on the left side of the heart. This is accomplished by administering antihypertensive drugs, diuretics (to reduce the volume of blood that must be pumped by the heart), and medications that increase the storage capacity of the circulatory system (e.g. nitroglycerin). Close attention to sodium balance is extremely important, and daily sodium intake must be restricted to two grams. For heart failure caused by rapid or slow heart rate, drugs are administered to decrease or increase the heart rate respectively.

Chronic Obstructive Pulmonary Disease (COPD)
COPD is a chronic, progressive condition characterized by airways obstruction that does not change markedly over several months or years. Today, most cases of COPD are the result of cigarette smoking. The alveoli or small airsacs and bronchioles of the lungs of a chronic smoker become damaged from years of smoke inhalation. Initially, COPD may not impair oxygenation, but after ten to twenty years or more of smoking, blood oxygen levels gradually begin to fall. Ultimately, the ability to remove carbon dioxide from the blood becomes impaired. As CO_2 accumulates, it causes breathlessness and the patient must compensate by breathing more rapidly. At the same time, the brain stem becomes less sensitive to carbon dioxide and ultimately unresponsive. The urge to breathe then switches from being stimulated by CO_2 excess to being stimulated by oxygen deficit. People who have progressed to this stage of COPD require supplementary oxygen, but the rate of administration must be carefully controlled. If oxygen is administered at a rate exceeding two liters per minute, the oxygen drive may be suppressed, causing breathing to cease.

COPD patients are particularly challenging to manage in a community setting and teaching them better self-care management is a primary part of their treatment. Against their natural instinct, patients must learn to slow their breathing and to decrease the inspiratory (inhalation) phase of their breathing while increasing the expiratory phase. It takes training, self-discipline, and commitment to control one's breathing while experiencing the dyspnea (air hunger) that associates with COPD.

COPD patients need reassurance and support. They are prone to severe anxiety as shortness of breath and anxiety usually go hand in hand. Anyone who begins breathing in rapid shallow breaths will automatically begin to feel anxious. Conversely, anticipating an anxiety-provoking situation usually increases heart and respiratory rates automatically. The shortness of breath and dyspnea on exertion that characterize COPD are both a cause of and a result of the normal anxiety that accompanies this illness.

Life becomes a series of paradoxical activities for COPD patients. They must train themselves not to breathe hard when they feel the need for oxygen. They must work at calming themselves despite the natural tendency for their labored breathing to cause anxiety. Their anxiety and depression may seem intractable. Caregivers may feel impotent as the patient constantly expresses disappointment and shows evidence of depression, anxiety and anger.

COPD patients will frequently develop opportunistic infections. These patients often require repeated treatment for pneumonia and other exacerbations of their condition. Steroid treatments are commonly used to decrease bronchial inflammation. The benefit of steroid treatments is balanced against the many potentially serious side effects. Skin gets thinner, blood vessels become more fragile, and patients can become puffy and moon-faced. Patients may develop purple lines (striae) on their abdomens, and their abdomens may enlarge. Muscles atrophy. Patients may develop the appearance of someone suffering from severe malnutrition, which can contribute further to their emotional decline. Most important is that steroids markedly hasten the development of osteoporosis.

Spinal Cord Injury
A spinal cord injury can be one of the most devastating injuries the human body can sustain. The loss of functioning that can result depends upon the level of the spinal injury; the higher the injury, the more impaired the patient will be.

The spinal vertebrae encase the spinal cord. Each of the vertebrae are classified by region—cervical, dorsal, lumbar, sacral, and coccygeal—according to the vertical positions they occupy. Beginning at the base of the skull, in descending position, there are seven cervical, twelve dorsal (or thoracic), five lumbar, five sacral, and four coccygeal vertebrae—thirty-three in all. Injuries to the spinal cord sustained at the upper C vertebral levels C1, C2, C3, C4 are the most immediately life-threatening as they affect nerves that relate to the functioning of the respiratory system (C1, C2) and the diaphragm (C3, C4). These injuries can paralyze all extremities (a condition known as quadriplegia) and impair bowel and bladder function. Injuries below C4, while potentially disabling, will not affect respiration or use of the arms. They may paralyze the lower extremities (a condition known as paraplegia) and affect bowel and bladder function as well.

Spinal cord injury patients are difficult to maintain in a home care setting. Bowel and bladder regimens need to be strictly adhered to. This may require several hours of personal care assistance to ensure regular evacuations and volume monitoring. Numerous other problems may occur due to loss of mobility, including skin breakdown, especially if the patient is bedbound. Safety concerns such as helplessness in a fire, injury from falls, and so on, are of paramount importance. Quadriplegics and paraplegics are especially vulnerable to respiratory infections, pneumonia, ulcers, and pressure sores.

Autonomic dysreflexia sometimes occurs with spinal cord injury patients. It is a rare condition precipitated by either a bowel or bladder obstruction. Pressure builds if the bowel becomes distended due to an obstruction or loss of function, or if urine is not totally drained. This may stimulate the fight or flight response in the autonomic nervous system. Patients become suddenly severely hypertensive as their blood pressure spikes and their heart rate decreases, increasing their risk for stroke, heart failure or myocardial infarction.

Understandably, spinal cord injury patients tend to be depressed, especially in the acute phase following the spinal cord injury. Their mobility impairment and personal care dependency is experienced as a loss of identity. Their sudden incapacity affects their ability to sustain intimate relationships and to continue relationships with friends and family whose lifestyles have not been altered. They have difficulty finding and retaining new employment or vocational training opportunities. Psychological and vocational counseling as well as intensive rehabilitation can mitigate these early reactions to loss, and many patients with spinal cord injuries are able to lead happy and productive lives. The recent interest in spinal cord injury research has created the hope that eventually we will be able to reverse the damage done by spinal cord injuries, but a final answer is most likely several decades away.

Multiple Sclerosis (MS)

Multiple sclerosis (MS) usually afflicts people in the third or fourth decade of life. It affects more than 350,000 Americans and is the most frequent cause of non-traumatic disability in early to middle adulthood. It afflicts more women than men, Caucasians more than other racial groups, and populations in temperate climates more than those in tropical ones.

Diagnosing MS can be somewhat difficult. Newer technologies including Computed Tomography Scan (CT or "CAT" Scan) and Magnetic Resonance Imaging (MRI) have facilitated diagnosis of this condition. Spinal fluid analysis may also be helpful.

Multiple sclerosis is so named due to the development of hardened (sclerotic) patchy lesions at several sites on the white matter of the brain and spinal cord. The primary clinical challenges for health care professionals treating those with multiple sclerosis are maintaining skin integrity, managing mobility and preventing falls, and slowing the progression of the disease. As the illness progresses, MS sufferers become increasingly dependent on appliances (braces, et cetera) and assistive devices as they struggle to maximize their independence. MS presents its victims with a unique set of adjustment challenges because of its mid-life onset. MS usually strikes at a time of life when careers are maturing, when child rearing is a primary focus, and when being the caregiver rather than the person needing care is the norm.

Overall, multiple sclerosis usually progresses slowly. A patient's ability to function can deteriorate steadily or precipitously and then level off; it may even improve for extended periods of time. Those who struggle with MS find themselves teased with temporary improvements, then relapses, and then periods of stability. This can make psychological, emotional, and lifestyle adjustments all the more difficult. Adjustment-to-loss counseling and psychotherapy are nearly always indicated.

A popular theory concerning the cause of MS implicates the immune system. Numerous treatments to reverse or retard the progress of MS have been tried, the most helpful being drugs that modulate the immune response. To date, however, there has been no cure for MS. Symptomatic treatment of muscle spasm, bladder dysfunction, and depression, and prevention of contractures and pressure ulcers remain important aspects of care.

As the condition progresses and the patient's ability to function declines, it becomes increasingly important to provide daily personal care assistance. Family members commonly provide much of the personal care. Because of the long course of MS, it is especially important to identify caregiver issues and to provide for regular respite care to enable the primary caregiver time to recover energy and motivation.

Diabetes

Diabetes occurs when the beta cells in the pancreas fail to produce enough insulin or when tissue sensitivity to insulin decreases (or both). Insulin is the hormone that facilitates the passage of glucose from the blood into cells throughout the body. This metabolic process provides energy to the body; if glucose is unable to enter the cells due to lack of insulin, the cells lose a critical source of energy and blood sugar levels increase. If the body cannot get enough energy from the conversion of glucose, it will begin to break down its own stores of fats and proteins, resulting in weight loss and, eventually, in the development of acidosis (increased acidity of the blood).

At the same time, when the level of glucose in the blood increases too much, it causes changes in the body's proteins, including those that comprise the walls of capillaries. These changes can occur in the blood vessels of primary organs such as the kidneys, the heart, and the central nervous system as well as in other structures such as the skin (especially in the lower extremities). Damage to capillary walls results in compromised microcirculation and end organ pathology. Thus diabetics are at risk for severe damage to multiple organs. To prevent such damage, it is necessary to maintain the blood glucose within a narrow range and to prevent hypoglycemia (low blood sugar) and hyperglycemia (high blood sugar).

There are two forms of diabetes—Type I or insulin-dependent diabetes mellitus (IDDM) and Type II or non-insulin-dependent diabetes mellitus (NIDDM). People with NIDDM either produce too little insulin or are insensitive to the insulin they do produce. Their treatment includes administering medications that cause the pancreas to produce more insulin or that make the body more sensitive to its own naturally produced insulin. People with IDDM either produce no insulin at all or produce so little that they must receive their insulin artificially by daily injection.

Diabetics must manage and monitor their condition very attentively, a requirement that applies to the caregiving team as well. Diabetics must be capable of sticking to a restrictive diet and adhering to a daily regime of medication compliance, diet monitoring, and maintenance of therapeutic blood sugar levels. They must be able to make the necessary lifestyle changes and to develop and adhere to strict routines that compensate for their illness.

Diabetics are full partners with their physicians in the management of their care. Their success in managing their diabetes depends upon their mutual investment in this partnership. They face an ongoing educational challenge. Eating and drinking habits must be monitored and modified and a high degree of motivation must be maintained to ensure compliance with the diabetic regimen. It is easy to appreciate that cognitively impaired diabetics–those with advancing dementia, mental retardation, et cetera–are extremely difficult to manage in a home care setting unless there is a responsible caregiver to provide the needed oversight. If there is no caregiver willing to assume the responsibility, institutional care often becomes necessary for cognitively impaired individuals who are unable to manage their diets and adhere to a rigorous medication regime.

Hypertension (HTN)

Hypertension is commonly defined as a blood pressure that exceeds 140/90, although other limits have been proposed for older people which may be twenty-five points greater or less than this number. The upper number is called the *systolic*, the bottom number the *diastolic* blood pressure. Systolic hypertension is thought to result from decreased elasticity of blood vessels that occurs as a person ages. Hypertension may precipitate end-organ failure, or be caused by it, as in the case of renal disease.

Hypertension is measured in increments of severity–mild, moderate, and severe. Screenings now begin in childhood, and early intervention and treatment have been shown to reduce morbidity and mortality.

There are many causes of hypertension, but heredity and lifestyle play important roles. Blood pressure depends upon both cardiac output and peripheral resistance. It has been suggested that increased peripheral resistance develops via structural narrowing of blood vessels. Any explanation of the cause of hypertension must account for this structural change. Other causative factors include kidney disease, hormonal influence, and autonomic nervous system effects.

Hypertension is best managed by a combination of medication, lifestyle change and diet restrictions, complimented by psychological/ emotional therapies. Medication compliance is often problematic because patients with hypertension may be asymptomatic, and many anti-hypertensive agents have unpleasant side effects, such as lack of energy and impotence.

Myocardial Infarction (MI)

Myocardial infarction, or a heart attack, is the destruction of the heart muscle (myocardium) caused by an interruption of its blood supply. Tissue is damaged or killed (infarcted) on the "down stream" (distal) side of a blood clot. The infarcted tissue loses its ability to function due either to tissue death (necrosis) or lost elasticity. Myocardial infarction is the leading cause of death in the United States. Five primary risk factors are associated with MI: excess weight or obesity, smoking, sedentary lifestyle, stress, and a genetic predisposition or a family history of hypertension or arteriosclerosis. Primary and secondary prevention strategies exist for each of the major risk factors. Smoking cessation, weight reduction, and pharmacolgic and dietary control of hypertension and blood lipid abnormalities can have a significant impact on the risk of coronary artery disease and, ultimately, myocardial infarction.

Although prevention is always the preferred approach to treatment of arteriosclerotic cardiovascular disease, preventive measures are difficult for many people. Even when high compliance is achieved, heart disease may still progress and result in myocardial infarction.

Injury to the muscle of the left ventricle impedes the ability of the heart to pump blood to the entire body (with the exception of the lungs) and results in left-sided congestive heart failure (see above). Damage to the right ventricle causes right-sided congestive heart failure. Extensive damage from infarction produces a condition called ischemic cardiomyopathy. People with this condition experience significant restriction in their physical capabilities. They are characteristically weak, fatigued, mobility-impaired, and short of breath. In extreme cases, cardiac transplantation is the only treatment option. In less severely affected people or in people for whom cardiac transplantation is inappropriate, symptoms are managed pharmacologically.

Aside from its obvious physiological significance, the "heart" has deep cultural significance as well, and a heart attack often has far-reaching psychological and emotional effects. A damaged heart may be experienced as damaged self-esteem. It confronts us suddenly with our own mortality, and the identity crisis that results often triggers a grief reaction in the heart attack victim. The challenge for family members and counselors alike is to avoid pathologizing the depression that often follows a heart attack and/or cardiac surgery. It may be more productive to normalize the experience and help the heart attack patient to acknowledge the loss of identity associated with many of the symptoms of heart disease. The patient's self-care challenge is to adopt lifestyle changes that prevent further episodes, or to accommodate them if they occur.

Managing the post-MI patient in a home care setting presents an array of challenges. Heart attack victims are frequently enervated, discouraged, and depressed. Treatment compliance is sometimes difficult to achieve and sustain. Their mobility may be impaired, which puts them at risk for falls and additional injuries. Treatment must involve the full interdisciplinary care team, and a detailed care plan must be implemented and careful follow-up coordinated to ensure compliance and improvement.

Cancer

There are many different types of cancer and each type affects individuals differently. Cancers are treatable by chemotherapy, surgery, or radiation, depending on the organs involved. Their lethality also varies depending on both the type of cancer and the organs involved.

Cancer is a major cause of death, and over 50 percent of new cases occur in those aged seventy or older. As life expectancies increase, the number of older people with cancer can also be expected to increase. New treatments will improve outcomes and ensure prolonged life for increasing numbers of elderly cancer patients.

Cancer prevention for older people requires both primary and secondary prevention approaches. Examples of primary prevention include changes in lifestyle, exercise regimen, and diet; all of which can help one avoid developing cancer. Secondary prevention involves screening tests and examinations that can detect cancer early and increase the chance of cure and the disease-free interval following therapy. People over age sixty-five are most commonly affected by cancers of the prostate, stomach, colorectum, pancreas, esophagus, breast, and lung. The incidence of breast and lung cancer is higher in early old age, but declines in late old age.

Cancer is not always fatal, though most people believe that it is. When developing long-term care plans, care managers must account for the possibility of either gradual or precipitous change in the client's health status. Plans must be adapted to the individual, highly flexible, and especially sensitive to medical treatment options. What is relevant one day may become irrelevant the next, and vice versa.

A cancer diagnosis may present all the possible home health care challenges, including maintaining the patient's skin integrity, safety, medication compliance, and provision of adequate personal care assistance. Hospice and palliative care have become increasingly important over the past twenty years for cancer victims who have exhausted their treatment options. The lifespan of a cancer patient may be more predictably terminal as compared to the more gradual decline for other chronic illnesses such as congestive heart failure or chronic obstructive pulmonary disease. It may be easier for a physician to certify that the cancer patient has less than 6 months to live, which is a primary criterion for hospice eligibility.

Cellulitis

Cellulitis (infection of the tissues), usually of the lower extremities, is a common disorder in elderly people. People who have limited mobility and sit in one position for much of the day are at higher risk for developing this condition. Such people frequently experience edema (swelling) of the lower extremities, which interferes with blood flow and the mobilization of interstitial fluid.

Any breach of skin integrity permits the entry of pathologic organisms that infect compromised tissues. Curing the infection is often complicated by the fact that circulatory problems may have precipitated the cellulitis. When blood circulation is impaired, antibiotics are delivered less efficiently to the infection site. It is also more difficult to reduce the inflammation caused by the pooling of fluid.

Treating cellulitis requires a three-pronged attack. First, infection and inflammation must be treated. Cellulitis tends to take hold and develop within twenty-four to forty-eight hours and requires treatment with appropriate antibiotics. Second, good circulatory return must be promoted to reduce venous pooling. Elevation of the extremity and the judicious application of warmth are helpful adjuncts to antibiotics. People with recurrent cellulitis may benefit from taking prophylactic antibiotics and wearing compressive elastic stockings. Third, patient compliance with special diet and mobility restrictions must be ensured, and adequate personal care assistance must be provided. This caregiving protocol may appear simple, but psychosocial issues such as depression, cognitive decline and memory impairment, social isolation, and caregiver inadequacy often complicate it.

In addition, since most cellulitis sufferers are either elderly or physically disabled, they are already at greater risk for injury and infection. In the absence of an adequate caregiver and advocate, cellulitis can result in nursing home placement.

Urinary Incontinence

Urinary incontinence is the loss of bladder control. It can be caused by genitourinary pathology, age-related changes, other illness, environmental obstacles, or some combination of these. Although urinary incontinence may not be a normal part of aging, as we age we often lose bladder tone and, as a consequence, urinary control. Incontinence can be classified as transient or established. The causes of transient incontinence can be remembered by the following mnemonic:

DIAPPERS

Delirium or confused state
I nfection
Atrophic vaginitis or urethritis
Pharmacologic agents that impair cognition, mobility, fluid balance, or sphincter function
Psychological disorders such as depression or severe psychosis
Excessive urine output due to diabetes, diuretics, CHF, et cetera
Restricted mobility from acute and chronic disorders
S tool impaction.

Established incontinence has four main causes:
1) Bladder muscle hyperactivity with impaired contractility
2) Failure of sphincter mechanisms
3) Impaired muscle contractility or outlet obstruction such as prostate enlargement, cancer, stricture, cystocele
4) Inability or unwillingness to toilet due to physical, cognitive, or environmental factors.

A careful evaluation is fundamental to making an appropriate diagnosis and implementing corrective therapy. The evaluation consists of a comprehensive history and physical examination, the results of which are used to select appropriate tests. Generally, treatment can be classified as behavioral or pharmacologic. Catheters, which fall into neither of these categories, should be used only when patients have problems with chronic urinary retention or non-healing pressure ulcers, or when they are requested by patients and families to promote comfort.

Urinary incontinence markedly increases the bed- or chair-bound patient's risk of skin breakdown and infections that can result from pressure sores (decubitis ulcers). When the skin is constantly wet, it is susceptible to irritation and breakdown, and bacteria can take hold and grow. This in combination with constant pressure can lead to ulcers. Ulcers can progress to sepsis or blood infection, and the patient's condition can become life threatening as a result.

For the home care patient, regular monitoring of skin integrity can prevent complications of urinary incontinence. Adequate personal care assistance is a must. It is probably the most cost-effective way to prevent institutional admissions among those with both urinary incontinence and mobility impairment.

Urinary incontinence can impose considerable limitations on an individual's lifestyle. It is nearly always an embarrassing blow to one's self-esteem. It limits mobility in terms of both the distance one can travel and the outing's duration. It may make the individual totally homebound.

Urinary Tract Infections

The urine of elderly people commonly contains bacteria; a condition called asymptomatic bacteruria. In one study in Finland, 20 percent of the population over age sixty-five had significant bacteruria, and women outnumbered men six to one. When asymptomatic bacteruria becomes symptomatic and the concentration of bacteria increases to more than 100,000 per cc, treatment with antibiotics is warranted. In patients with indwelling foley catheters, treatment of urinary tract infections is reserved for those who have such symptoms as fever, chills, blood in the urine (hematuria), or other signs indicative of invasive infection. Premature or unnecessary treatment of urinary tract infections can lead to antibiotic resistance, rendering future treatment problematic.

The clinician's challenge in a home care setting is to overcome the infection while keeping patients hydrated adequately and not compromising their cardiopulmonary system. Infections in the urinary tract can become serious if they back up into the renal system. Urinary tract infections can become life threatening if the infection spreads from the urinary tract into the bloodstream and causes urosepsis. Urosepsis might manifest itself in a sudden change of cognitive status. Patients can become confused and anxious. They may become dehydrated and hypotensive. These symptoms can easily be mistaken for other syndromes or disease processes.

Alzheimer's Disease and the Dementing Illnesses

Years ago, elderly people who experienced marked cognitive decline were described as senile. Today, dementia is the more commonly used term. It describes several different types of senility. The common characteristic among all dementias is significant memory impairment. Alzheimer's-type dementia has perhaps become most familiar because of the debilitating nature of the illness and the growing number of elderly people afflicted with it.

Alzheimer's disease can strike as early as age forty, though most commonly it manifests in the later years of life. It is diagnosed by determining that a patient has a consistent pattern of progressive symptoms that can include both short-term and long-term memory loss, impaired cognitive functioning, emotional lability, impulsive and sometimes antagonistic behavior, disorientation, paranoia, and even psychosis. Alzheimer's disease is progressively debilitating and progressively difficult to manage in a home care setting not only because of personal care and safety issues, but also because of the high rate of caregiver burnout.

Patients with Alzheimer's disease, even in the early stages, almost always need twenty-four hour supervision to ensure their safety. Their inability to make good decisions, their inclination to wander and lose their way, and their impaired memory and inability to comply with treatment recommendations make them unsafe to be left unsupervised. Eventually they become legally incompetent and/or incapable, and in need of a guardian to protect them from harm and exploitation.

Physiologically, Alzheimer's disease destroys gray matter (brain tissue). These changes affect not only cognition but also physical functioning. As the disease progresses, Alzheimer's patients lose bowel and bladder control. Their mobility and equilibrium become impaired. If they live long enough they lose mobility all together. Alzheimer's disease has been described as "regressive." Over time, Alzheimer's patients regress through the developmental stages, back to a condition that approximates infancy.

The Alzheimer caregiver's experience is a "long good-bye." Slowly but surely, Alzheimer's patients fade away while their bodies remain. The person who was once spouse, companion, or parent no longer behaves as such, despite the fact that he or she may look like the same person. The emotional drain of caregiving and witnessing the patient's decline takes its toll on even the most committed of caregivers.

Few conditions require more attention to housing adaptations than Alzheimer's disease. The patient's living environment can either ease or exacerbate the patient's frustration, confusion, and anxiety, depending on its design, the furniture in it, the wall hangings, or the room's color schemes. Since long-term memory is affected later in the progression of the disease, familiar objects and pictures from a person's past are important anchors and should be present in the living environment.

Many different types of housing options have been developed in recent years in response to the growing Alzheimer's "market." They include residential dementia programs in specialized units within nursing homes or assisted living facilities. People with various types of dementia often reside in Alzheimer's facilities. Early stage Alzheimer's patients may fit well enough into other types of seniors' communities, but will need either higher levels of care and supervision as the disease progresses or to be transferred to an Alzheimer's care facility.

Alzheimer's facilities are specially designed for Alzheimer's patients. They facilitate residents' ability to find their way around by use of colors and environmental cues, providing for safe indoor and outdoor wandering. Furniture is grouped to encourage social interaction. Lighting is even and ubiquitous. Alzheimer's programs accommodate residents' varied sleep and eating patterns and have higher staffing ratios.

In considering an Alzheimer's facility, family members are usually eager to find one with a resident population with which their loved one shares similar traits. Given their loved one's incapacity, it is important for family members to believe that residents will be treated with dignity and respect and that their rights will be protected. Advance directives such as a durable power of attorney, a health care proxy, and a Do Not Resuscitate (DNR) order are very important to ensure that the patient's and family's wishes concerning medical treatment are followed.

If home care is chosen for the Alzheimer's patient, home safety is of primary concern. Caregiver support is also a priority. The high level of stress associated with caring for an Alzheimer's patient may necessitate respite services for the caregiver. These often include adult day care, high levels of personal care assistance, and short-term nursing home placements.

Although safety is always the primary concern, it should be noted that restraints of all types can have a destabilizing effect on those with Alzheimer's dementia. Even tranquilizers and sedatives must be seen as restraints. All forms of restraints can be harmful to the health and well being of those incapacitated by dementia. But when they are necessary to ensure the safety of either the patient or others in the same environment, every effort should be made to develop creative alternatives that protect the patient's dignity. The importance of environmental design cannot be overstated—environmental boundaries that do not feel like restraints are always preferable.

Judicious use of behavior-modifying medication may be indicated when the health, comfort and safety of the patient and caregiver(s) cannot be assured by non-pharmacologic means. Depression also occurs in up to 40 percent of all dementia patients and may accelerate a patient's decline if left untreated. Non-anticholinergic antidepressants such as trazodone, SSRIs, bupropion and mirtazipine can be tried after careful evaluation for depression. For agitation, neuroleptics such as haloperidol, rispiridone, and olanzapine can be cautiously introduced, but the patient must be closely monitored to detect impaired balance and increased risk of falling. As with all medications for older people, the rule is "start low and go slow."

The common goals when caring for Alzheimer's patients are to protect and foster the patient's dignity, to reduce the risk of injury from falls and/or combative behavior, to maintain skin integrity, and to minimize emotional distress. Alzheimer's disease is not yet curable. The disease progresses in stages that caregivers must understand if they are to maintain their motivation as well as their patience. Treatment for Alzheimer's disease, with the exception of sedatives to protect patient safety and reduce anxiety, is mostly non-medical. The primary focus of treatment should be on maintaining psychosocial well being. Currently available Alzheimer's drugs such as donepezil (Aricept) and tacrine (Cognex) have a minimal effect on symptoms. Their main value is in retarding the advance of dementia. They are quite expensive, and at best, they slow cognitive decline by about one or two years.

Fractures of the Hip and Knee

Fractures have especially devastating consequences for frail elderly people. Indeed, they are the leading cause of nursing home placement today. They are among the most preventable long-term care problems, but their prevention is often more easily described than accomplished.

Knee and hip fractures can cause permanent disability. They often result from falls and inevitably lead to hospitalization, protracted inpatient rehabilitation, and sometimes nursing home placement. In rare instances surgical repair is infeasible, and individuals may become bedridden as a result.

Knee and hip injuries can lead to what has been termed the cycle of deconditioning. Bedbound patients—prone to problems with elimination, skin breakdown, infection, and pneumonia—lose muscle tone and strength. Depression may develop, precipitated by expectations of continued disability, dissatisfaction with the institutional environment, or disappointment with a slowed rate of recovery. Depression-induced inactivity causes additional deconditioning. As long-term care expenses mount, hope and motivation can wane and depression can deepen. The cycle of deconditioning continues.

Many knee and hip fractures can be repaired but it is sometimes possible to avert them altogether by joint replacement surgeries. While joint replacements are not nearly as debilitating as the fractures they prevent, they are not always entirely successful either. After the surgery, patient compliance with mobility restrictions and physical therapy often determines rehabilitation potential. A knee replacement patient with osteoarthritis may have difficulty complying with exercise regimens following surgery. Perhaps excess weight was an underlying cause of the degradation of the knee joint to begin with. If excess weight cannot be shed to sustain the viability of the repaired joint, it may not be possible for the patient to make a full recovery.

We emphasize, however, that the prognosis for recovery among those receiving hip or knee replacements is generally very good with appropriate preoperative evaluation and selection. Hip, pelvis, or knee fractures need not mean the end of independence for frail elders. Intensive rehabilitation can succeed for many, and full function is often restored. The prospects for recovery are best if the person possesses the three Ms—mentation, motivation, and muscle. Successful rehabilitation requires that a person be capable of reasonably normal mental activity in order to understand and implement the prescribed treatment. Motivation is critically important to completing a prolonged, difficult and sometimes painful rehabilitation program. Lastly, the person's muscle and neurological functions must be near normal to enable progress. Without these three Ms, it is doubtful that rehabilitation will be successful.

Fractures are perhaps the most preventable of disabling conditions. Thus, it is critical that frail elderly patients be screened and treated for osteoporosis, that their risk of falls be reduced through modifications to their environment and provision of adequate personal care and supervision, and that medications that might impair their stability and balance are avoided.

Osteoarthritis and Rheumatoid Arthritis

Arthritis is the most common cause of disability in people over seventy-five years of age. The two most common forms of arthritis are rheumatoid arthritis and osteoarthritis (degenerative arthritis).

Rheumatoid arthritis is a chronic inflammation of the membranes surrounding the peripheral joints. The inflammation occurs at the point of bone intersection (articular) or in the area surrounding the joint (periarticular). The cause is unknown. Most people with rheumatoid arthritis are over the age of sixty. Rheumatoid arthritis with an onset in old age tends to be more severe than rheumatoid arthritis that begins before the age of sixty.

Osteoarthritis causes erosion of the cartilage at the weight-bearing or stress-bearing joints. Lifestyle and physical type have an impact on the development of osteoarthritis. Thus, degenerative joint disease tends to develop among those who are obese or those who worked for extended periods of time in jobs that placed increased stress on the joints of the lower extremities.

Arthritis is progressive and disabling. As mobility and manual dexterity become impaired, safety issues inevitably need to be addressed as the risk for falls increases. Rheumatoid arthritis sufferers may become severely disabled and unable to perform even the basic ADLs (Activities of Daily Living) due to the loss of function of hands as well as legs. Early intervention with this type of patient is extremely important to identify future dependent care needs. Managing chronic pain is also a primary challenge in helping arthritis sufferers maintain their quality of life. Pain can be both a physical and psychological obstacle to the maintenance of function.

Treatment of osteoarthritis currently focuses on reducing inflammation and pain through the use of non-steroidal anti-inflammatory drugs, physical therapy, joint replacement, and bracing. For rheumatoid arthritis, non-steroidal anti-inflammatory drugs, steroids, penicillamine, methotrexate, cyclosporine A, and injectable gold salts have been effective for symptomatic relief and to delay progression. Physical therapy, joint replacement, podiatric care, and bracing are also frequently useful in the treatment of rheumatoid arthritis.

Cerebrovascular Accidents (CVA or Stroke)

CVAs can be classified into four clinical categories: transient ischemic attacks (TIAs, which resolve within 24 hours), reversible ischemic neurologic deficits (which resolve within one week), stroke (occlusive or hemorrhagic), and cerebral multi-infarct states (cortical, subcortical, or diffuse).

There are three basic mechanisms for strokes, each of which results in the interruption of blood flow to the central nervous system:

1) Thrombus or blood clot formation in an artery of the central nervous system
2) Embolization (foreign substance or blood clot obstruction) to an artery of the central nervous system due to a clot from a site outside the central nervous system
3) Rupture of an artery in the central nervous system with resulting local hemorrhages.

Interruption of the blood flow to the central nervous system results in insufficient oxygenation of tissue (anoxia) and subsequent rapid destruction of the affected tissue. Recently, the use of recombinant tissue plasminogen activator (rt-PA) has been shown to be of benefit in reversing acute ischemic symptoms if used within the first hour after the onset of symptoms. But preventive interventions must be employed to reduce the risk of stroke. Primary prevention methods such as good nutrition, moderate salt consumption, and regular exercise, and secondary prevention methods such as treatment of hypertension, normalization of lipid disorders, and surgical correction of carotid artery narrowing and aneurysms of the cerebral arteries have been shown to be effective methods of reducing the risk of stroke.

Once irreversible damage to the central nervous system has been sustained, rehabilitation is the primary focus of treatment. Substantial improvement is possible within six weeks of a stroke and additional improvement occurs over the ensuing five months. Physical therapy, speech therapy, and occupational therapy are the primary rehabilitation modalities and should be employed early and intensively during the initial six-week period following the stroke. Thereafter, maintenance rehabilitation should be employed as needed. Evaluation of the patient's living environment by a qualified occupational therapist can be extremely helpful in assisting the stroke patient to return to an independent lifestyle. Structural modifications to the kitchen, bathroom, and access routes to the home can substantially reduce or eliminate dependence on personal care providers, reducing the cost of ongoing care in the home.

Depression associated with a normal grief reaction is to be expected in the stroke patient. The patient who has lost his or her ability to walk or speak may also suffer an identity crisis. While the grief reaction associated with loss should not be pathologized, clinical benefit can often be gained by utilizing antidepressant drugs early in the stroke patient's rehabilitation program. Antidepressants are particularly helpful for patients whose depression is due to biochemical aberrations brought on by the stroke. Time is of the essence for the stroke patient's recovery. Antidepressant therapy may overcome reduced motivation that accompanies the grieving process. The precious opportunity for rehabilitation that immediately follows the stroke should be aggressively exploited. As noted for hip and knee surgeries, rehabilitation is most successful if the patient has the three Ms–mentation, muscle, and motivation. Depression can markedly impair motivation and thus reduce the effectiveness of rehabilitation.

Ocular Disease
Severe visual impairment is much more prevalent in people over the age of sixty-five than in younger people. Strategies for preventing visual impairment include biennial ophthalmic examinations for people with normal vision, and semiannual ophthalmic examinations for people with established eye problems. The most treatable, as well as most preventable eye disorders are glaucoma, diabetic retinopathy, macular degeneration and cataracts.

Glaucoma, or increased pressure inside the eye, causes impaired peripheral vision that can advance to total blindness. African Americans and the elderly are most at risk for this disease. Treatments include both surgical and pharmacologic interventions.

Diabetic retinopathy results from damage to the retina caused by elevated blood sugars. These lesions consist of microaneurysms, hemorrhages, and proliferative retinopathy. The primary method of prevention is careful control of blood glucose. Treatment consists of laser photocoagulation of severe retinopathy.

Age-related macular degeneration (ARMD) causes atrophy of the cells of the macula, the central area of the retina that is utilized when we look at something in a focused way, for example, when we read. A person with ARMD experiences a hole in the middle of their visual field. Risk factors for ARMD include age and exposure to sunlight. Certain forms of ARMD may be treated with laser photocoagulation. Magnifying lenses and electronic magnification devices are helpful in aiding patients to read printed material.

Cataracts cause clouding and, ultimately, opacification of the lens of the eye. Risk factors include age, sun exposure, smoking, steroids, and diabetes. Treatment consists of replacement of the damaged lens with a plastic implant. The procedure requires about one-half hour and is usually an outpatient procedure.

Individuals who have lost some or all of their vision are likely to have significant psychological adjustment problems. Sight is the most utilized of the five senses. Ninety-five percent of the information processed by the brain is "downloaded" through the eyes. Our eyes are also intimately expressive. Through them we make contact with other people, and they with us. Loss of eyesight is both immediately disabling *and* a critical blow to our relationships and our identities.

Care managers must appreciate how significant the loss of eyesight can be. Care planning for those with vision loss must include the acquisition of adequate personal care assistance, assistive devices and community supports. As addressed in chapter 4, dealing with a client's personal adjustment issues almost always precedes the care planning effort. Local associations for the blind can assist with special training and devices to enable blind people to rebuild their lives and to become functional and productive once again.

Osteoporosis

Osteoporosis is a condition characterized by low bone density and an increased risk of fractures. Women are at greater risk for this disease, especially if they are post-menopausal. Other risk factors include low calcium intake, physical inactivity and lack of weight-bearing excercise, smoking, and excessive alcohol consumption. Those who receive pharmologic treatment with corticosteroids, heparin, and certain antiepileptic drugs (e.g. phenytoin) may also be at greater risk.

Preventive interventions include adequate calcium intake (1500 mg per day in women if given with estrogen, 1000 mg per day in men), 400 to 800 IUs per day of vitamin D, weight bearing physical activity, estrogen or raloxifene, and 5 mg per day of alendronate (fosamax).

Treatment is essentially the same as prevention except for the addition of 200 IUs of Calcitonin daily by nasal spray. Calcitonin not only increases bone density, but also reduces the pain due to vertebral compression fractures. In treating osteoporosis, the primary goal is to prevent painful and costly fractures of the spine, hip and wrist and to reverse the cycle of fractures, pain, and inactivity that invariably accompanies the disease.

Parkinson's Disease (PD)

Parkinson's disease is a neuro-degenerative disease and motor-system disorder. It is characterized by cell death in the substantia nigra, the region of the brain that produces the chemical dopamine, which is critical to the direction and coordination of muscle activity. Dopamine enables the substantia nigra to communicate with another area of the brain, the corpus striatum, to produce coordinated, deliberate movement. Parkinson's disease was named after James Parkinson, a British physician who in 1817 described it as the "shaking palsy." The cause of PD is unknown.

There are four primary symptoms of Parkinson's disease: tremor of the extremities and face or jaw; general stiffness of the extremities and the torso; bradykinesia or slowness of movement; and mobility impairments such as disequilibrium and discoordination. In most patients, PD first manifests in "pill-rolling" tremors of the thumb and forefingers. Rigidity also develops, as opposing muscles remain constantly tensed or contracted due to the disturbed brain function. Activities that were once performed automatically and quickly, such as dressing or washing, may take several hours to perform (bradykinesa). Marked disequilibrium manifests as retropulsion (uncontrolled backward steps), propulsion (uncontrolled forward leaning movements) and festination (increasingly rapid forward steps apparently to maintain balance). Parkinson's sufferers can experience broad functional decline that also includes difficulty swallowing and chewing, speech changes, urinary problems and constipation, dyskenesias (involuntary twitching), sleep disorders and skin problems. Dementia occurs in almost half of PD patients, and emotional instability, swallowing dysfunction, and depression may develop as the primary disabling aspects of the illness.

Treatment for Parkinson's disease usually begins with less powerful anticholinergic drugs or amantadine. As the disease progresses, the present standard treatment is the administration of levodopa (L-dopa). Nerve cells are able to use L-dopa to manufacture dopamine and replenish the supply that has been reduced by the deterioration of the substantia nigra. Levodopa is usually combined with carbidopa, which delays the conversion of levodopa into dopamine until the chemical reaches the brain. After a few years of treatment, L-dopa's efficacy may diminish such that many PD patients experience an arbitrary, on-again/off-again response.

L-dopa has reduced the need for surgery for PD; however, some PD patients who do not respond to drug therapies still benefit from surgery. One procedure, cryothalamotomy, involves the insertion of a super-cooled metal probe into the thalamus to destroy this tumor-producing area of the brain. Neuralgrafting may hold promise for the treatment of Parkinson's disease. To date, this procedure of implanting nerve cells from fetal brain tissue from the substantia nigra into the brains of animals with Parkinson's has enabled damaged nerve cells to regenerate. These procedures are still experimental and it is too early to evaluate their outcomes. Advanced diagnostics, made possible through Positron emission tomography (PET) scanning, have greatly advanced knowledge of the disease. PET scans produce images of chemical changes in the brain and enable researchers to monitor the sequence of changes in the progression of PD.

Approximately 50,000 Americans are diagnosed with Parkinson's disease every year, and a half million are currently afflicted. Many Parkinson's disease patients mistakenly believing their symptoms are part of normal aging and are not diagnosed until late in the course of the illness. Early symptoms may be minor and can include fatigue, malaise, difficulty standing, shakiness, handwriting changes, problems with word finding, irritability or mild depression. Loved ones may notice a flattening of affect and abnormalities of movement. Other conditions may also produce symptoms similar to Parkinson's disease, further confusing diagnosis. Parkinson's affects men and women equally and tends to strike later in life—the average age at diagnosis is 60. Parkinson's disease is the fourth most common neuro-degenerative disease for the elderly.

Regular exercise is important for the PD patient, especially as the illness progresses and motor function becomes impaired. Physical therapy may help re-establish physical conditioning and teach adaptive strategies. Home modifications and increasing levels of personal care assistance should be considered to reduce the potential for falls. Diet is important since physical inactivity and drug use, as well as the disorder itself, can lead to impaired bowel function. Protein significantly reduces the absorption of L-dopa and meals and medication should be carefully timed to avoid reduced drug effectiveness.

Suggested Readings and References

Holloway, Nancy. *Medical Surgical Care Planning*, Second Edition. Spring House, PA: Spring House Corporation, 1993.

The Merck Manual, 16th ed. Rahway, NJ: Merck Research Laboratories, 1992.

The Merck Manual of Geriatrics, 2nd ed. Rahway, NJ: Merck Research Laboratories, 1995.

Pick, T. Pickering, Robert Howden, and Henry Gray. *Gray's Anatomy*. New York, NY: Gramercy Books, 1977.

Reuben, David B., George T. Grossbert, Lorraine C. Mion, James T. Pacala, Jane F. Potter, Todd P. Semla, *Geriatrics At Your Fingertips*. 1998/99 edition. Belle Mead, NJ: Excerpta Medica, Inc.

Thomas, Clayton, L. *Taber's Cyclopedic Medical Dictionary*, 18th ed. Philadelphia, PA: F. A. Davis Company, Publishers, 1997.

CHAPTER 6

Housing For CLCP Clients

No CLCP task is more important than helping clients determine where they want to live and whether it is feasible for them to live there. Where we live is a reflection of who we are. Our homes matter to us personally, not just practically.

Housing options are determined by four primary considerations—affordability, acceptability, availability, and appropriateness. CLCP clients often confront a bewildering array of housing choices, none of which may be *perfectly* suitable. Assisted living isn't for everyone and neither is home care. Care managers who are well informed about the advantages and disadvantages of different housing arrangements can provide valuable, unbiased decision-making assistance.

AFFORDABILITY

Affordability must be the care manager's first concern when addressing housing alternatives. There is no point in considering what the client cannot afford. For our purposes, "affordable housing" is the kind clients can pay for out of their fixed income and without a reduction in their liquid assets. By this measure, most assisted living residents probably can't afford to live where they live. But this does not mean that assisted living has been inappropriately chosen. Most CLCP clients will make tradeoffs between quality and quantity when nearing the end of life. Two years in an assisted living facility may represent 75 percent of the rest of an 81-year-old client's life. If the socialization and recreational opportunities available in assisted living are attractive enough, despite the financial risk, then who is to say that the "unaffordable" choice is not the right one?

Many CLCP clients will chose to live only where it is affordable for them on a permanent basis, while many others are priced right out of many housing alternatives from the start. Monthly maintenance fees (assisted living facilities don't use the term "rent") in most assisted living facilities are well out of reach of the average Social Security beneficiary with a fixed income of approximately $800 per month. So, too, are the costs of independent living facilities and continuing-care retirement communities. Government subsidies do exist, for example, through an SSI waiver (Supplemental Security Income) that gives income- and asset-eligible seniors an income boost as well as a state supplement to live in so-called Group Adult Foster Care facilities. But these placements are limited in those assisted living and intermediate care facilities that dedicate relatively few units to this population. We expect this option will grow considerably in the coming years.

Determining affordability is easy enough for care managers who are proficient at analyzing income and assets and developing cost-of-living budgets. The housing complex or assisted living facility costs X, and the client's income will or won't cover it. If the client's income, along with other family members' contributions, is sufficient to cover the cost of housing, the care manager can quickly go to the other three considerations—acceptability, appropriateness and availability. Thereafter, the decision-making effort need not address the affordability issue unless the client wants to spend *less* than what he or she can afford on paper.

Lower income CLCP clients wishing to remain in the community can avail themselves of housing options that mimic assisted living and continuing-care retirement facility lifestyles. The carpeting may not be as new, the cuisine as delicately prepared, the recreational facilities as state of the art, or the apartment size as commodious, but congregate-care and subsidized apartment options for thousands of low- to average-income individuals exist all across the country. They have been built in converted elementary schools as well as once grand hotels. These apartments are usually restricted to senior citizens and people with disabilities. They are nearly always handicapped accessible and are subsidized by federal and state governments. Living is "assisted" by visiting nurse agencies under Medicaid waiver programs and other chronic-care programs, as well as the same Medicare home health care benefits also enjoyed by more affluent seniors. The price is also right—usually 30 percent of the eligible senior's or physically disabled person's income. Assets may not preclude eligibility unless they are so high that they generate too much income.

Affordability may also turn on family resources. Many adult children are willing to contribute financially to their aging parents' care, especially if that contribution can make the difference between nursing home placement and continued residence in a community setting. This is a sensitive area for care managers to tread, but one they should not shy away from. The risks and consequences in raising this issue are addressed in greater depth later in this chapter.

ACCEPTABILITY

Making a housing decision is rarely simple. It is complicated by two general, but sometimes competing concerns—practicality and client preference. Care managers should anticipate client resistance when living arrangements that appear tailor-made to meet a client's medical, social, environmental, and spiritual needs might not appeal to the client at all. While the care manager's job may be to try to find a happy medium, he or she must also remember that the housing arrangement that is unacceptable to the client is usually the wrong housing choice. Client dissatisfaction will supercede pragmatism every time. Remember the importance of client support for the care plan.

Care managers must understand how difficult the housing decision can be for the client. Few issues press a client more immediately than home modification or relocation. It is far easier for family members, health care professionals, and facility staff to make long-term housing decisions for clients than it is for the clients to make the decisions themselves. Too often, clients are pressured into deciding in favor of the preference of others. Many go to nursing homes because nursing home placement is the easiest, safest, and quickest way to solve a client's chronic care problems for everyone—with the possible exception of the client. Housing alternatives may not even be discussed in the effort to minimize risk for an elderly, but perfectly competent individual. With the best of intentions, clients are persuaded to do what is "best" for them (translated least problematic for all else concerned). Care managers need to remember their purpose is to serve the client.

If we are unhappy in our homes or in a residential facility *everything* feels wrong. The care manager must always advocate for the housing choice most acceptable to the client except when that choice puts the client at unacceptable risk. This may put the care manager at odds with several influential people in the client's life. The care manager's greatest value may be his or her objectivity and willingness to advocate on behalf of a client's right to folly.

This does not mean the care manager should support bad decisions. As suggested earlier in chapter 4, care managers should try to persuade the client to the safest, best housing alternative while suspending the frustration that often accompanies watching clients make choices that may not be in their safest, best interest. It may be useful for the care manager to ask him or herself a simple question—"What would my reaction be if my client was 45 instead of 85-years-old?" For a younger person, the care manager or family member might not be so concerned. But what is the difference if the client is competent and has been educated to the risk? Age-ism is a double-edged sword. It can be wielded by well-meaning caregivers as an excuse to make decisions for an aging, but capable parent, and it can also be used manipulatively by elderly clients themselves.

The care manager can advocate on behalf of a client's housing choice while disagreeing with the client as to its appropriateness. Over time the client may agree that he or she is not choosing appropriately, but this will not happen unless the client has had time to adjust. One again, we see the importance of a care manager's familiarity with the counseling and engagement skills of CLCP.

AVAILABILITY

Having evaluated affordability, it is essential that the care manager make sure the type of housing that appears best suited for the client can actually be acquired. Care managers do not want to create false hope for clients and their families if the housing option they recommend has no vacancies.

In most areas of the country, assisted living and its no-frills cousin, independent living, is readily available for those who can afford it. Indeed, there appears to be no end in sight to the construction boom in assisted- and independent-living facilities. Most middle- and upper-income elders can rest easy knowing that an efficiency apartment in an assisted living facility, replete with long hallways, social and recreational opportunities, decent meals, and medical support services, is coming to a town near them—if it isn't there already. Assisted living and independent living facilities have sprung up everywhere. They are both desirable *and* profitable, and the paysource for them is as secure as the Social Security program itself.

Such may not remain the case for publicly subsidized housing for seniors and those with disabilities. Public subsidies for alternative housing compete for the same tax dollars as Medicare, Medicaid, and all other government programs. Care managers exploring these options on behalf of lower- to middle-income clients must make preliminary inquiries of local housing authorities to determine apartment availability and eligibility criteria. Clients may encounter waiting lists for the most desirable locations. There may be restrictions on eligibility that can be overcome, but that may require advance estate planning. In some states applicants must have sold their own home prior to taking up residence in a subsidized seniors' apartment complex or congregate-care facility. This requires planning and coordination. Some states allow the resident to retain home ownership after he or she has moved into the subsidized unit. The former home is then considered an income-generating asset if the homeowner rents it after relocating. CLCP clients are well advised to consult with an accountant ahead of pursuing this strategy as there can be significant tax consequences when a primary residence becomes an investment property and may lose capital gains tax exclusions.

Sometimes what appears *not* to be available may become available with some digging. The waiting list at one subsidized housing facility may be shorter than the list at the client's first choice. Less preferable alternatives may also become attractive as a client's circumstances change. This is especially true for family-care options. The son or daughter of a client may regard housing modifications in his or her own home as impossible to make (and therefore "unavailable") and the client may also resist this option. But things may change when a medical problem threatens nursing home placement. Suddenly housing options that were unavailable and/or unacceptable become very attractive. Under emergency circumstances, housing issues can become a pivotal estate planning concern. In long-term care planning, nothing focuses the mind like a looming $6,000-per-month nursing home placement.

APPROPRIATENESS

Affordability, acceptability and availability do not necessarily make a particular housing arrangement the best choice. The most appropriate housing alternative is the one that best suits a client's safety and medical treatment needs. For the frail, the disabled, and the chronically ill, safety and medical stability is *the* bottom line. These should be the first concern in evaluating a placement's appropriateness.

For *most* CLCP clients, *most* safety considerations can be addressed by providing adequate amounts of supervision and personal care assistance. Environmental design can be very important, but it is rarely as important as the caregiving itself. Selecting appropriate housing is therefore inextricably linked to affordability. For example, assisted living facilities generally provide no more than thirty minutes to an hour of daily personal care assistance as part of a resident's monthly maintenance fee. Additional personal care help is nearly always available from the facility, but residents must usually pay by the hour for it. The facility may be appropriate given the resident's ready access to personal care help, but it may be more expensive in the long run as personal-care fees add up.

An inappropriate placement is one in which a client's safety or medical stability is *unnecessarily* placed at risk. It is conceivable that a nursing home, purportedly the safest long term-care placement, may put a disabled client at greater risk than home care *despite* the 24-hour presence of medical and personal care staff. The nursing home resident with assets over the Medicaid limit can expect to pay up to $6,000 per month for nursing home care. For this cost, the most important service the resident receives is personal care assistance from a certified nurse's aide (CNA), often at the ratio of twelve residents to one aide. Sometimes the ratio is as high as twenty to one, as when a CNA fails to show up for work one day and fill-ins cannot be located. Because of this staffing ratio, it is not unusual for a bedbound resident who needs to use a commode to wait up to thirty minutes or more for transfer assistance. If the CNA is not able to respond in time, the *best* that happens is the resident wets his or her bed. The worst that happens is he or she tries to make it to the commode alone, falls, and fractures a hip.

Alternatively, with a care manager's administrative assistance and for the same $6,000 per month or less, many CLCP clients can acquire adequate private duty care, with private duty RN supervision, and receive 1:1 personal care and supervision, 24-hours per day, in their own homes. For clients who can be maintained at home with competent medical care management, the latter arrangement can actually be safer and more appropriate than nursing home placement.

HOUSING OPTIONS

Disability Modifications

A person's home may need to be adapted to compensate for different types of disability. Impairments in mobility, dexterity, and perception must often be accommodated by changes in living environment design and by acquisition of durable medical equipment. Aside from improving the client's quality of life, comfort, and emotional stability, housing modifications for CLCP clients generally focus on achieving two medical stability goals—preventing falls and maintaining skin integrity.

At the risk of over simplifying the issue, when considering environmental redesign, care managers must remember that we are all mostly skin and bones. A sophisticated medication regime may be able to postpone complications from congestive heart failure, cellulitis, and chronic obstructive pulmonary disease. Adept counseling may reduce anxiety for a stroke patient and, thus, reduce the risk for further cerebrovascular accidents. But in the scheme of things, nothing is more important to keeping a frail CLCP client safe at home than the prevention of falls. The same holds true for bed bound, incontinent, chronic-care clients at high risk for medical problems without adequate skin care.

The care manager who is successful in persuading a client and his or her family to modify the caregiving environment to support these two goals does the client a great service. A seven-inch riser (or step) may be an insurmountable barrier to a physically disabled individual. A 30-inch door opening into a long, narrow bathroom may prevent a wheelchair-bound CLCP client from taking a tub bath or shower. Care managers must understand how these and other barriers can be overcome to promote safety, maximize a client's independence, and maintain medical stability in a home care setting.

Ramps

Ramps offer easy access and egress from homes or apartments. The decision whether or not to install a ramp turns on a clinical assessment that is often best performed by a physical therapist, preferably one with home health care experience. Sometimes ramps are contraindicated because they discourage stair climbing and the physical exercise it entails. When a ramp is appropriate, the client must have adequate resources to pay for the ramp's installation, whether from personal or community sources, as well as adequate space on the exterior of the home.

The building code for ramps in most localities requires that they have adequate railings, that they be sturdily constructed, and that for every inch of rise they be one foot in length. Most steps are approximately seven inches in height. Thus, if the first floor of a home is three steps above ground level, the ramp will need to be 21 feet in length. Usually ramps require an exterior landing or a deck wide enough for the wheelchair to clear a storm door. The ramp then proceeds down from the deck. If a ramp is feasible, a competent carpenter may be all that is needed to create an accessible home or apartment.

Most ramps are built from pressure-treated lumber supported adequately by pillars fixed in concrete footings embedded in the ground below the frost line. Ramps are usually affordable for CLCP clients—material, labor, building permits, and so forth may total no more than a few thousand dollars for a 20–30 foot ramp. But complications may arise. Walls may need to be removed, interior doors widened or perhaps installed in new locations. The ramp itself may be made of more expensive materials such as aluminum or poured concrete, or it may have to be portable. Clients who own their home but lack the funds to install a ramp may find support through a community residential rehabilitation program. An example of such a residential rehabilitation program is provided in Appendix C.

Ramps are important to protect the safety of clients and their caregivers. Assisting mobility-impaired individuals with ambulation and transfers (from wheelchair to shower or from wheelchair to car seat) can be hazardous work. Back injuries are common among nurse's aides and home health aides. A ramp affords a measure of safety that protects the client and the home health aide from the injuries that either of them may sustain when the client loses his or her balance and falls. In northern climates ramps may compensate for ice problems as well.

Many CLCP clients in need of a ramp will resist having them installed. They may be concerned about the impact the ramp will have on the home's appearance or that it may broadcast to the entire world—"Disabled Person Within!" They see the ramp as a flag for their disability and fear it will draw the attention of the criminal element looking for easy prey. Their resistance may also stem from the normal difficulty many have adjusting to disability. Accessibility design is a growing specialty that can address client resistance by creatively solving the cosmetic and safety issues. As the "disability market" expands, more homes will be built or retrofitted for improved access in ways that do not appear unusual or stigmatizing. Care managers can help clients overcome their resistance to accessibility modifications by teaching the critical importance of preventing falls and by helping clients recognize how barrier modifications promote safety.

Accessible Bathrooms

Any nurse, physical therapist, or nurse's aide who has ever worked in a long-term care venue, whether in a nursing home, rehabilitation facility, or home health care agency, knows that running water is good for skin. A bath or a shower beats a bed bath any day, especially for someone who is mobility-impaired, incontinent, and otherwise at risk for skin breakdown.

CLCP clients may face obstacles getting in and out of a bathtub or shower. An upstairs bathroom may by inaccessible to the CLCP client who cannot walk. The wheelchair-bound client may be unable to transfer into a bath and needs a roll-in shower instead. The client who is prone to falling may be able to access the bath or shower with assistance, but what if the bathroom is so narrow the home health aide cannot escort the client into it safely?

Accessible bathrooms also facilitate toileting. For the purposes of this section we will focus on accessibility for bathing as opposed to toileting since the latter is always made easily accessible with the acquisition of a portable commode. This is not to suggest that portable commodes are always an acceptable option. However, they are relatively easy to acquire and use, and can serve in place of an inaccessible bathroom.

Building codes are specific with regard to the term "accessibility." Every bathroom fixture and dimension is regulated for the word "accessible" to pertain. Here we are less regulation-specific than conceptual. For our purposes, an accessible bath is the kind that the client can use safely. Every client's bath-access requirements are going to be different, but the concept remains the same–the fewer obstacles to bath or shower the better.

The primary considerations in deciding whether or not to make a bathroom accessible are space and cost. Most homes or apartments have the space to make bathing accessible to someone in a wheelchair. The Soden's are a case in point.[1] In developing their care plan, we were concerned that the space was so small that their personal care attendants would get cabin fever in the winter. The Soden's home is no bigger than a doublewide trailer. Installing an accessible bath did not appear to be feasible. And if lack of space wasn't problem enough, Mr. Soden was stubbornly set against the idea of modifying anything–inside *or* out.

But a more accessible bath was desirable to compensate for Mrs. Soden's high risk for skin breakdown. She was wheelchair-bound and incontinent of bladder and bowel. The solution was not to modify the

---

[1] The Soden case is illustrated in depth in Appendix F.

bathroom at all, but rather to install an overhead shower in the rear entranceway on the opposite side of the bathroom wall. The care manager who recommended the Soden's simple roll-in shower "design" understood that walls hide pipes. The water supply and the drain needed for the Soden's shower were in the wall and under the floor right next to the rear foyer. This simplest solution turned out to be the only one that was workable given Mr. Soden's resistance to any home modification. The "accessible" shower was nothing more than a drain in the floor and a showerhead protruding from the common wall between bath and entranceway, all of which was surrounded by a privacy curtain. The total cost was approximately $250 (the Soden's nephew was friends with a plumber).

Not every accessible bath will be as small or as inexpensive as the one in our example. Some clients will want marble tiles with brass fixtures. Others will have to install a full bath where there is none, as in the case for those whose only full bathroom is on the second floor. The concept remains simple, however—*skin likes running water*. And most CLCP clients can run hot and cold water lines and a drain to some accessible location in their home.

Handrails

Caring for frail elders and physically disabled individuals is a little like walking on a flagstone sidewalk while balancing an egg in a teaspoon. Everything is fine so long as you don't trip or shake. Then, very quickly, everything is not fine

Most mobility-impaired clients are at risk for a fall because of disequilibrium or weakness in the lower extremities—feet, ankles, legs, or hips. Most of them *can* grasp, however. Visit any assisted living facility or nursing home. All of the hallways have ledges or handrails that lead to rest areas in strategic locations. They are designed to prevent falls. For our purposes, "handrails" means *anything* the client can grab either to prevent a fall or to facilitate walking. A walker, a quad cane (a 4-pronged cane), grab bars in the shower, handrails in the hall, and so on—all can prevent injury from a fall by giving the client something to grasp and lean on.

Walkers and handrails are usually anathema to CLCP clients. Accessible baths and ramps may be unpopular, but they may not be as vigorously resisted as the ever-present walker, cane or handrail, simply because they are not encountered every time the client wants to move.

Mobility-assistance devices are a constant and immediate reminder of disability. Care managers will repeatedly hear their clients say "I hate that *!@# walker", or "I can't wait to get rid of those ugly railings."

It is important for care managers to understand that when clients resist the use of devices or home modifications, it is normal and in many respects even healthy. But care managers must work to minimize the risk that lost mobility entails. They do so by counseling and by building relationships with clients that enable them to let go of their fear. When this does not happen right away, care managers should not interpret the client's difficulty adjusting to dependency as the care manager's failure. Care managers should perceive this resistance for what it is—an expression of the client's will to survive and hold on to the life he or she has known. Letting go is not easy.

The Technology Wave

Most environmental adaptations are decidedly low-tech. When combined with adequate personal care help, ramps, handrails, and other inexpensive modifications will usually compensate for most of the mobility problems encountered by a physically disabled person.

But assistive devices are changing and improving all the time. The increased number of disabled people has spurred demand for durable medical equipment. Care managers should regularly visit medical equipment suppliers to keep abreast of new and useful products. Any device or machine that improves client safety or reduces a caregiver's burden is bound to reduce the rate of hospitalization and nursing home placement among the chronically ill. This is true for all illnesses and disabilities, especially for the dementing illnesses where client supervision is made easier by video technology, motion sensors, and tracking devices (in case those with Alzheimer's disease or mental retardation wander).

We have also seen information technology make amazing advances in just the last few years. Monitoring and communication devices simplify the supervision and ongoing assessment of long-term care clients. Telemedicine now allows us to check a patient's blood pressure, blood sugar level, blood oxygen level, heart, lung and bowel sounds via telephone hook-up. Soon, telemedicine hook-ups will be commonplace.

For care managers, Internet access is a must. The Internet is fast becoming the most powerful technological support for CLCP. It already enables communication within the care planning team. And it has opened up a valuable information stream for professionals, family caregivers, and clients alike. Whether a client wants to know about Medicare benefits, find a care manager, evaluate an assisted living facility, or keep everyone in the family apprised of a care plan via email, the Internet is the place to be. It will continue to develop additional technological supports in the form of secure medical, legal, and financial information capabilities. These communication advances along with an array of sophisticated machines—from computerized medication dispensers to conveyor belt beds—will serve the CLCP effort.

Technology extends our reach but it does not eliminate the need for human relationships or human touch. We should be prudent in our reliance on machines to do our caregiving. Computers and machines cannot adapt or learn, and they certainly cannot feel. Indeed, the limitations of technology make human attention even more important to the success of the caregiving effort.

No matter how powerful a computer program may be at making a medical diagnosis, writing an estate plan, or giving financial advice, its accuracy turns on the data it is given. The "garbage in, garbage out" phenomenon limits the software's utility and the accuracy of automated recommendations. Then there is the liability factor. For example, an Internet-based medical diagnostic service must err on the side of caution if only to protect the Internet company's liability for fear that *actual* decisions will be made based on the information people acquire. This begs the question—what is the real utility of the service if out of self-protection it becomes so simplified as to be useless?

The answer may be that automated information services that help with the care-planning and care-management effort are probably most useful for the professionals—the doctors, lawyers, financial planners, and care managers themselves. In fact, this is the premise for telemedicine. The patient does not interpret his or her own clinical status based on the computer's measurements—the doctor or nurse does. The machine reduces the cost of the assessment; it doesn't *replace* the professional.

Relocating to Alternative Housing

When deciding whether or not to relocate, those of advanced age may have to say goodbye to their beloved homes (and perhaps a big piece of themselves), but they also may confront the question—Is my new home the last residence I will have before I die? The experience is one of actual loss *and* anticipated loss.

There are many reasons why CLCP clients choose to relocate.

Their current home may be too difficult to maintain or may have become too expensive following the loss of a spouse (and the loss of the spouse's income). They may wish to be nearer to their adult children or may have lost the ability to drive. They may be lonely and wish to live in a residential community that enables more frequent social contact, or they may need the cash that is locked up in the equity of their home to pay for their long-term care.

Here we offer several examples of housing alternatives. This list is not all-inclusive, but covers those most likely to be explored by CLCP clients at the present time. The fast-changing elder housing industry assures that many others will soon be available.

Assisted Living Facilities

"Assisted living" is what it sounds like–help with the challenges of daily living. Assisted living facilities offer medical support services such as personal care help, nurse consultation, and medical assessments, as well as homemaking (shopping, cleaning and laundry services), meals, socialization, recreation, transportation, and educational opportunities for their residents. As residential facilities, they offer direct supervision of daily routines such as medication taking, personal hygiene, and meal attendance. They also afford supervision by association–people are bound to be noticed (or missed) when they live with other people. Assisted living facilities are usually "environmentally correct" and are designed to accommodate mobility impairment and to help residents recover from it. Long, flat hallways enable long walks in all kinds of weather.

Assisted living facilities may have an "entrance fee" (or purchase price) or they may charge only a monthly "maintenance fee" (or rent). They usually have minimum entrance criteria–residents must be able to get themselves to and from the dining room and must be relatively stable medically. After moving in, a resident's apartment becomes his or her home. If additional personal care assistance becomes necessary, aides can be hired, either privately or from the assisted living facility staff, or they can be acquired by community supports.

States consider assisted living facilities to be "community settings." Residents are still eligible for community support services that are enjoyed by people living independently in their own homes. They are also protected by the same landlord/tenant rules that pertain to other renters in most states. Medicare may not cover the cost of ongoing medically remedial services that may be offered to assisted living facility residents; however, residents can still qualify for skilled care under the Medicare home health care benefit. Some residents of assisted living facilities may quality for SSI-G income and Medicaid support if the assisted living facility has also qualified as a "intermediate care" facility for Group Adult Foster Care residents. Some assisted living facilities may be required to serve a minimum number of Medicaid residents as a condition of their license or charter. Many accept both young adults with disabilities and elderly residents.

Independent Living Facilities

Most independent living facilities look and feel like assisted living facilities. They may offer social and recreational opportunities, long hallways, communal dining, laundry services, and so on. They differ from assisted living in that they do not offer medical support services as part of a resident's maintenance fee. They are staffed by non-medical facility managers who can call for help in a crisis, but who cannot provide emergency medical treatment or personal care. They are usually less expensive than assisted living facilities or continuing-care retirement communities. They may feature apartments as well as individual cottages and may have small kitchens in which residents can prepare their own meals if they so desire. They may also accept both young-adult disabled and elderly residents.

Continuing Care Retirement Communities (CCRCs)

CCRCs, sometimes referred to as "lifecare communities," offer a continuum of care within a single-campus community. The continuum may even exist under one roof with a nursing home on the fourth floor, assisted living on the third floor, independent living on the second and recreational and dining facilities on the first. The community has a contractual relationship with the resident that determines the amount of care it will provide based on the resident's health status.

The cost of residency in a CCRC may be set in a fashion similar to the cost of an automobile. The "base model" costs less, but residents will be responsible for all additional health care costs on an as-needed basis. The "premium model" costs a bit more, but doesn't include everything. Residents may receive discounts on health care services or a lower private pay rate in the nursing care facility. The "luxury model" is the most expensive and usually gives residents lifetime access to all health care services. With some qualifications, these residents receive no increases in monthly maintenance fees regardless of their venue of care. Residents in this category may also be eligible for nursing home placement for life at the CCRC assisted-living rate so long as admission to the nursing care facility is not associated with treatment for a pre-existing condition. "Pre-existing condition" may be defined by the CCRC as any medical problem for which the resident received treatment any time within two years prior to entering the CCRC. Some CCRCs may even require that residents purchase long-term care insurance policies before admission. Anyone considering moving to a CCRC should scrutinize the lifecare contract very carefully to avoid any misunderstanding as to what the community will and will not provide, and what it will cost.

Congregate Care Facilities (CCFs)

CCFs are independent living facilities for income-eligible seniors and people with disabilities. Local or state housing authorities often subsidize these programs. They may have adult day health programs attached to them. They usually offer communal meals that are also subsidized by public funds, and may be staffed by a housing manager on a 24-hour basis who can respond to emergencies but who does not offer medical services. CCFs may not be as well appointed as assisted living or independent living facilities, but they offer similar support services for considerably less money. They may also offer recreational activities, housekeeping, religious services, laundry and health monitoring. They may be publicly or privately owned.

Subsidized Apartments for the Elderly and the Disabled

Nearly every town in the country has an apartment complex set up to provide housing for income-eligible senior citizens and physically disabled people. These apartments are usually subsidized through the US Department of Housing and Urban Development (HUD). Rental cost is typically 30 percent of a tenant's income. Subsidized apartment complexes are supported under the Federal Section 8 Housing Program. The housing subsidy attaches to the apartments within the facility, but does not follow the resident if he or she decides to relocate. Section 8 also makes rental vouchers available to qualified individuals and families that enable them to rent independently from landlords who are willing to qualify their rental properties for the Section 8 program. Care managers will usually find that apartment availability for their elderly or physically disabled clients is greater in subsidized facilities than it is through the voucher program. Most voucher programs have long waiting lists.

Apartments that are restricted to the elderly or physically disabled offer many features similar to assisted living facilities and CCRCs. Apartments are likely to be wheelchair accessible. Housing complexes usually have a few units that are specifically designed for their mobility-impaired residents. These apartments may feature roll-under sinks, accessible showers, wider doorways, specially designed door handles, and so on. The housing complex itself also affords socialization opportunities otherwise unavailable to individuals living in a separate apartment or home. The building is likely to be located conveniently for shopping and may even be a dedicated public transportation stop.

The Family Care Option

In the last fifty years, financing structures and caregiving institutions that didn't exist prior to the creation of Medicare and Medicaid have come to provide a great deal of chronic-care services. The Medicaid program alone pays for more than half of the institution-based care in nursing homes and intermediate care facilities in this country. But if Medicaid and Medicare cuts are inevitable, then the resources of long-term care consumers and their families will have to fill the gaps.

As highlighted in the chapter 3, family members and friends are an abundant long-term care resource. But family caregiving is about to undergo a renaissance. In greater numbers than in recent years, aging parents will move in with their adult children (or vice versa) and pooled family resources will forestall nursing home placement for the elderly and physically disabled.

It is perhaps inaccurate to suggest that we will *return* to family-based and community-based long-term care giving. Indeed, we never really left it to begin with. In their comprehensive report on the state of continuing care, *Chronic Care in America: A 21st Century Challenge*, the Robert Wood Johnson Foundation highlighted that most of the chronic care provided in the United States is still given by family, friends, and neighbors—85 percent by their measure. If they are reasonably accurate, then long-term care still remains well within the purview of the extended family.

Few long-term care issues are more emotionally charged than reconstituting extended families to live under one roof. Care managers must be sensitive when addressing this option. A deep sense of guilt, even shame, may accompany a family's inability to either bring aging parents to live with them or to move back into the family homestead. Conversely, the parents may feel they are a burden on their children, something they never wanted to have happen.

But if the question is never asked then many who are in a quandary over this issue will never address an option that *can* work very well. Most often families appreciate the opportunity to address this issue head-on with an objective, professional advisor. The discomfort the family may feel is usually better dealt with directly so that, after all is said and done, they can safely say they looked at *all* the options. CLCP is a decision-making service that can rule out alternatives as well as help develop them.

For some clients and their families, in-home family caregiving is the *least* stressful option. Living with an aging parent or disabled relative eliminates one of the greatest obstacles to successful Community LifeCare Planning–geographic distance between family caregivers and the person needing care. The importance of family member proximity to elderly or disabled relatives cannot be over emphasized. For CLCP clients who feel vulnerable, just knowing a family member is at hand can mitigate emotional distress, as well as the confusion, sleep, and appetite disturbance that often go along with it. Common sense holds that chronically ill and disabled people are likely to feel better if they feel those who love them most are close by.

For family caregivers, the lifestyle adjustments of living with a relative needing care can be less stressful than when they lived apart. Bi-weekly visits to an elderly parent to balance the checkbook, help with the insurance claim, provide personal care help, or simply share a meal, can become a chore. The hour and a half visits (let alone the non-emergency "emergency" calls) plus the 50-minute roundtrip in the car can be a significant commitment, especially for middle-aged working parents. "Visiting" is a lot less work when the person needing attention already lives with you in your home or in an apartment attached to your home. It also reduces the guilt that family caregivers may feel when they do not meet their self-imposed or culturally sanctioned expectations of the "dutiful-child." By caring for the aging parent at home, the adult child fulfills this role and may feel more personally fulfilled in the process.

Care managers must be careful not to communicate a bias with regard to family caregiving. Many families cannot and should not try to manage their aging parents' or disabled relatives' care at home. Everyone has limits. Family caregivers seeking to fulfill their self-defined, dutiful-caregiver role may do so at their aging parents' expense. Here the care manager's help can be invaluable, either in alleviating the intractable guilt a family caregiver feels when he or she simply cannot take his or her parents home, *or* to give the family the confidence they need to experiment with a family-care plan.

Last, but certainly not least, there can be a considerable financial benefit to in-home family caregiving for each of a family's generations. Many middle-aged couples who are also rearing children can benefit greatly from the sudden influx of their parent's Social Security Retirement and pension income that suddenly helps pay the mortgage, the tuition, the car payments—*the bills!* And the parents can benefit by avoiding nursing home placement. Nighttime assistance provided by family members may make home care an option that would otherwise be unaffordable. Resources may then be sufficient to pay for a minimum of private duty assistance during the day. For those CLCP clients who do not need a nurse available on a 24-hour basis, much personal care can be done in a home care setting by less skilled family caregivers.

More often than not, when family care plans work, everything becomes more affordable. Estate planning options may also be created, as when a family caregiver establishes residency with the aging parent and the home can be gifted to the caregiver exempt from Medicaid transfer rules. Finally, the family's future can be assured as inheritances are protected rather than spent down on nursing home care.

Family caregiving need not be a do-it-yourself effort. Care managers can lend valuable support with planning, decision-making, staffing, counseling, ongoing supervision and consultation services. Family members look to the care manager for guidance as each generation adjusts to the caregiving routine as well as their new and sometimes confusing role reversals. But, lest we forget, families have been caring for their elderly and disabled family members throughout human history. As complicated as life has become, the basics of life today are the same as they were for our ancestors. Family caregiving is not simple, but it needn't become overly complicated either. As system supports diminish, families will do what they have to do and have always done—take care of their own.

CHAPTER 7

Community Care Planning Resources

The term "community" derives from the Latin *com*, (with) and *munus*, (obligatory services, duties), or *communis* (shared by all or many, i.e. common). Communities exist in concentric circles–a smaller social group is contained within the next larger one. Communities are collectives which share responsibility for the commonweal.

The term "community" implies "family" and "home." We recognize the family as the smallest, most essential communal unit. Individual families combine into small or large groups of families, neighborhoods, churches, and recreational groups. These extended families and groups combine into towns. Towns often set up relationships with one another, developing communities that exist collaboratively within the same concentric circle. These groups of towns combine into counties that form broader community organizations within *their* concentric circle. Counties combine into states. States make up the nation.

Communities all offer resources and support, in one form or another, to individuals or families. They may provide recreational opportunities, counseling, information and referral services or any number of other resources to meet virtually every vital need. Community members that are eligible for and in need of help can turn to their community-organized support groups, agencies, and organizations. A care manager or "community lifecare planner" cannot fully offer decision-making support or help with access to community services without a working knowledge of a community's resources.

As described in chapter 3, long-term care is supported by one or all of six resources–health insurance, income/assets, community resources, the home, family/friends, and the client. For many who lack health insurance, financial resources, family supports, or housing, the community steps in to offer health care and long-term care resources. Accessing the resources of the community requires specific knowledge and skills. It is not enough to know that the resource exists or simply to provide information to a client that he or she may be eligible for X,

Y, or Z benefits. The care manager must have the resource acquisition skills without which the client may never receive the benefits at all.

COMMUNITY RESOURCE ACCESS

Communities try to regulate their largesse in clearly delineated terms. But all regulations are subject to interpretation. Benefit guidelines may be interpreted differently by prospective beneficiaries (clients) than they are by those who process the resource requests (social service workers).

The people who administer access to community support services are a little like shoe sellers. If they're good, they will help with the shoehorn, tie the shoe for you, have you stand up and walk around, measure whether you have enough room, and so forth. If they're not so good, they will put the shoebox on the floor, watch you fumble putting it on, allow you to decide it doesn't fit, and watch you leave the store to go elsewhere. One community service worker may say, "I helped the applicant understand eligibility and service options, made the referral to the person that could help her best, and she got the benefits." Another may say, "You're not eligible. Next!"

A care manager seeks out and establishes relationships with civil servants in Medicaid application units, Social Security offices, housing assistance programs, and elsewhere. A helpful civil servant is worth his or her weight in gold for the benefit he or she can develop for a CLCP client. These relationships can pay handsome dividends. Many civil servants have worked in different units administering different types of benefits. A worker in the Medicaid unit may know someone in the Disability Services unit and can expedite a referral or an application across the boundaries of different programs. People, not machines, staff the bureaucracies that provide for the common good. The key to navigating a bureaucracy effectively is to connect personally with the people who staff it.

No one can know everything about all of the community support programs that are out there. An effective care manager is skilled at finding the people who know the most about the services his or her client needs. Having actual knowledge of resources *is* relevant, however. There are three basic areas of concern regarding community resources with which the care manager must be familiar. They are:

- Community Resource Benefits
- Benefit Eligibility Rules
- Benefit Eligibility Strategies

Community Resource Benefits

Community resources come in the form of either goods or services. The goods may include food, clothing, shelter, assistive devices, barrier modifications, medications, or even cash. The services may include personal care assistance, counseling, skilled nursing, chore services, transportation, and so forth. Whatever the goods or services offered may be, the care manager must be able to interpret their benefit to the client in clear, unambiguous terms. If the care-planning client does not understand the benefit, he or she will not support the often-strenuous application/acquisition process.

Nothing destroys a client's confidence more effectively than dashed expectations. When a care manager creates the expectation of benefit by referring a client to a community support service, he or she must be very clear as to the nature and amount of the goods or services offered. If after a lengthy referral and application process, the client fails to acquire the promised benefit, the client will be dissatisfied not only with the community program, but also with the care manager.

Therefore, it is in the best interest of the care manager to investigate both the quality and the availability of a community support service prior to a referral. Community support programs very often have waiting lists. Most community support programs are not entitlements—the budgets governing their operation and provision are limited. Thus, eligibility does not ensure availability and, in any case, availability does not ensure quality. Neither the client nor the care manager benefits from a service that fails to meet the client's need; what looks good on paper isn't always good enough.

The care manager must investigate how programs actually work as opposed to how they are supposed to work. There is often a significant difference between policy and reality. Take, for example, the Medicare home health care benefit. At the time of this writing, the Medicare home health care benefit authorizes up to thirty-five hours per week of skilled nursing, physical therapy and home health aide assistance. The eligibility criteria for this highest level of care are open to fairly liberal interpretation. In reality, there are very few Medicare home care patients today receiving anything close to this amount of service, despite their eligibility for it. It may be that the agency providing the home care is unable to find enough home health aides to provide this level of care, or it may be the agency's unwritten internal policy is never to provide this level of care in the first place. While this may not be formalized, it is effectively how the game works. Another example of the difference between policy and reality is in the way the Medicaid dental benefit works. While nearly all Medicaid beneficiaries are entitled to dental treatment, it is often very difficult to find a dentist who accepts assignment under Medicaid. The insurance is there, the provider isn't!

There is no substitute for experience, and in determining the actual benefit a client will receive from any community resource, care managers rely on experience—either their own, or that of others. But favorable experience is no guarantee either, since a great program today may not be such a great program tomorrow. Still, decisions must be made and experience is the best informer. When relying on the experience of others, it is important that the care manager investigate the truth of the report. Having exercised due diligence in investigating a resource, the care manager can then convey the referral to the client with the caveat that there is no risk-free care plan. Where community resources are concerned, the expectation should always be that anything can happen.

Benefit Eligibility Rules
Community resources are limited. Community-sponsored assistance is available only to those who qualify. This generally excludes individuals and families capable of meeting their own needs. The standard by which this capability is determined varies from program to program and community to community. The amount of goods and services made available through similar programs also varies from state to state and region to region.

In Massachusetts, for example, at the time of this writing there is only one, very restrictive Medicaid waiver program. It is available to elders at risk for nursing home placement but applies strict income guidelines. Step over the state line to Connecticut and there are several Medicaid waiver programs with relatively liberal income guidelines. They serve not only elders at-risk (and not necessarily clients of any particular state agency), but also people with traumatic brain injury, disabled children, and the physically disabled under age 65. Head south again and New Jersey adds people with AIDS to the waiver eligible group list.

Not all community supports are designed to serve only the poor. A broad array of home health care and residential rehabilitation services are available to middle class homeowners with assets as high as $80,000 or more, and incomes up to $1,500 per month. In many states the criteria may be even more liberal. (Eligibility criteria for two such programs are illustrated in Appendix C at the end of the book.) The Home Care Program for Elders (Appendix C) can provide over $3,000 per month in home care supports for residents of Connecticut who are both income and asset eligible and who may require nursing home placement without such supports. Medicaid may also be part of the package. The Residential Rehabilitation Program (Appendix C) makes either low-interest or interest-free loans available to income-qualified homeowners in many small cities under the Small Cities Block Grant. This federally funded home modification program assists people with disabilities of all ages in making homes more accessible and in correcting code violations.[1]

In these two examples, eligibility depends upon a mix of health status, financial status, and housing status. Subtleties exist in the administration of these rules that do not emerge at first glance. For example, the Home Care Program may disregard up to nearly $80,000 in assets for the applicant's spouse, but appeals to have higher amounts disregarded may succeed.

Conversely, the consequences of accepting benefits may not emerge from the eligibility rules at first glance. Depending on their level of income, there may be a co-pay for Home Care Program clients. Additionally, the same consequences of receiving Medicaid benefits that exist for institutionalized beneficiaries also exist for community-dwelling beneficiaries. The state has a right to recover the cost of the care from a beneficiary's estate, whether that care was provided in a nursing home or a community setting. The same may also be true of the Residential Rehabilitation Program. The home which has been repaired may subsequently have a lien placed upon it. This can affect homeowners' ability to borrow against their property should they need money to pay for their care. It may also restrict their ability to transfer the home as an estate planning measure.

---

[1] The actual benefits under these two programs may differ from those that existed at the time of this writing. Readers should interpret these as examples only, and do their own research before advising clients or families based on the benefits represented here.

Thus, in addition to an eligibility determination, the care manager should also do a "consequence determination." The client must understand the trade-off inherent in acquiring a community resource. Community resources are both vital and plentiful, however, "free" services may not be so free.

Benefit Eligibility Strategies

No one is always and forever ineligible for a community support program. In most states, any billionaire could gift all of his or her money to a friend and become eligible for Medicaid in three years and one day, noncancellable income notwithstanding. Today's ineligible client may become eligible tomorrow if the correct and legal strategy is followed.

But the agencies administering community resources rarely teach eligibility strategies. Indeed, many people who could easily become eligible are denied access to community support services despite relatively minor obstacles. For example, an individual may be disqualified for having too many assets, yet by creating a $5,000 irrevocable burial contract with a licensed funeral home that person could reduce his or her assets to within eligibility limits. Removing an applicant's name from a relatively small bank account he or she owns jointly with a spouse may also do the trick, or perhaps a small gift to a relative would make a client eligible within a month or two.

Whatever the strategy, it is often the case that for lack of guidance and planning many people never acquire the community supports that could postpone institutionalization. For some the postponement may be only temporary. For others it can be indefinite. There can be little doubt, however, that many who might have avoided placement are currently residing in nursing homes. The cost of their residence to the states is often far greater than their community-care option might have been had they received guidance in meeting community resource eligibility requirements.

Estate-planning and elder law attorneys with specialized knowledge of community resources are often the referral-of-choice for a care manager trying to access community support services on behalf of an apparently ineligible client. Lawyers working in concert with financial planners can develop long-term care options otherwise unavailable without their involvement. The care manager's role is often to teach the client the value of engaging the help of resource management teams that can include these professionals. Once the client understands the value of such a team, care managers can then help find the professionals willing to work together to support the client. The care manager also informs the resource management team of the client's life circumstances including health status, long-term care prognosis, family care options, adjustment issues, and so forth, as well as the client's financial and insurance status. Resource management is not strictly a matter of calculating the mathematics of eligibility.

COMMUNITY-BASED CAREGIVING

Diminishing government subsidies will force us to develop caregiving alternatives, or in many cases to revive traditional caregiving strategies. Communities are the wellspring from which these alternatives will be nourished. Slowly but surely the word is getting out. Families, the essential basis of all communities, must now restructure themselves to care for their elders. As families go, so go communities. Recently, we have seen a boom in the assisted living industry. We should also anticipate the proliferation of co-housing, communal housing, senior foster care, and elder roommates among the growing number of lifecare alternatives. In addition, we will also see the resurgence of to the time-honored, real McCoy–elders living with their children and grandchildren.

Care managers must perceive the community for what it really is. Communities develop from the same simple, but utterly compelling human instinct–the need to express compassion. Community caregiving, offered through programs such as those below, expresses our compassion and defines our humanness. Ultimately, our humanness may be our *only* resource. Let's look at how we care for one another through community organization and service.

THE COMMUNITY RESOURCE SPECTRUM

Here we provide a glimpse of the broad spectrum of community support services. We have highlighted four categories of community support for purposes of illustration. It is well beyond the scope of this book to provide readers an exhaustive list of the services available across the nation. Comprehensive resource lists can be acquired from many municipal, state, and federal agencies. Many social service and health care professionals are effective individual referral sources. And slowly but surely, the Internet is becoming the ultimate place to go for community resource information. Everyone is now a fast, search-engine ride away from becoming a community resource expert.

Federal Resources — Three Examples
Social Security Disability Income (SSDI)

The Social Security Administration offers a variety of benefits to those who have contributed to the Social Security Retirement system, as well as to many who have not. Social Security Disability Income (SSDI) is the income support program for people who have made sufficient Social Security contributions and who have become disabled prior to being eligible to collect Social Security Retirement Benefits (currently age 62 for early retirement, 65 for standard retirement). Dependent children, spouses caring for dependent children, and a disabled widow or widower may also qualify for benefits on the disabled beneficiary's record. To be eligible, claimants must have worked long enough and recently enough while making contributions to Social Security. Eligibility is determined on a credit system. Each Social Security contributor earns a maximum of 4 credits per year, one for each quarter, so long as his or her quarterly wage contribution is sufficient. The amount of earnings required for a credit rises each year as general wage levels rise. Generally, applicants must have earned 20 credits during the forty tax quarters (ten years) prior to the date of disability. The number of total credits needed also rises with age, illustrated as follows:

Born After 1929, Become Disabled at Age	Credits Needed
31 through 42	20
44	22
46	24
48	26
50	28
52	30
54	32
56	34
58	36
60	38
62 and older	40

Since SSDI is disability insurance, those who qualify can elect to receive Medicare benefits as well. At the time of this writing, the Medicare option for SSDI beneficiaries begins two years after the first disability income payment. Since income payments do not start until five months after the established date of disability, Medicare cannot begin for SSDI beneficiaries until approximately two and one-half years after that date.

SSDI eligibility is determined following an application and disability determination process. The date of disability is set at the last date of gainful employment and not the date the applicant first received treatment for a disabling illness or injury. Disability must be affirmed by reports from all of the treating physicians that the individual applying for benefits will not be able to return to gainful employment of any kind within one year, whether in the occupation he or she had prior to the disability or in some other type of suitable work, or if the disability will result in death.

This does not mean that anyone receiving SSDI benefits can never return to work again. Indeed, beneficiaries are encouraged to retrain and return to work, and are allowed a nine-month trial work period (not necessarily consecutive) while retaining SSDI benefits following their return to employment. A trial work month is any month the beneficiary earns more than $200. After the trial work period ends, if average earnings do not exceed $500 per month, benefits will usually continue. If average earnings exceed $500 per month, benefits will stop after a three-month grace period.

Today, disability reports are almost entirely completed by Social Security Administration employees. Care managers can be advocates for their clients by requesting that they be permitted to review their disability report and make appropriate modifications. The care manager can prompt physicians to submit reports in a timely manner to expedite the disability determination process. Additionally, the care manager can maintain contact with the disability determination and medical review units of the Social Security Administration, usually located in a large city near the applicant's residence.

The care manager must be cautious and remember to maintain the delicate balance between responsible advocacy and being too pushy. He or she should find ways to work *with* the disability determination worker, and to create opportunities for the worker to experience the human side of his or her job. For the moment, the determination worker on the other end of the phone is in control of the client's application—interpreted literally—the client's *life!* The care manager must be delicate but must also be firm in dealing with benefits workers. What transpires between client, care manager, and worker could have significant consequences for the client's opportunities. The application may get processed in twenty minutes or in two weeks depending upon the worker's "discretion." The purpose of advocacy is to engage the worker to help your client, not to alienate him or her at your client's expense.

Medicare Coverage of Therapeutic Footwear for People with Diabetes

Medicare offers coverage for therapeutic footwear to individuals with diabetes who qualify under Medicare Part B. Individuals may qualify for up to $300 in assistance for depth-inlay shoes, custom-molded shoes, and shoe inserts. For diabetics, all foot problems are potentially dangerous. For the Medicare program they can also be very expensive. Diabetic foot problems can lead to lower-limb ulcers, costly hospitalizations, surgeries (including amputations), and subsequent rehabilitation and home health care expenses.

To qualify for this benefit the physician must certify that the individual has diabetes, is being treated under a comprehensive diabetes care plan, and needs therapeutic footwear because of diabetes. Claimants must have one or more specific conditions including a history of partial or complete foot amputation, foot ulceration, pre-ulcerative callus, peripheral neuropathy, poor circulation, or foot deformity.

Qualified individuals are limited to one pair of depth-inlay shoes (plus inserts) or one pair of custom-molded shoes (plus inserts) per calendar year. The certifying physician must sign a "Statement of Certifying Physician for Therapeutic Shoes." The prescribing physician then issues a prescription for them. The supplier—podiatrist, orthotist, prostetist, or pedorthist—then submits the Medicare claim to the durable medical equipment regional carrier. Medicare pays 80 percent of the payment amount allowed. The patient may pay more than 20 percent if the dispenser's fee is higher than the allowable Medicare rate or if the dispenser does not accept Medicare assignment.

Third Party Query Form (TPQY)

The Third Party Query Form or "TPQY" is a powerful affidavit that is available for free to all recipients of Social Security Retirement, Survivors, Disability or Supplemental Income (SSI) benefits. The TPQY can be obtained from any Social Security office or by calling Social Security's 800 number (at the time of this writing the number is

1-800-772-1213). Anyone can request the TPQY on behalf of a Social Security recipient, however, it can only be given or mailed to the individual receiving the benefits.

The TPQY verifies four very important pieces of information—the client's Social Security number, date of birth, income from Social Security sources, and legal address. The TPQY can expedite all sorts of community resource applications for clients who may not have their birth certificate, their Social Security card, or evidence of their income or residence on hand. The form usually takes no more than four or five days to arrive in the client's mailbox.

Two caveats are in order when requesting the TPQY. First, the form is dated, and therefore, if it is going to be used as proof of client information, it should be promptly obtained and attached to all benefit applications (e.g. Medicaid waivers, home modification programs, et cetera). Second, the Social Security Administration may be the single most efficient federal bureaucracy of all (and the author does not intend this as a facetious statement—how many organizations get almost 45 million checks out the door every month, on time, every time?), but some of its employees *are* newly hired. If either the care manager or the client call the Social Security 800-number to request the form, he or she should be prepared to make a second, or even a third phone call if the Social Security representative who answers the call does not know what the TPQY is.

The best strategy in this case is *not* to educate the Social Security worker about the TPQY! It is better to politely hang up and redial until the voice on the other end of the phone confidently responds, "the Third Party Query Form? No problem! I'll have that in the mail for you today!" The extra few minutes this additional call may take is often time well spent. If the client receives the wrong Social Security form he or she will have lost a minimum of two weeks in submitting the community support application that the form was supposed to expedite. Delays can also cost clients additional hours of the care manager's time.

Care managers should also anticipate that the applications worker to whom the form is being sent might not be aware of the TPQY's validity. The care manager should prepare the client for a preliminary denial of benefits and/or a letter from the community program applications worker requesting a birth certificate, Social Security number, proof of address, and proof of income despite the submission of the TPQY. After this request, the care manager will educate the applications worker about the validity of the TPQY, possibly by referring him or her to a supervisor for instruction. Community LifeCare planning is an educational process–for everyone!

State Sponsored Programs — Three Examples
Personal Care Attendant (PCA) Programs

Nearly every state in the country subsidizes a recently-developed approach to helping people with disabilities remain independent of the institutional care system. Many disabled individuals, whether disabled by a congenital condition (such as spinabifida or cerebral palsy) or by a disabling injury, are in need of relatively low-skilled assistance with their Activities of Daily Living (ADLs) and/or Instrumental Activities of Daily Living (IADLs). ADLs include bathing, dressing, using the toilet, eating, and mobility transfers. IADLs include telephone use, laundry, shopping, bill paying, and so forth. While disabled or chronically ill individuals often need a nurse or a physician supervising their personal care, they may not need these skilled clinicians on a daily or even weekly basis. Personal care attendants provide a broad array of chronic-care supports at relatively low cost under state subsidy.

Personal Care Attendant (PCA) programs have been developed to offer people with disabilities two very valuable opportunities. First, the programs pay for PCAs to provide home health aide and homemaking services. They make a critical contribution to the prevention of hospitalizations and nursing home placements among this most vulnerable population. Second, since disabled individuals are authorized as employers, they experience the dignity of being in control of the hiring, training, and ongoing service supervision. PCA programs are structured to approximate the kind of relationship between chronic-care consumers and caregivers that is enjoyed by those individuals who have the means to pay privately for this type of care. The states usually will set up fiscal intermediaries to handle issues of workers' compensation, tax withholding, and household employer liability considerations. All other "normal" employer/employee issues pertain.

Through PCA programs, the disabled individual or his or her surrogate locates the prospective employee, whether by word of mouth or by running an ad in the local paper. It is the program beneficiary's responsibility to find, hire, and train his or her employee, no different than if he or she was paying privately. The disabled individual or surrogate then pays the PCA from payroll deposits made by the state to his or her personal checking account. Under these programs PCAs may not need to be certified, however, the employer (disabled person) has the right to require any level of experience or certification to meet his or her own standards.

Eligibility for PCA programs is usually means-tested at the state's Medicaid eligibility level. It is also disability-tested. Applicants must need a certain minimum amount of "medically necessary" or "medically remedial" personal care assistance to qualify. The amount of care needed by any individual is determined by a medical professional, usually a nurse or physical therapist, who performs a clinical assessment as part of the application and ongoing case management process. The rule of thumb is that if in the opinion of a competent medical authority, the applicant is in need of nursing home care, the applicant's disability is sufficient to qualify him or her for this nursing home placement *prevention* program.

Pharmacy Support Programs

Most states offer limited pharmaceutical assistance to qualified individuals. Eligibility is means-tested, age-tested, disability-tested and/or diagnosis-tested, depending upon the program. There may be annual caps on the amount of money available under the benefit. Limitations as to the types of drugs the program will and won't pay for may also apply. As with all state-funded programs, applicants should determine whether or not the state has the right to recover the costs it incurs by providing these subsidies from the beneficiary's estate following his or her death. Pharmaceutical assistance programs do not normally investigate an applicant's asset transfer history. Those in need of pharmaceutical assistance who have transferred assets as part of a Medicaid acquisition strategy may qualify for a medication subsidy program sooner than they would qualify for Medicaid. Tax returns are normally requested during the application process to verify the difference between a former and a current year's income.

Pharmaceutical assistance programs can often make the difference between independence and institutionalization. Many chronic-care clients do not have the ability or the desire to pay for medications. In providing medication subsidies for these individuals, the states figure they will save money in the long run by preventing hospitalization and subsequent nursing home placements that might have been precipitated by medication non-compliance.

Home Care Services for the Elderly

States provide for the needs of the elderly through specific government offices or departments. Home care funds flow through the state to the local agencies that contract with the state to provide certain social and health care services. In most states these services include the following:

- Information and Referral – Various types of questions are answered by telephone. For example, seniors may receive decision-making assistance concerning supplementary health insurance policies available to them in their state of residence.
- Home Care Supports – Seniors may acquire home care supports provided by the access agency. These may include medical alert services, personal care assistance, case management, home delivered meals, chore services, and so forth.
- Protective and At-Risk Services – These are advocacy services for seniors who are at risk in community settings. "Protective" services cover those at risk due to their inability to protect themselves from abuse, exploitation, neglect, or abandonment. "At-Risk" services are for those who are placing themselves at risk through their own questionable judgment and decision making, despite the fact that they are considered legally competent.
- Ombudsman Services – Social service and health care professionals perform a "watch dog" service in nursing homes, investigating allegations of resident/patient abuse and nursing home compliance with state licensure regulations.

Local Programs

Local governments often administer services otherwise partially or wholly supported by grants from either state or federal sources. Counties and towns may administer local welfare benefits, including food stamps, housing subsidies, residential rehabilitation programs, adult day care, handicapped transportation, food pantries, and community companion programs, to name a few. Sometimes two or three municipalities will join together to set up a single administering entity for their respective town residents.

Although the importance of the services they provide should not be minimized, local budgets are limited. Care managers should not expect that local programs will provide the staples of long-term care. More often than not they supplement the more expansive services individuals acquire at the state or federal level, or that they find and pay for themselves.

Churches, Charities, Volunteer Groups, Professional Organizations and the "Societies"

Considerable support is offered to those with chronic illness and disability and their families under non-governmental auspices. Churches and volunteer organizations make small and large contributions to the long-term care security of many people struggling to maintain their independence. Here we offer a few examples of this type of assistance. These supports often serve as vital links in the chain of community resources.

Retired Seniors Volunteer Program (RSVP)

Important services are available from the growing cohort of elders themselves. Many senior citizens engage in a broad array of volunteer activities organized through volunteer groups such as the Retired Seniors Volunteer Program (RSVP). Senior citizens volunteer their time as friendly visitors to hospital and homebound patients. They organize and staff food pantries, sponsor support groups, provide socialization and recreational opportunities, provide transportation assistance, and so forth.

The American Cancer Society (ACS)

Aside from its national education and advocacy mission, the American Cancer Society (ACS) maintains a thriving volunteer organization that offers a variety of support services for community-dwelling, chronically-ill individuals—and not only for those with a cancer diagnosis. ACS organizes caregiver support groups, volunteer transportation services (for example, to and from medical appointments), and pharmaceutical discounts.

The Pharmaceutical Manufacturers Drug Assistance Program

Pharmaceutical manufacturers offer free medications for income-eligible individuals receiving chronic-care medications. Enrollment in the program usually requires that a physician make application on behalf of his or her patient. Medications are delivered in bulk to the homes of program beneficiaries. Income guidelines are fairly liberal. Many individuals with less than $25,000 income per year can qualify. Not all pharmaceutical manufacturers take part in the program, however. Prospective applicants must confirm that the manufacturer of their medications participates in the program, and that they fit within the manufacturer's eligibility guidelines. Brochures describing the program are available from the following address:

Pharmaceutical Research and Manufacturers of America
1100 Fifteenth Street, N.W.
Washington, D.C. 20005

The St. Vincent dePaul Society

From time to time, charity is needed to bridge a small gap between needs and resources. The St. Vincent dePaul Society gives small cash disbursements for specific, short-term needs.

Care managers are likely to encounter problems that have relatively simple, low-cost, quick solutions. On more than one occasion, one-time disbursements from this and other charitable groups have covered the costs of a home care patient's prescription while the application for a medication subsidy was pending. This help can be crucial for patient and pharmacy alike. Pharmacists regularly find themselves subsidizing customers whose prescription benefits have lapsed, but for whom sickness will surely result if they miss even one dose of a maintenance medication (insulin, for example). Admittedly a last resort in the arsenal of community resources, charities can play a critical role in sustaining the medical stability of those at risk.

COMMUNITY LIFECARE PLANNING IN A COMMUNITY HEALTH CENTER

CLCP is not just for wealthy or middle-class clients. The following service model and proposal describes an alliance between an inner-city community health center, serving primarily Medicaid patients, and a private, care-management company. This alliance offered CLCP services in conjunction with a monthly podiatry clinic held in the common room of subsidized seniors' housing apartment building. The care manager performed a longitudinal survey during six months of the program's operation. The findings indicated below are actual and clearly demonstrate the portability of the CLCP approach across social, financial, ethnic, and geographical boundaries. The report highlights the importance of community-sponsored resources and the value of creative, independent, aggressive care planning and care management advocacy for those in need. It is hoped that this proposal will be funded to provide similar services throughout the state.

Community LifeCare Planning:
Preventing Institutionalization of Community Dwelling, Chronically Ill Medicare/Medicaid Eligible Seniors

Submitted by: Joseph A. Jackson, LICSW, CCM

Program Description

Springfield Southwest Community Health Center, Inc. (SSCHC) recently undertook a study of unmet need among community-dwelling, chronically-ill senior citizens living in subsidized housing in Springfield, MA. The project combined the provision of preventive medical treatment with Community LifeCare Planning services.

The study utilized SSCHC's monthly podiatry clinic, conducted for three hours a month in the common room of a seniors-restricted housing complex, as a platform and opportunity to provide care planning services for clinic patients. The circumstances created were ideal in terms of both patient availability and receptivity to care planning and counseling assistance.

The aim of the study was to identify opportunities for the prevention of nursing home placement and hospitalization among the residents of seniors restricted-housing. Foot clinic patients became a captive audience for continuing-care needs assessments. These assessments were performed by a care manager who is a licensed, masters-level, medical social worker with extensive home health care experience, whose services were contracted on an hourly basis from an independent care-planning company, ElderCare Advisors, Inc.

The needs analysis and counseling service, provided in tandem with preventive medical treatment, proved to be a reliable patient/customer access strategy. In six consecutive monthly clinics, 23 continuing-care needs assessments were performed. *Not one foot clinic patient refused an interview with the care manager!* This remarkable 100 percent response rate is likely attributable to several factors. They are:

1) The "group effect:" Receptivity to the care-planning interviews is significantly increased by association with others who have taken part in such interviews. No single group member was isolated as more needy than another was. This created a common experience among those in the room who already share a common residence. The environment in which the clinic and the interviews took place enhanced this effect. Interviews were conducted in the same room as the podiatry clinic itself—a large common dining area with several cafeteria style tables and chairs. At one end of the room sat eight to ten clinic patients soaking their feet, awaiting either physician or nurse practitioner attention. One-to-one interviews were conducted at the other end of the room between the client/patient (who had just completed his or her foot care) and the care manager.

2) The "trust effect:" The inherently trusting relationship between the patient and the clinic physician, nurse practitioner, or clinic nurse facilitated patient receptivity to the planning effort. The physician-patient relationship was utilized as an icebreaker for engaging patients in considering their long-term care needs.

3) The "captive audience effect:" It is difficult to refuse to speak with someone with whom the others in your group are willing to speak, who is introduced by someone you trust, and who is already in the room where you must remain for half an hour as your feet soak!

Demographic and Clinical Profile

The following tables illustrate both the demographic and clinical profiles of the clinic patients interviewed by the care manager.

Total Clients		65-75 Y/O	75-85 Y/O	85+ Y/O	Married	Widowed	Single	Divorced
	Male	2	1	1	4			
	Female	4	10	5	4	13	2	

Income and Net Worth	
Individuals with less than $1,000 per month	15
Individuals with $1,000–1,500 per month	0
Individuals with more than $2,000 per month	0
Couples with less than $1,500 per month	3
Couples with more than $1,500 per month	1

Savings (Couples and Individuals)	
Savings of less than $4,000	19
Savings of $4,000–10,000	3
Savings of more than $10,000	1

Chronic Health Problems by Diagnosis	Female	Male
Congestive heart failure	1	
Arthritis	8	1
COPD	6	1
Recent fracture: a) Hip b) Arm c) Other (leg amputee)	2 1	
CVA	1	
HTN	1	
Cancer Hx	1	
Cardiac Hx (MI, CABG, et cetera)	8	1
Diseases/Infections of the skin	2	
Diabetes	4	1
Sensory impairment: a) Hearing b) Sight	3 6	 1
Hx and/or current symptoms of psychological/emotional disorder	3	
History of falls	9	1
Other (Polio, Neuropathy, PVD, Osteoporosis, Phlebitis, Muscular Dystropy	9	2
Family Supports		
Individuals/Couples with adult children a) At least one child living within one hour travel time b) All children beyond one hour travel time Individuals/Couples without adult children		 16 3 4
Veterans		2

Unmet Need

Of the 23 individuals interviewed, all had *significant* unmet need (unmet need that could precipitate an institutional admission) for either skilled services (medical and/or personal care), home care resources, meals on wheels, homemaking, pharmaceutical assistance, transportation, mental health counseling, or financial resources. Some had significant unmet needs in all of these categories. Many lacked not the resources, but the information needed to access them. One of those interviewed was anxious that she might miss a scheduled appointment with her physician the following week because her brother, who usually drove her to her medical appointments, was himself sick. Alarmingly, she did not know that as a Community Medicaid beneficiary she had medical transportation benefits available to her. Neither did she have any recollection of ever having been advised of this by the Medicaid enrollment center, her senior services case manager, or the home health care agency serving her. We emphasize that she may not have remembered that she was eligible for this service, rather than that she had never been informed about it by the other agencies involved.

The following table illustrates the level of unmet need among those interviewed at the Seniors Housing Complex.

	Unmet	Inadequately Met
Transportation	12	2
Homemaking	5	8
Pharmaceutical Assistance	12	2
Skilled Services	3	2
Durable Medical Equipment	1	
Counseling Support	8	
Underinsured and/or No supplementary Insurance	5	
Socialization	4	
Home Furnishings	2	
Chore Services	1	
Advance Directives (POA/proxy)	17	1
Other		

The Care Planning Solution

When the needs of people with chronic conditions go unmet they wind up in hospitals and nursing homes. As illustrated above, community-dwelling, low-income, frail-elderly and/or physically disabled individuals need medical as well as non-medical assistance. They need meal preparation assistance. They need homemaking assistance (e.g. shopping, cleaning, laundry). They need financial assistance. They need transportation assistance. They need companionship and emotional support. They need personal care at the home health aide level—on an ongoing basis. They need periodic supervision of their personal care and assessment of their medical condition. Above all, they need education, guidance, and encouragement if they are to effectively manage the often complex, but also sometimes simple challenges they face. And when they lose their health to illness or injury, as inevitably they will, they need medical treatment and discharge planning. It inevitably helps with their discharge if they have been linked with chronic-care supports prior to their admission.

For each of the above-referenced unmet needs a resource was available to meet them despite the individual's low financial resources. The connection to that resource can be made through the Community LifeCare Planning process. Very often, the connection can only be made through care planning. Eligibility assessment is not enough. In case after case we saw foot clinic patients who were also visiting nurse agency patients as well as senior services clients, but who were not receiving guidance toward resources in a proactive, prevention-minded, creative way. Here are some examples:

1) A seventy-eight-year-old unmarried woman is receiving bath and homemaking services through the Senior Services Home Care program. She has no medication assistance, no transportation assistance, and no regular personal care assistance despite a history of falls (one within the last month), and severe edema in her legs due to cellulitis. She reveals that she is ineligible for MassHealth as she is slightly over income and has $5,000 savings, making her $3,000 over the asset limit. She believes she is ineligible because a worker at the MassHealth enrollment center advised her that her income and assets were too high.

In a single twenty-five minute interview, the care manager acquired the above information, as well as additional information about her medical history, family involvements, social/emotional status, and so on. He then instructed the client regarding allowable asset exclusions for Medicaid eligibility, including the irrevocable funeral contract ($8000 limit) and a revocable burial account ($1500 limit) as well as spend-down strategies that would enable income eligibility. It was determined that money currently being spent on a Medigap policy and for prescriptions and private duty personal care assistance was more than sufficient to enable the client to satisfy eligibility spend-downs early in any six month period, and to sustain them on an ongoing basis. The care manager was further able to instruct the client as to her eligibility for the Personal Care Attendant program and the Home Care Initiative, following her acquisition of MassHealth, which would provide significant amounts of personal care assistance as well as companionship and socialization opportunities. Perhaps the single greatest benefit to this patient would prove to be the medical transportation available to MassHealth beneficiaries.

2) A sixty-five-year-old married white male is a disabled veteran with approximately $1,300 per month in income. He receives clinic services, free prescriptions, adult day care, and socialization opportunities subsidized by the Veterans' Administration. He is at significant medical risk due to a recent heart attack and the implantation of cardiac monitoring instruments. Indeed, his life expectancy is very short. His wife, eight years his senior, has a variety of chronic conditions including chronic obstructive pulmonary disease (she is a heavy smoker and has had part of her left lung removed), carpal tunnel syndrome, arthritis and severe neuropathy in both upper and lower extremities. In addition to, and (to a great extent) because of her medical problems she is extremely anxious and depressed. Her apprehension manifests in sleep and appetite disturbance, obsessive thinking, inattentiveness, shortness of breath, and so on. She is afraid of her husband's imminent death and also fears she will face eventual nursing home placement. Her fear is as disabling as her medical conditions. She has no medication assistance and worries excessively about the cost of living. She is regularly non-compliant with medication therapies.

In his meeting with her, the care manager recognized that her income, $424 per month, makes her eligible for the MassHealth 2176 waiver program if she becomes a senior services' client and if she meets the level of need criteria for admission to the program. Both she and her husband acknowledge that they had interviewed with a senior services case manager. However, because of the husband's income, their co-pay would have been too great for personal care assistance, so they declined home care services. The care manager was able to describe the advantage of becoming a senior services client, despite the co-pays for Meals on Wheels and personal care assistance, given the fact that by becoming a senior services client, the wife could become eligible for the 2176 waiver. He further explained that once on the Medicaid waiver, she would receive medication assistance, transportation assistance and, eventually, personal care assistance through the Personal Care Attendant program for which she could only become eligible by acquiring Medicaid. This would more than compensate for the home care program co-pay.

In addition, neither the husband nor the wife was aware that mental health services were covered under Medicare Part B, separate and distinct from the Medicare Part A subsidized home health care services. The care manager, himself a Licensed Independent Clinical Social Worker, recognized the wife's emotional problems as more than situational and referred her to a Medicare-certified mental health clinician willing to visit her in her home.

3) A seventy-four-year-old, married, white male has an income of $795 per month from Social Security. His wife, eight years his junior, has $650 per month in Social Security income. Neither is receiving senior services assistance. The wife does all the shopping, cooking, cleaning, laundry, and personal care assistance for her mobility-impaired husband. He is an insulin-dependent diabetic without prescription assistance. The care manager advises him of his eligibility for the Senior Pharmacy Program (which gives qualified seniors $1250 per year in medication subsidies) and also advises him of eligibility for the Qualified Medicare Beneficiary program that would enable him to save an additional $45.50 per month on his Medicare B deductions from Social Security income. The care manager refers the client to the Social Security Administration to obtain a Third Party Query Form (TPQY) as legal verification of age, Social Security number, address and Social Security income. This facilitates the Senior Pharmacy Program application, as the client, in this case no longer in possession of his birth certificate, is able to submit the TPQY as evidence of eligibility. He submitted the Senior Pharmacy Program application within a week of meeting with the care manager.

4) An eighty-seven-year-old widow recently fell while boarding a bus she was taking to the grocery store. Her fall did not result in debilitating injury, however, she stayed overnight in the hospital for observation and has experienced occasional lower back pain ever since. Aside from the physical trauma, she is understandably wary of shopping by herself anymore. Since the episode she has complained of sleeplessness, anxiety and depression to her physician who prescribed antidepressant therapy. She has become socially isolated and has withdrawn from her normal interactions with other housing complex residents.

The care manager inquired as to her family situation believing that some companionship and emotional support, aside from a mental health referral (to which she was resistant) might be useful. Her granddaughter lived nearly an hour away and was mostly too busy to spend time with her. It was clear that the client felt considerable rejection by her granddaughter as well.

The care manager referred this client to the Retired Seniors Volunteer Program for a volunteer companion. This referral was meant to address the social, emotional, and psychological issues that the client suddenly had to face because of her lost independence. It was hoped that the volunteer would develop enough of a relationship with the client to accompany her on her routine bus runs.

Proposal

As described above, the provision of Community LifeCare Planning services in conjunction with community health clinics is easily reproduced and monitored. Program success turns on four key factors. These factors are:

1) Immediate client engagement in the care-planning process.
2) The care manager's competence in determining clients' continuing-care needs and educating clients and their families about the community, personal, and familial resources available to meet them.
3) Effective, short-term casework and referrals provided by the care manager.
4) Care manager training.

Care managers should be competent, experienced medical social workers, nurse case managers or physical therapists, preferably with home health care experience. They must be capable of interacting fluently with the medical treatment community; familiar with the broadest constellation of community resources; skilled in counseling therapy (individual and family) and casework; and knowledgeable about the "lifecare" professions such as legal services, financial planning, insurance, and the like. The program is based on the following rationale:

1) Neither the federal government (through Medicare) nor the states (through Medicaid) can continue to subsidize the provision of medical treatment or long-term care services at anywhere near the current levels.
2) Nearly 70 percent of all medical treatment provided in this country is provided to those with chronic conditions.
3) The most powerful opportunity for maintaining wellness among the chronically ill and reducing the burden of health care costs for society lies in improving the self-efficacy of those who manage chronic conditions every day, around the clock–the chronically ill themselves. The first, most important step is engaging those most at risk for hospital and nursing home placement in the process of improving their own long-term care prospects. Those with chronic conditions are their own single greatest resource in the effort to create a new health care approach. More than any system fix we know of, their empowerment, their improved self-care management ability, their self-efficacy, and their ability to acquire and manage the resources they need to remain well in the community will determine whether health care and long-term care will retain an acceptable measure of quality, let alone improve.

Enhancing community-based long-term care options through prevention planning, education, strategic resource acquisition and utilization is immediately achieved in the Community LifeCare Planning model described here. This approach has shown itself to be 100 percent efficient at engaging clients in the assessment, education, and planning process when provided in tandem with preventive medical treatment. When performed correctly, a continuing-care needs assessment can determine the level of need for skilled medical support services, social/emotional support services, advocacy, casework services, family support services, and so on. It can then identify the available resources, whether personal or community-based, to link clients to the help they need.

The potential to prevent far more expensive hospitalizations and nursing home placements, and to do so cost effectively, is very high with such a program. The health status and medical stability of most frail-elderly and physically-disabled people is, by definition, very fragile. A seemingly insignificant need can snowball into an avalanche of medical problems. Resource connections must be made *ahead* of the time they will be needed. Care-planning services decrease the likelihood of hospitalization and nursing home placement by linking chronic-care clients to the resources needed to maintain wellness.

Program Costs and Benefits

The costs of this program fall into two categories. They are:

1) Community LifeCare Planning service costs
2) Increased public program enrollment costs resulting from care manager referrals. In Massachusetts, such a service might increase enrollment in the Senior Pharmacy Program, Community Medicaid, the Personal Care Attendant program, the Home Care program, the Enhanced Care Options program, Residential Rehabilitation Services, and so forth. It is therefore conceivable that a reduction in medical treatment costs that might otherwise have been borne by the federally-funded Medicare program will be paid for by *state*-subsidized programs such as those described above. On the other hand, Community LifeCare Planning will contribute significantly to the prevention of nursing home placements, the expense of which would ultimately be paid for by the states under Medicaid.

In six months, SSCHC's Community LifeCare Planning service cost less than $2,000. This represents three hours per month assessment, information and referral services, and three hours per month of casework provided by a masters-level care manager. Twenty-three senior's housing residents were served. Seven were referred to the Senior Pharmacy program. Four were successfully referred to the Qualified Medicare Beneficiary program. Four were referred for community

Medicaid, either directly or through the 2176 waiver program. Three were referred to the Personal Care Attendant program. Four were referred to the senior services' Home Care program. Three were referred for volunteer companion services. Three were referred for mental health supports. Seven family members were contacted and educated about a long-term care planning option for their senior relatives. Five clients were referred for transportation services they either did not have or did not know they already had. Three were referred to the Pharmaceutical Manufacturers Association Drug Subsidy program. Last, but certainly not least, all twenty-three clients and all medical clinic staff were educated about prevention-minded, community-based, long-term care planning approaches.

Discussion

A valid measure of the hospitalization and nursing home placement prevention effects of Community LifeCare Planning (CLCP) would require a longitudinal comparative analysis of both a sample group that receives CLCP and a control group that does not. The groups would need to be made up of similarly afflicted chronically-ill individuals with similar demographic profiles, and they would need to be of statistically adequate sample sizes. Such a study could test the hypothesis that CLCP services, when provided in conjunction with preventive medical treatment, significantly decrease nursing home and hospital placements among low-income, chronically-ill, frail-elderly, and physically disabled individuals.

We submit that such a study is unnecessary. If such a study were conducted and proved the hypothesis (or "failed to disprove" in statistical parlance) that planning works, it might finally lend validity to the adage "a stitch in time saves nine." However, we believe that even the most exacting of scientists would be willing to stipulate that planning is a prerequisite to the success of any endeavor, including the prevention of illness and injury among the chronically ill and those with disabilities. We believe, therefore, that a study should be constructed not to determine *if* planning is of significant value, but rather *which approach* to planning, and performed by *which type of professional* is most effective.

The model described here has been shown to be 100 percent effective at engaging clients in the assessment process. Perhaps more effective interview methodologies, needs-assessment instruments, casework approaches, or information and referral strategies exist. If so, they should be compared by survey and testing.

It is entirely plausible that the money spent for the above-described care-planning service, plus the added cost to state programs resulting from the referrals it generated, has already paid off. What is the value of the programs to which people were referred as a result of the care-planning services if not to prevent more costly medical treatment and long-term care placements? We cannot flatly state that the CLCP service has saved "X" thousand dollars for Medicare and "X" thousand dollars for Medicaid. We can state, however, that the likelihood of savings to both the Medicare and Medicaid programs has greatly increased by virtue of the links made to less costly chronic-care programs, and that the Community LifeCare Planning program herein described provided the necessary linkage services cost effectively. We can also state that despite the involvement of social service and home health care agencies, the care-planning needs of low- to mid-income senior citizens living in subsidized housing are not currently being adequately addressed.

A new approach to prevention planning among the chronically ill is called for. It must pull together the best prevention professionals and utilize the best prevention services from the public and private sectors. The above-described program does just that. It combines the community health maintenance efforts of an inner city, community health center with a highly skilled, private sector care-planning/care-management service. The combined effect is very powerful.

CHAPTER 8

Estate Planning
For Care Managers

Not long ago, frugal living and hard work were how we ensured that our lives would end comfortably, and our children and our grandchildren would receive an inheritance. Owning a home, saving money and investing wisely was everyone's estate plan. At the end of our days, we could rest easy; wills had been drafted, we had some money in the bank, and we lived with our kids and their extended families. Our legacy was assured.

Today, if we live long enough (and more of us will), it is a near certainty that we will need to do more planning if we wish to provide for ourselves and our progeny. Proper estate planning covers a lot of territory, including wills, trusts, tax planning, asset protection, advance directives such as powers of attorney and health care proxies, and so on. But most people still view estate planning in a negative light or consider it too expensive. They think, "Estate planning is just rich people hiding their money" or "I'm not wealthy, so estate planning isn't for me." Unfortunately, many have paid a dear price because of their failure to plan.

Estate-planning assessments and community resource assessments follow similar paths. An estate-planning attorney begins with an assessment of a client's resources, looking both at what is available and what is missing. Estate planning supports CLCP by sorting out the resources that are needed to develop long-term care security and by developing strategies for their acquisition. This cross-disciplinary, comprehensive approach has emerged as a uniquely potent combination in the long-term care planning effort.

AN EXAMPLE OF CREATIVE LAWYERING

In the same way everyone's health care needs are different, everyone's estate-planning needs are different. Consider Gladys; at ninety-four years old she is incompetent due to advanced dementia. She has been living in a nursing home for two months. She has fifteen thousand dollars in savings and eight hundred dollars per month in Social Security income. She owns a duplex worth forty thousand dollars. Her seventy-six year-old son, who has recently also been diagnosed with Alzheimer's Disease, lives in the half of the duplex that Gladys resided in, and her daughter, herself in her late sixties, lives in the other half with her husband.

Medicare, supplemented by Gladys's Medigap policy, is about to stop paying for Gladys's nursing home stay. Gladys cannot sign a deed, has no power of attorney and no health care proxy. Gladys could spend her fifteen thousand dollars on her long-term care and apply for Medicaid; a lien would be put on her home or the state in which she resides could force the sale of the house. But who has legal authority to sign checks or sell the duplex?

It became clear that Gladys had been receiving personal care assistance from her daughter for ten years prior to her nursing home admission. In this case, the "caregiver-child exception" that exists under federal and state statutes enabled the transfer of Gladys's home to her daughter without Medicaid penalty. In order to do that, however, the estate-planning attorney needed to have a guardian appointed for Gladys, given her incompetence. In this case, although it took three thousand dollars in legal fees to file for the court-ordered guardianship and to do Medicaid planning, the money was well spent, as it protected the home and the balance of the cash for Gladys's children.

This is an example of how estate planning may benefit even those with a relatively low income and few assets. While the legal fees incurred may represent the largest bill this family will pay in their lifetime, the alternative was total impoverishment. The care manager was a critical link in the planning, having provided them with the key advice regarding the caretaker-child exception that allowed them to save the family's home, and having referred them to the estate-planning attorney.

GOALS OF ESTATE PLANNING

Whatever the circumstance, estate planning addresses one or all of four general goals. First, estate plans focus on the here-and-now. They can be geared to ensure that our lifecare needs are met throughout our lifetime and that income and assets are protected while we are alive. Second, estate plans may ensure that wealth is transferred to the persons or organizations we designate, with a minimum of administrative expenses and that the state and federal tax bite will be as little as possible. Third, estate plans enable us to select the person(s) who will handle various administrative and management functions on our behalf. Estate plans designate the health care agents, trustees, powers of attorney, or guardians who can serve while we are still living. They also provide the vehicle for the designation of executor(s) and trustee(s) to manage our estate after death. Fourth, estate planning allows us to make arrangements that can provide for our family's needs after our death, and into the future.

BASIC STRATEGIES OF ESTATE PLANNING

Estate-planning strategies often involve more than just executing a will. They can include making arrangements for the accumulation and handling of assets while we are alive and upon our death; drafting *inter vivos* or living trusts to manage our assets during and after our lifetime to support dependent children until they are of age, and to shelter the estate from taxes; giving assets or cash as gifts to people or charities to reduce taxes; incorporating life and disability insurance into the estate plan to provide liquidity; and more. By following a number of strategic planning steps, estate planning minimizes or even eliminates estate taxes and settlement costs while ensuring that our assets are distributed according to our wishes both before and after our death. A description of these steps follows.

Goal Evaluation

In the goal evaluation phase of estate planning, we determine who we want to inherit our assets and how we choose for our property to be distributed. Once these objectives are clear, we can develop strategies designed to help meet our individual goals. In determining goals, estate-planning attorneys may ask clients to address several questions, including, "Do you want any of your assets to go to charity or for your children's education?" or, "Who would be a good candidate to serve as your personal representative and as the guardian of your children?" and, "If something were to happen to your entire immediate family, what would you want to happen to your property?"

Estate Inventory

After goal evaluation, the next step in estate planning is to list all of an individual's holdings, including his or her home, jewelry, stocks and bonds, bank accounts, insurance, retirement plans, and real property, and to note how they are owned. A fair market value is then placed on the assets. Next a similar inventory of debts and liabilities is created. This can be done by using a comprehensive estate-planning questionnaire, similar to the Initial Consultation Checklist utilized by care managers. (See Appendix A. Estate inventories utilized by attorneys may be more detailed.) Subtracting debts from the value of assets determines the actual gross estate value. This is the amount we could leave to our heirs.

At this stage, the individual begins to consider the tax ramifications of the estate plan, and ways to minimize estate shrinkage. The best vehicles to carry out the plan, including wills, trusts and other estate planning tools, can then be chosen.

Estate inventory questionnaires are designed to elicit the information needed by both estate-planning attorneys and care managers to systematically gather critical information without overlooking crucial facts. The caretaker child, the disabled child, the recently transferred asset and many other variables can have a significant impact on life-care planning options. One missing piece of vital information can lead to an inappropriate care plan, resulting in the loss of significant assets, independence, or both.

Will and Trust Preparation
A will or a revocable trust is often the cornerstone of an estate plan. These two instruments determine who will receive assets and how those assets will be distributed.

Family Gifts
Lifetime gifts to family members can reduce the taxable estate and provide personal satisfaction. At the time of this writing, an individual can give up to ten thousand dollars each year, to as many individuals as they choose, without reporting the gift or paying taxes on it. Gifting in excess of this ten thousand dollar limit to any individual in any given year does not automatically impose taxes on the overage, but it does reduce the tax-free allowable amount an individual can leave to his or her heirs after death.

For the years 2000 and 2001, the limit for federal and state tax-free inheritance is $675,000 for an individual estate. For example, if an individual gives a daughter fifteen thousand dollars in one year, that individual must declare the gift. The five thousand dollar excess would reduce the individual's tax-free inheritable estate limit to $670,000 ($675,000 less the $5000 reported excess).

Charitable Giving

Contributions to a qualified charity can be made gift-tax free and may result in a current-year income tax deduction. These contributions may also reduce estate taxes.

THE GOALS OF ESTATE PLANNING HAVE EVOLVED

People are beginning to realize that a lifetime of saving is not enough to protect their standard of living or pass on an inheritance to their children. Several factors have combined to threaten what once was a relatively secure method of providing for our heirs and ourselves. Two stand out—more of us are living longer and the cost of chronic care is rising.

Not long ago relatively few people lived into their seventies and eighties, much less their nineties. Today these life spans are becoming commonplace. Our longevity is a triumph of modern medicine, but our success has its price. The longer we live, the greater the likelihood we will develop chronic illnesses that require chronic care. The more severe our chronic conditions become, the more expensive our care and treatment becomes. Thus nursing homes, home health care agencies, assisted living facilities, and so on, have multiplied in recent years and are thriving. In short, chronic care has become big business.

The Social Security program covers some of the cost of long-term care by providing income to the elderly and the disabled. Medicare's rehabilitation and home health care benefits provide a modicum of protection against long-term care costs. For most people, however, these two programs are not enough to ensure coverage of more than a short nursing home stay or a few hours of daily, disability care in the home, and only for a short period of time. Depending on the level of care one receives, nursing homes can run anywhere from four thousand to eight thousand dollars per month. It doesn't take long for such an expense to deplete most people's life savings.

It is possible to plan for long-term care costs and to avoid having taxes consume one's life savings. We may not be able to forestall the need for long-term care, but we may gain peace of mind from knowing that our savings are working most effectively for us and are also protected for our progeny. This peace of mind can make a huge difference in our quality of life at the most critical time—the end of our lives.

The carefully constructed plan of an elder law attorney, developed in concert with a care manager, can help protect savings against long-term care costs. A comprehensive estate plan can prevent hospitalization and nursing home placement by creating community-care options that might not otherwise be possible. Planning strategies often do not require one to "spend down" or give assets away but may simply require one to change the "asset class" or the type of asset in which one invests.

Many people are understandably concerned about the cost of the estate planning itself. The plan's complexity usually determines the cost of the services, for the obvious reason that the more time an attorney and/or care manager spends evaluating the estate plan and care-planning options, the costlier the plan will be. Clients must therefore understand the value of the activity before they hire an estate-planning attorney.

Generally, one can determine whether estate-planning services are necessary by answering the following four questions:

1) Are my life savings at risk if I need either a nursing home or long-term home care services?
2) Is it likely that I will need expensive chronic care?
3) Is it critically important to the well being of a spouse, child, or other dependent that my estate be protected for their welfare?
4) Am I interested in seeing my life savings transferred to my children and grandchildren, provided my health care and long-term care options are preserved?

If these questions are answered in the affirmative and the client has taken no steps to protect assets or does not have a power of attorney, a health care proxy, a will, or other necessary legal documents, the advice of an estate-planning attorney should be sought.

When we develop an estate plan we are betting that our planning efforts will pay off. There is always the possibility that the plan will never be needed. Many estates are protected by the simple fact that some people die suddenly, without high chronic-care expenses. But the odds are generally not in our favor that this will happen; three out of every four deaths in the United States are from chronic illnesses.

The estate-planning process may be emotionally stressful. Estate planning compels an objective evaluation of sometimes limited alternatives and consideration of the possibility of a crisis or death. But the goal of estate planning is to reduce stress, not increase it. It does this not only by preserving a client's assets, but also his or her decision-making autonomy. As public supports for chronic care continue to subside, people with chronic illnesses and disabilities will need to use their own resources creatively to meet their chronic-care needs. CLCP and estate planning can be cost-effective ways of protecting our assets and options and buying some peace of mind. If the money paid to an estate-planning attorney is less than the amount the estate plan protects, estate planning is usually worthwhile even for the smallest estate. More importantly, for many, estate planning can often protect a family's future and a family's dreams.

ESTATE PLANNING OPTIONS

Wills

A will is one of the most effective ways to direct the distribution of property according to one's own wishes. However, many individuals assume that wills are only for very wealthy people, or are only for people who want to set up trusts or protect their assets from estate taxes. The fact is that whether someone is young or old, married or single, a parent or not, if he or she has financial assets, he or she generally should have a will.

Unfortunately, three out of four Americans die without leaving a will, probably because no one enjoys contemplating his or her own death. The primary reason for making a will is to provide instructions on how assets are to be distributed among beneficiaries after one's death. A will is a written document that fulfills the following functions:

- A will outlines a person's wishes for the distribution of his or her assets and specific gifts of tangible personal property.
- A will designates an executor or personal representative who is responsible for taking inventory of the decedent's property, preserving the estate, paying creditors, administrative expenses and death taxes, and disposing of the remainder of the decedent's property among the beneficiaries.
- A will appoints Guardians for minor children in the event of the death of both parents.
- In special circumstances, a will establishes trusts that can protect assets.

Wills can be used to establish testamentary trusts (also called a "trust under will") to ensure that assets are held, managed, and distributed in the manner one specifies. The trustee manages certain assets for the benefit of the decedent's family and/or other beneficiaries, and distributes trust income and principal at specific times and in the manner set forth in the will. For example, if one is concerned that one's spouse may remarry after one's death, a trust can be created that provides income and principal for the surviving spouse during his or her life, but preserves the remaining principal for one's children upon the spouse's death. Likewise, if assets are left to children, a trust can ensure that they do not receive the funds until they reach a certain age or level of maturity, and then only for certain specified purposes such as support, maintenance and education.

Without a will, the court will appoint a "personal representative," or "administrator" of an estate. This may be a relative if one is willing and able to serve; or the court will appoint an administrator of its choice. Since a personal representative will cost an estate a percentage of the estate assets in commissions, most people find comfort in selecting someone they know and trust to oversee the administration of their estate.

A will is financially advantageous for the decedent's family. Dying intestate (without a will), without the benefit of any tax planning, leaves the estate open to federal and state death taxes.

Probate and Non-Probate Assets

Most estates include probate assets and non-probate assets. Care managers should be aware of the impact of both. Probate assets are those owned in an individual's own name (a bank account or residence titled in the client's name alone). After the individual's death, court determination is required as to where the assets should go. Non-probate assets are those that transfer automatically to another person or designated beneficiary upon the individual's death. Examples of non-probate assets include assets held in a revocable living trust; assets held jointly with a surviving spouse or as joint tenants with a right of survivorship; proceeds of an insurance policy in which beneficiaries other than the estate are named; balances of retirement plans, individual retirement accounts, or Keogh accounts and tax-deferred annuities that may be payable to designated persons rather than to the estate.

For those assets that go through probate (or court administration), two procedures are involved. First, the surrogate's court in the county where the individual resides determines whether a particular instrument is a will and whether it will be held to be valid to transfer the decedent's assets. If the individual dies intestate, the court determines legal heirs according to the applicable state law on intestate succession. Second, the court oversees the process of settling an estate, including supervising the actions of the personal representative named as either executor or administrator, ruling on the legitimacy of any creditors' claims against an estate, supervising the transfer of remaining property to the beneficiaries named in a will or to legal heirs if the individual died without a will, and overseeing a guardian's use of any property that is left to minor children until they reach the legal age of majority (eighteen years of age in most states).

Court supervision of the probate process helps ensure that the directions left in a will are carried out properly. The probate process can take as little as several months or as long as several years (for example, if a will is contested or if the decedent owned additional property in states other than the one in which he or she lived). A properly drafted, current estate plan will minimize probate delays and expenses. It can provide for the prompt appointment of Executors, Guardians and Trustees, payment of expenses and taxes, and the settlement of claims. With an estate plan, business interests can continue and Will contests and unsubstantiated claims can be avoided.

Avoiding Probate

It may be desirable to avoid probate out of a desire for privacy. Trust documents are generally not filed with the court, but there are some exceptions, such as when a "pour over" will is used (see glossary for definition). If property is owned in more than one state, an expensive "ancillary" administration in the second jurisdiction may be required if probate is involved. People may prefer to avoid probate so that they can be sure that management of their assets will continue uninterrupted. Depending on the size of the estate, it may be preferable to avoid certain probate expenses and undue administrative delays, and certainly, knowing that everything has been taken care of prior to one's death can provide a tremendous sense of relief.

An effective way to avoid probate is to employ an *inter vivos*, or living trust, which can provide for the management of assets during an individual's lifetime and for the proper disposition of those assets upon the individual's death. The terms of the trust may change or be revoked at any time and may designate anyone—a professional manager, a spouse, or a child—as trustee. This person can be a co-trustee, but in most states it is advisable also to appoint an independent co-trustee. This type of trust is also useful if the individual becomes incapacitated and/or incompetent, because the trustee will be able to manage assets and provide for the person's needs without court intervention.

Power of Attorney

An essential part of current estate planning is the appointment of individuals known as fiduciaries to act on one's behalf. In a will, a fiduciary is called an executor, and in a trust, the fiduciary is called a trustee. In addition, there are several other methods to appoint individuals to act on one's behalf during one's lifetime, as the need arises. Through a power of attorney (POA) an individual is appointed to transact business on behalf of and in the name of the person granting the POA authority. A general power of attorney gives an agent, known as an Attorney-in-Fact, the authority to conduct banking, real estate business, and all other transactions in the grantor's name. A durable power of attorney grants authority that lasts beyond any disability or incompetence the grantor may suffer, so that if those events do occur, an individual has been appointed to manage a person's affairs when most needed.

Typically powers of attorney are assigned to trustworthy relatives. Power of attorney gives an individual authority to act on the behalf of another in order to manage that person's general affairs or for certain specific purposes. A power of attorney may be designed so that it is for a limited period of time or for the life of the grantor (as in the general and durable POA). It can become active immediately or "springing" (activated at some future time). The springing power of attorney can identify the trigger, usually a medical crisis, whereupon if the individual's physician determines that he or she is no longer capable of managing his or her financial affairs the powers of attorney are activated. The "power" is therefore available when needed, but not before, as a way of protecting funds from being pilfered should that be a concern.

Health Care Proxy and Living Will

Health care decisions cannot be made by an attorney-in-fact. A health care proxy should be appointed or a living will should be executed for those who wish to have someone available to make health care decisions in the event that they are unable to do so themselves.

Appointing a health care proxy (in some states they are called health care agents or health care surrogates) is a crucial step in developing advance directives. Consider the case of an elderly couple whom we will call Mr. and Mrs. Jones. Mrs. Jones suffered a stroke that put her in a persistent vegetative state, and she was admitted to Helpful Hospital. Mrs. Jones had no advance directives such as a living will or health care proxy. The hospital refused to terminate life support. Mr. Jones sued the hospital to terminate life support, and won the case at the trial level in which all of the family members testified that it was clearly not Mrs. Jones's intent to be kept alive by artificial means. The hospital appealed the decision, but the family won again at the appellate level, and life support was mercifully removed, allowing Mrs. Jones to die naturally. But the hospital wasn't through, and it sued Mr. Jones for the cost of his wife's care during the course of the legal proceedings. The hospital won on the grounds that they were justified in challenging the family's request to terminate life support in the absence of any advance directives. The idea of assigning a health care proxy becomes much more compelling after hearing this story.

State laws differ regarding powers of attorney, health care proxies and living wills, and it is essential that a qualified elder law attorney be consulted in the client's home state. Statutes and forms can vary widely, and advisors (especially those counseling the elderly) must be certain that the documents being recommended are appropriate, thorough, and properly executed.

New York is one example of a state that has passed legislation regarding health care proxies. Effective January 1, 1991, New York state residents are authorized to designate an agent to make health care decisions on their behalf. In the event that an individual becomes incapacitated or incompetent, as determined by his or her physician, the health care agent would be authorized to make any decisions regarding treatment, including discontinuation of treatments that would unnecessarily prolong life or terminate artificial life support when there is no hope of recovery. There are a number of procedural safeguards built into New York State's law, which protect people from having unwanted or unauthorized decisions made. New York (as well as many other states) does not have any statute recognizing a living will, although the courts have stated that if an individual leaves "clear and convincing evidence" of his or her intention to have artificial life support terminated, then the court may direct a physician or hospital to discontinue such treatments. A living will should constitute "clear and convincing evidence," but because there is no agent appointed in the living will, a health care proxy should also be executed.

A single document can serve as both a health care proxy and living will. The following is an example of a document that gives instruction to a health care agent and declares the intent of the individual signing the health care proxy.

In the event that I sustain substantial and irreversible loss of mental capacity, and there is doubt as to whether or not life sustaining treatment is to be administered to me, I direct that my health care agent, and all physicians, hospitals and other health care providers, abide by my decision that my life not be artificially extended by mechanical means, and to resolve any such doubt in favor of withholding or withdrawing life sustaining treatment.

Without limiting the generality of the unrestricted authority conferred by my health care proxy, I affirm that I do not draw a distinction between nutrition and hydration and any other kind of life-sustaining treatment, and I expressly authorize my health care agent, in his or her unrestricted discretion, to direct that nutrition and hydration be withdrawn or withheld from me when my agent believes that it is in my best interest to do so.

Furthermore, I hereby state my instructions, and direct that my health care agent communicate said instructions, that if there is no reasonable hope that I will regain mental capacity, all life sustaining treatment (including, without limitation, administration of nourishment and liquids intravenously or by tubes connected to my digestive tract) shall be withheld or withdrawn, whether or not I am conscious or free from pain, and that no cardiopulmonary resuscitation shall thereafter be administered to me if I sustain cardiac or pulmonary arrest. I recognize that when life-sustaining treatment is withheld or withdrawn from me, I will surely die of dehydration and malnutrition within days or weeks. I further state and direct my said health care agent to communicate my instructions that all available medication for the relief of pain and for my comfort shall be administered to me after life sustaining treatment is withheld or withdrawn even if I am rendered unconscious and my life is shortened thereby.

I have made this instrument while in full command of my faculties in order to state my intentions, and to furnish my health care agent with written instructions, in clear and convincing language, of the strength and durability of my determination to forego life sustaining treatment in the circumstances described herein, and in any circumstances whereby my health care agent determines that I would wish to do so. It is my firm and settled conviction that I am entitled to forego such treatment in the exercise of my right to determine the course of my medical treatment, and my belief that my right to forego such treatment is paramount to any responsibility of any health care provider or the authority of any Court or judge to attempt to force unwanted medical care upon me.

TRUSTS

What is a Trust?

Under a trust agreement an individual selects someone, known as the trustee, to hold and manage property for the first individual's beneficiaries. The individual, as grantor, settlor, or creator of the trust, dictates the terms of the trust, and the trustee is responsible for carrying out written instructions as set forth in the agreement.

Thus, a trust is a legal arrangement by which property is given to a trustee to be managed and used for the benefit of those named by the creator of the trust. There are two main types of trusts: testamentary trusts, which go into effect when the grantor dies, and living (*inter vivos*) trusts, which take effect during the individual's lifetime. Living trusts may be revocable or irrevocable.

Inter vivos trusts should generally be prepared in conjunction with a "pour-over" will. Such a will ensures that assets remaining in an individual's name upon death, which are inadvertently left outside the trust, will be transferred into the trust for distribution to designated beneficiaries in accordance with the individual's wishes, and as expressed in the trust instrument.

Transferring the title to all or a portion of a person's assets into the trust name funds the living trust. The trust "owns" the assets. If the trust is revocable, the individual retains complete control of the assets and can change the terms of the trust at any time. If it is irrevocable, all rights to the property are forfeited and the terms of the trust cannot be amended.

Advantages and Disadvantages of Living Trusts

A trust arrangement generally offers several advantages over a will. It can help manage and protect assets during one's lifetime, provide continuity in the management of one's affairs after one's death, control how and when assets are to be distributed, avoid the costs and delays of probate, ensure privacy in the handling of one's affairs, and, when properly designed, it can reduce taxes and/or expenses. It also keeps control of the assets in the trust in the hands of the grantor who can revoke it at any time.

While there are many benefits to trusts, they can also become disadvantages. Most trusts, and particularly trusts that cannot be revoked, involve some degree of loss of flexibility or control over assets. Many trusts are initially more expensive to prepare and implement than wills given their complexity and the labor-intensive process of drafting them.

Types of Trusts
The following are more detailed descriptions of some common types of trusts.

Revocable Trusts
For clients who are at risk due to physical or cognitive impairment, the revocable trust is a useful asset protection tool. Trustees of a revocable trust are held to a higher standard than attorneys-in-fact as they are entrusted with the management of assets outside the grantor's immediate knowledge or control. A revocable living trust can protect an individual's personal and financial security in the event that he or she becomes incapacitated during his or her lifetime. A successor trustee is designated to make decisions and act on the behalf of the creator of the trust should he or she become incapable of making management decisions. In addition, use of a revocable trust allows an individual to appoint a professional manager, to maintain complete control over the trust property, to receive income from the trust, to transfer property to heirs, to provide privacy for his or her family, and to reduce estate settlement expenses.

Irrevocable Trusts
Irrevocable trusts are a way to transfer ownership of assets without giving the recipient unbridled access to the money or property. If an individual relinquishes all rights to income and principal from the trust, as well as the power to change the trust agreement in any manner, the asset will not be considered part of his or her taxable estate. The individual creating the trust names the recipient of the income generated during the life of the trust, as well as the beneficiary of the trust when it is terminated. Because the transfer is considered a gift to the trust, a gift tax may be imposed unless the transfer qualifies for the gift-tax annual exclusion (As mentioned previously, at the time of this writing, the total amount of any gift is limited to ten thousand dollars per year, per individual gift for the gift to be excluded from the taxable estate).

Irrevocable Life Insurance Trust

One popular use of an irrevocable living trust is to have the trust own the individual's life insurance policies, thereby removing the proceeds of such policies from the taxable estate. If the death benefit proceeds are not included in the taxable estate, they will be available to provide liquidity to accomplish estate-planning objectives. This cash may be used to buy non-liquid assets from the estate or loan money to the estate, thereby eliminating any need to sell estate property or borrow excessively in order to pay estate taxes.

Marital Trust

A marital trust can provide for a surviving spouse without leaving property directly to the spouse from the decedent's estate. A third individual may be appointed to act as trustee for the surviving spouse, who is the beneficiary. If certain technical requirements are met, the trust assets will qualify for a marital tax deduction.

QTIP (Qualified Terminable Interest Property) Trust

With this form of trust, a person can dictate how his or her property will be distributed upon the death of a surviving spouse. This trust is generally used in second marriages when the testator may wish to provide for his or her spouse for life, but pass the remainder of the estate to children of a first marriage. The surviving spouse must receive the income from the trust for life and may receive some rights to principal, but the trust agreement must be carefully drafted to satisfy a myriad of highly technical legal requirements to enable the property transferred to the trust to be eligible for the unlimited marital deduction.

QPRT (Qualified Personal Residence) Trust

This mechanism allows an individual to transfer his or her residence or a vacation property to a trust and still collect income or use the property for the term of the trust. This type of trust is often used to freeze the value of estate assets for estate-tax purposes.

Minor's Trust

If both parents die, a testamentary minor's trust can hold assets for the children until they reach a certain age, provide management of the assets, and pay income and principal as directed for such purposes as their support, maintenance and education.

Charitable Trusts

Charitable Remainder Trusts can help an individual obtain income tax deductions, diversify an investment portfolio without incurring an immediate capital gains tax, increase cash yields generated by assets, and decrease the size of an estate. They work best for older individuals who have charitable giving objectives and find themselves holding low yielding, highly appreciated assets. Assets are transferred by an individual to a trust and then sold to be reinvested in higher yielding assets. Generally, an individual and perhaps a spouse receive income for life, with the remainder of the assets going to a charity after the death of the last income recipient. The value of the property given to the trust is often replaced for the heirs with a life insurance policy in an irrevocable life insurance trust. A charitable lead trust provides a charity with the income from an investment's principal, paid over a certain amount of time, after which the remainder of the assets pass to an individual's heirs at greatly reduced transfer tax costs.

Medicaid Trusts

A popular planning technique for asset protection is to transfer assets into a "Medicaid" trust, retaining the income for the grantor and preserving the principal of the assets for the children or other beneficiaries. As part of its eligibility determination process, Medicaid will disregard assets when applicants transfer those assets into a qualified trust. When properly drafted, this sort of trust will provide asset protection and significant tax benefits, including the avoidance of gift taxes, and the elimination of capital gains taxes. In addition, trust assets will avoid probate. The trust allows the trustee to access the principal of the trust for the beneficiaries during the grantor's lifetime, although the trustee cannot give the principal directly to the grantor. Most grantors choose to maintain the right (called a "special power of appointment") to change the ultimate beneficiaries of the trust, by reappointing the assets to different family members at a later date. This power allows the grantor to maintain control, and prevents transfers to the trust from being treated as taxable gifts.

A properly drafted "income-only" trust that gives a trustee no discretion to distribute principal to the grantor-beneficiary, or to his or her spouse, is considered a viable long-term care-planning tool. Therefore, a senior may keep his or her income from an irrevocable, income-only trust, while in some states (not all) the remainder principal can be distributed to specific beneficiaries, and the grantor can qualify for Medicaid. The state does not consider the assets of such a trust to be available to pay for the cost of long-term care.

The Medicaid trust may not be the most advantageous instrument for a sixty-five year old estate-planning client who is not yet disabled or impaired by a chronic condition. A good estate-planning attorney will be reticent to create a Medicaid trust for such a client when there is sufficient income to finance long-term care insurance, life insurance, privately paid personal care, living expenses, and so forth. Those concerned about both asset preservation and long-term care costs may find the resources they already have can create both more opportunities and more control over their long term care options.

MEDICARE ADVOCACY AND INSURANCE APPEALS

Appealing the denials of benefits under Medicare and private insurance is an increasingly active area of elder law and estate-planning practices. As health care costs continue to climb, and claims continue to grow in number, both public and private health insurers are changing their minds about what health care treatments are and aren't covered. Clients/patients who have been receiving a benefit for two or three years may suddenly find that their health insurance policy no longer covers that benefit. Coverage for durable medical equipment, in-home care, even surgical procedures is being reduced or discontinued altogether. Semantics have become very important in government and insurance industry efforts to cut costs. For example, different interpretations of terms such as "medical necessity," "homebound," and "personal care" can lead to home care benefit denials. Such denials may be overturned on appeal, but often, legal action must be taken.

Appellants of Medicare decisions must pay for an attorney's time, but not for filing fees and other court costs. Lawsuits brought against private health insurance entities are a different story altogether. Because there is no mandatory arbitration clause in any of today's private health insurance policies, the client/patient has no informal forum to pursue an appeal.

Private health insurers who suddenly deny coverage for services they have always covered must usually be sued in the state Supreme Court. This requires that the client hire an attorney to prepare an action. The client must pay court filing fees and retain the attorney for as long it takes the to wend its way along the Supreme Court track to conclusion. If the client is a frail elder he or she may not even survive the sometimes-lengthy court process.

Insurers cannot be sued for medical malpractice because they are not considered to be medical providers. An insurer's decision to terminate coverage is not considered to be a medical decision. But some states have found a way around this protection. Individuals have successfully sued managed care companies for decisions to restrict coverage for prescribed medical treatments. Courts have found favorably for plaintiffs by charging insurance companies with breaching the "standard of care" when the denied treatment might have kept the patient alive or lead to a cure.

In this situation, an elder law attorney's role in acquiring health care and long-term care resources and in maintaining medical stability is more sophisticated than standard estate-planning activities. Clearly, a specialized approach to legal advocacy for the elderly, the infirm, and the physically disabled is necessary.

GUARDIANSHIP

Care managers must be familiar with both the caregiving needs of incapacitated individuals and the legal system's response to the need for protection of the person and his or her estate. Few issues are more complicated or more stressful for CLCP clients and their families, let alone for our social service and legal institutions. Community support services face unique and often-complicated challenges when no legitimate decision-maker can be found for someone who has lost the ability to think for him or herself.

Consider the case of another couple whom we will call the Smiths. Mrs. Smith suffered a massive, incapacitating stroke and was placed in a nursing home by her husband. Mrs. Smith's daughter objected to her placement and wanted her brought home. This would have required hiring a private caregiver, which Mr. Smith was unwilling to allow, much less pay for. The daughter sued for guardianship and Mr. Smith contested his daughter's right to guardianship of his wife. The case was tried for seven full days over the course of four months. Mr. Smith was eventually appointed guardian and kept Mrs. Smith in the nursing home.

In most cases the courts are not equipped to deal with these issues. In many states, these cases are not heard in family court, but in the Supreme Court, by judges who also deal with medical malpractice and product liability issues. Cases involving disputes over guardianship of incapacitated elders are heard along with damage claims against insurance companies. This is likely to change over the next few years as the number of incapacitated elders grows dramatically. Some states have already begun to develop special guardianship divisions of their courts with judges who hear nothing but guardianship cases. The efficiency of guardianship proceedings will likely improve as the judges become more familiar with guardianship statutes and the problems of long-term care.

What is a Guardian?

A guardian is a person, institution, or agency appointed by the probate court to manage a ward's or an incapacitated individual's personal affairs. Individuals over the age of eighteen are presumed capable of managing their own affairs in all states, but guardians may be required to act as surrogate decision-makers for adults who are physically disabled or disabled by mental illness, developmental disability, or deterioration of cognitive capacity and who cannot make or communicate responsible personal decisions.

Guardianship laws vary among the states. Some are broader in scope than others. In Illinois, for example, a guardian may be appointed if, because of "gambling, idleness, debauchery, or excessive use of intoxicants or drugs," an individual "wastes" his or her estate, thereby leaving his or her dependents open to "want or suffering." Guardianship may be deemed necessary either to protect the incapacitated individual or to protect the interests of service providers or creditors.

The Guardianship Process

Guardianship always requires court involvement. Generally, before starting a court proceeding, the individual or organization seeking guardianship must obtain a physician's report describing the person's disability and explaining the need for a guardian. The report should address such issues as the nature and type of the disability and how the disability affects the individual's capacity for making decisions or ability to function independently. It should cite an analysis of the person's mental and physical condition performed no more than three months prior to the date of the filing of the petition, and it should explain why guardianship is indicated. Finally, it should make housing and treatment recommendations for the allegedly incapacitated individual.

Mental health and social service professionals and others may contribute to the report if the physician is not familiar with all the relevant aspects of the individual's life.

Attorney Representation and Other Protections
A person who is facing guardianship adjudication (the respondent) has the right to a court-appointed attorney and, in some states, a trial by a jury. The respondent also has the right to request an independent medical evaluation, which must be paid for from his or her own funds.

Guardians *ad Litem*
Most states require the appointment of a guardian *ad litem* (GAL) in all guardianship cases. A GAL may be a private attorney, a social worker, or another trained professional. Care managers often serve as guardians *ad litem*. The GAL is an independent expert advisor to the court who informs the court concerning the apparent need for guardianship. The GAL's duty is to provide ongoing independent reports to the court regarding the best interests of the respondent. In most states, if the GAL is not a licensed attorney, he or she must be a qualified advocate for individuals with the respondent's type of disability. The court may pay the GAL a standard fee for his or her services.

The GAL informs the respondent about the nature and intent of the guardianship proceedings and assesses the respondent's reactions concerning the evaluation and possible adjudication of disability. He or she evaluates the acceptability of the proposed guardian and educates the respondent concerning changes in residential placement and care that may result from the guardianship. The GAL then submits a written report to the court and appears in court at the guardianship hearing to testify as to whether it would be appropriate to appoint a guardian for the respondent. The GAL often discusses his or her testimony with the respondent or the respondent's attorney prior to the court hearing. The respondent has the right to attend the hearing; if he or she wishes to be in court but faces a significant obstacle to getting there, the court and the GAL should be advised so that special accommodations can be made.

Guardianship must be used with caution. Imposing guardianship is a profound abrogation of an individual's right to self-determination. It may permanently transfer control of an individual's personal and financial decisions to the guardian. It can be extremely difficult to revoke, even when the guardianship may no longer be necessary. Courts will generally require expert testimony to revoke a guardianship, and health care and mental health professionals may be hesitant to certify the appropriateness of the revocation. Generally, guardianship should be used only to protect the clearly incapacitated respondent against the ill effects of neglect (by self or others), exploitation, abandonment, and abuse, while promoting the highest degree of independence and autonomy possible.

MEDICAID APPEALS

Even when it appears unlikely that a client will be eligible for Medicaid coverage, an attorney who is willing to appeal the denial of coverage can often prevail. Two cases illustrate the possibilities. An elderly gentleman with two adult children owns a half dozen real properties. His several commercial buildings are heavily mortgaged, with tax foreclosures pending on a few of them. One of his sons is permanently physically disabled. With some persuasion, he assigns power of attorney to his well son. This enables him to transfer all six properties to the disabled son, allowing him to take advantage of the "disabled-child exception" whereby assets can be transferred to a disabled child, and thus be exempt from Medicaid recovery rules. The gentleman eventually qualified for Medicaid coverage in a long-term care facility but could not have done so without extensive legal assistance.

In other cases, legal assistance for a client already receiving Medicaid becomes crucial in order to acquire a higher level of care. An elderly blind woman in New York hires an estate-planning attorney to argue that her blindness qualifies her as an exception to the "physical assessment rule" under the Medicaid home care program. Exceptions to the physical assessment rule are controlled by federal standards. In this case, if a physician is willing to state that a nursing home will be detrimental to the woman's health, she would be eligible to receive twenty-four hour in-home personal care assistance paid for by the state of New York.

Such an exception is subject to the 90 percent fiscal assessment test; which holds that when the cost of home care is over 90 percent of the cost of institutional care, in-home care paid for by Medicaid can be denied and the patient can be institutionalized. With proper hardware, personal care, care planning and care management in place, in many cases the cost of care can be brought down to under 90 percent of the cost of a nursing home, and the Medicaid home care benefit may be granted.

Obtaining approval for this level of care through the Medicaid system requires the services of an attorney who is highly skilled at the Medicaid appeals process and who is also knowledgeable about federal and state statutes and the latitude of their interpretation. Accessing benefits and advocating for clients' rights are the specialties of elder law and estate-planning attorneys.

GENERAL ESTATE-PLANNING ADVICE

There is little that can be done after death to relieve an estate from taxes if an individual has not planned the disposition of his or her estate properly. Anxiety about estate protection rises when long-term care needs become central. Any time life circumstances change dramatically (especially when a health crisis occurs) estate plans should be established or reviewed and, if necessary, updated.

Care managers should be familiar with estate-planning options as they affect long-term care security. CLCP clients should be educated about the following general rules of estate planning.

- Business and personal affairs should be kept in order and an inventory should be maintained of all property.
- Personal representatives should be educated about the property and they should know where the estate inventory is kept.
- A will is effective until changed or revoked. A will may be altered by executing a new one or by adding a "codicil," which is executed with the same formalities as a will. Trying to make changes to a will by writing on the document itself may invalidate the entire will.
- Designating a beneficiary of a life insurance policy does not take the place of a will. Life insurance is but one asset that needs to be considered in an overall estate plan. Under certain circumstances, it is advisable to transfer ownership of a life insurance policy either to a trust or to a beneficiary.
- If an individual owns a house and checking account jointly with a spouse, those items will not need to go through probate, and the surviving spouse will have immediate access to them. This is not true for assets held individually.

- Married couples should work closely together in estate planning so that family objectives can be met regardless of who dies first.
- A beneficiary generally should not serve as a witness to a will. If the beneficiary is needed as a witness to validate a will, he or she may not be able to collect an inheritance.
- Generally, an individual may not exclude a spouse completely from a will without the spouse's consent. In some states, a surviving spouse is automatically entitled to at least an "elective share" of the estate, which is equal to one-third of the net estate, including testamentary substitutes.
- The best assets to give as gifts may be those that are gaining in value because future appreciation will be excluded from an estate for tax purposes.

SAMPLE ESTATE-PLANNING LETTER

An estate-planning letter dealing with long-term care issues is included in Appendix D. It is complex, but a careful reading will help you understand how the concepts described in this chapter support the long-term care planning process. It will also help you learn to communicate better with attorneys. It is enlightening to see how the elder law/estate-planning attorney must advocate in today's complicated long-term care environment.

Glossary of Estate Planning Terms

Administrator – A person appointed by the surrogate's court to manage the estate of a person who dies intestate

Beneficiary – A person designated to receive the income or principal of a trust or estate

Bequest – Personal property given to another by will; compare with devise

Codicil – A document that adds to or changes a will; its execution must comply with the formalities required for the execution of a will.

Decedent – A deceased person

Devise – Real property given to another by will; compare with bequest

Estate – Assets and personal property; also the legal entity that manages and distributes a decedent's property

Estate Tax – The transfer tax paid to the IRS and the state's Department of Revenue by the executor or administrator of an estate out of the assets of the estate itself

Executor – A person appointed by a testator in a will to carry out the provisions of the will; a woman acting in such a capacity is an executrix; a co-executor acts as executor together with another or others; see personal representative

Fiduciary – A person in a position of trust or confidence; fiduciary is bound by a duty to act in good faith. Examples of fiduciaries are trustees, executors and administrators

General Power of Appointment – The power to decide who should receive assets and when

Grantor – A person who makes a transfer of property; the term is commonly used to describe a person who establishes and transfers property to a trust. See settlor and trustor

Guardian of the Person and/or Property of a Child – A person legally appointed by the court to manage the rights and/or property of a minor; a guardian *ad litem* is appointed by the court to prosecute or defend an action for a minor

Heir – One who is entitled to inherit a part of the estate of a person who has died without a will; an heir may also be known as a distributee

Intestate – Without a will

Legacy – Personal property transferred by a will

Living (*Inter Vivos*) Trust – A trust that goes into effect while the settlor is alive

Personal Representative – An executor or administrator charged with marshaling assets, paying bills and taxes, and ultimately distributing an estate

Pour Over Will – A will used to transfer assets to a trust that is already in existence; very often it is used in conjunction with a revocable living trust to dispose of those assets not previously placed in the trust

Power of Attorney – A document in which you authorize someone to act as your agent; a durable power of attorney continues after a you become incompetent, and a springing power of attorney comes into existence only upon the happening of a predefined event or contingency

Probate – The administrative process by which the validity of a will is proven

Settlor – The creator of a trust; see grantor or trustor

Testament – A will

Testamentary Trust – A trust that begins after the Testator's death, and which is established by a will

Testator – A man who makes or has made a will; a testatrix is a woman who makes or has made a will

Trust – A legal entity by which property is transferred to and managed by a person or institution for the benefit of another

Trustee – The person or institution entrusted with the duty of managing property placed in trust; a co-trustee serves as one of two or more trustees. A successor trustee becomes trustee upon the happening of a predetermined future event.

Trustor – One who creates a trust; also called a grantor or settlor

Will – A legally executed document that explains how and to whom a person would like his or her property distributed after death, and that appoints personal representatives to carry out the management and distribution of assets

Suggested Readings

Clifford, Dennis, and Cora Jordan. *Plan Your Estate: Absolutely Everything You Need to Know to Protect Your Loved Ones.* 4th ed. Berkeley, CA: Nolo.com, Publishers, 1998.

Strauss, Peter J., and Nancy M. Lederman. *The Elder Law Handbook. A Legal and Financial Survival Guide for Caregivers and Seniors.* New York, NY: Facts On File, Inc., 1996.

The following three listings are published by state-specific agencies/publishers. All states have equivalent comprehensive references utilized by estate-planning attorneys and care managers. Care managers are directed to their county law libraries or to an elder law attorney in their area for assistance. Elder law attorneys can be found through the National Academy of Elder Law Attorneys' website at:

http://www. naela.com

Freedman, Donald N., and Emily S. Starr. *Estate Planning for the Aging or Incapacitated Client in Massachusetts.* Boston, MA: Massachusetts Continuing Legal Education, Inc., 1999 Revised Edition.

Kasle, Annette Levinson. *New York Elder Law Handbook.* New York, NY: Practicing Law Institute, 1999.

Regan, John J, J.S.D. *Tax, Estate & Financial Planning for the Elderly.* Albany, NY: Matthew Bender, 1998.

CHAPTER 9

Finance For Care Managers

Medicare eligibility is based on age or disabling illness or impairment. Most beneficiaries are over age sixty-five and receive Medicare as part of their Social Security Retirement benefits. But adults who have made sufficient contributions to the Social Security pension system and who become permanently disabled by either a mental or physical condition may qualify for Medicare regardless of age.

Understandably, since their eligibility for Medicare implies a certain vulnerability to illness or injury, Medicare beneficiaries consume the largest portion of health and long-term care services in this country. The Balanced Budget Act of 1997 (BBA) was geared to slow the growth of the Medicare program. As intended, its passage has forced health care providers to greatly reduce levels of service to Medicare beneficiaries. However, service reductions have resulted less from actual changes in Medicare benefits than from the fact that caps were imposed on the fees that providers are permitted to bill to Medicare. In response, health care providers have done the only thing they can to stay in business—interpret the language describing benefits far more narrowly, enabling them to reduce services and at the same time provide the levels of care to which Medicare beneficiaries remain entitled.

Care managers must have a working knowledge of asset and resource management, particularly in light of the recent changes in the Medicare program. People who are homebound with chronic health problems no longer enjoy the same levels of daily personal care assistance or chronic-care services, and they no longer receive the same number of home health care visits, however "medically necessary" these benefits may be. Those in need of long-term care support are being given a clear message from the government: What our entitlement programs no longer subsidize, you will have to pay for yourselves. Chronic-care consumers must now purchase the help they need.

Thus, the importance of financial planning as a primary component of Community LifeCare Planning cannot be overemphasized. For those with chronic conditions, strategic use of even the most limited financial resources can mean the difference between independent living and nursing home placement. Care managers must be able to help their clients enhance their chronic care purchasing power. Eligibility assessments and community support referrals are no longer sufficient. Care managers must be capable of investment portfolio analysis and they must be able to interpret how an individual's or a family's resources can best be used to support long-term medical stability in a residential setting, most often an individual's home. Care managers must be able to comprehend quickly the income producing capacity of their clients' assets–both actual and potential–and they must be able to see the long-term care options that open up as a result of these assets. They must also be able to communicate these options to clients, their families, and their professional advisors, and to make clear the importance of organizing financial resources. If no appropriate financial or legal advisors are involved, a care manager should be able to link clients with the best advisor for their circumstances.

To understand financial planning the care manager must understand the value of money and how it can be managed. No two financial plans are ever exactly alike. A client's life circumstances and his or her personal values also determine financial planning options.

Everyone's financial planning needs differ somewhat depending on their age, income needs, and estate-planning priorities. Additional factors are a client's personal values and life circumstances. Care-planning clients who grew up prior to or during the Great Depression are likely to be savers for the proverbial rainy day. Their frugality is usually accompanied by a vigorous sense of self-reliance. For these reasons, among others, nursing home placement is extraordinarily unattractive to them. However, if nursing home placement becomes necessary, advance financial and estate planning are critical. The sad reality is that despite the success of the Social Security program, two-thirds of all Americans over the age of sixty-five would be flat broke after thirteen weeks of privately paid nursing home care. Helping them manage their limited assets is at the core of the long-term care planning effort.

There are three different types of assets that care managers should understand. They are government benefits, personal assets, and retirement plans and insurance.

GOVERNMENT BENEFITS

Government benefits include state teachers' pensions, federal retirement programs, Social Security benefits, Railroad Retirement benefits, et cetera. These types of income benefits may cease at the time of the retiree's death. One notable exception is Social Security Survivors' benefits, which are assigned to minor and/or disabled children of deceased contributors. There are also cases in which the benefit amount received by a beneficiary is greater than the benefit amount received by his or her spouse, and in such cases the greater benefit is assigned to the surviving spouse. But income to a beneficiary's family following his or her death is reduced overall when, for example, a decedent's wife continues to receive her husband's often greater Social Security income, but loses her own lower benefit check in the bargain. Thus, this type of asset is not controllable. We have no say in whether or how it continues after our death.

Aside from the emotional loss, the economic loss caused by the death of a parent or a spouse can be great for a family. If a husband and wife are each receiving government benefits of $1,000 per month, and one dies at age sixty-five, the measurable economic loss over twenty-five years is $214,000. This assumes a 3 percent rate of inflation and a 6 percent after tax rate of return. These calculations demonstrate the advantage of government pension benefits, in this case Social Security, as mostly or even entirely tax-free.

PERSONAL ASSETS

Personal assets fall into several different categories or classes. The main asset classes are listed below.

Stocks

By purchasing shares in a company, one can participate directly as an owner, or stockholder in that company. People own stocks to increase wealth and generate income. This happens either because the value of the stock appreciates or the stock pays dividends that can be taken as income or reinvested. However, stocks are not guaranteed in terms of dividend reliability or stock value. If the stock appreciates, it represents a gain in capital, and if the stock depreciates it represents a loss in capital. This loss or gain is taken by either selling the stock outright or borrowing against it. Stocks may not be the investment of choice for elderly long-term care planning clients with relatively short life expectancies. The risk associated with price fluctuations may be greater than they can tolerate given the possible need for cash to pay for chronic care. Some stocks carry less risk for loss than others, depending on the nature of the company's business and the volatility of the market for its products.

Bonds

Bonds are loans to institutions or governments that are made by the investor. The institution that borrows the money is "bonded" to make fixed interest rate payments for the life of the bond, or length of maturity. Bonds are most often purchased for their income producing potential. Thus, bonds represent more secure investments for elders no longer in the accumulation phase of their investment life.

However, the value of bonds is also subject to appreciation or depreciation. The value of a bond (the price someone would pay to purchase it on the "secondary" bond market from the holder—as opposed to its original purchase price) is determined by comparing the bond's fixed interest payout and the prevailing interest rates of the day. For example, any type of bond purchased on January 1 would be worth less than its original purchase price by December 31 of the same year if overall interest rates in the economy had climbed by then. Why would anyone pay $10,000 for a 6.5 percent bond (the lower rate available on January 1) if interest rate increases meant that $10,000 could buy a 7 percent bond by December 31? The 6.5 percent bond would be priced at a discount because of its lower income generating potential relative to the prevailing interest rates of the day. Of course, the opposite would be true if interest rates declined in the year following the purchase of a bond. In that case, the bond could be sold on the secondary market at a premium because of its higher income generating potential.

Bonds mature in a fixed period of time between ten and thirty years from the date of issue. For example, a thirty-year bond issued January 1, 1980 would mature on January 1, 2010. On that date, the bond is guaranteed to be redeemable at face value from the issuer. Several different systems have been developed to rate bonds on the basis of the financial health of the issuing institution. The goal is to give bond investors some idea of the issuer's ability to redeem the bond and/or to make regular interest payments. Bonds may also be "callable," or redeemable at the issuer's discretion. Normally the call feature may only be activated after a date specified by the issuer at the time of purchase. For example, a 6 percent corporate bond issued on October 1, 1999 may have a call date of October 1, 2004. The issuing corporation therefore retains the right to redeem that bond at any time *after* October 1, 2004. In some cases, bonds may feature an ability to be converted to stock at the holder's discretion.

Treasury Bills and Notes

Treasury bills and treasury notes reach maturity more quickly than treasury or corporate bonds. Treasury bills mature at any time between three months and one year. Treasury notes mature at any time between one year and five years. Because of the shorter period of time until maturity, bills and notes are considered more liquid than bonds and extremely safe. The risk of interest rate changes is reduced by the short amount of time one has to wait before the entire face value is reacquired. Treasury bills, notes, and bonds can be bought directly from the United States Treasury or through brokers, as with corporate and municipal bonds. Unlike certificates of deposit (CDs) there is no early withdrawal penalty, although, as illustrated above, one may incur a loss for selling early if interest rates rise following the purchase of the bill, note, or bond. On the other hand, if interest rates decline, then there is a bonus for selling early. A new treasury issuance called the Treasury Issuance Protection Security, or TIPS, offers a guaranteed yield and the adjustment for inflation of both the principal and the payment on the principal. Typically TIPS offer even lower yields than Treasury bills, but with greater capital preservation capabilities.

Debentures

Debentures are unsecured loans that pay higher interest. These instruments are highly speculative. They enable small investors to become venture capitalists by investing into a pool of venture capital. In exchange the issuer of the debentures is bound to repay investors at very high rates. The problem with these instruments is that investors have no protection against the failure of the business into which the pooled venture capital is invested.

Commercial Paper

Commercial paper is an instrument that business institutions use to borrow money for a short period of time. A bank or lending institution may loan money to a corporation at one rate, then offer the loan as an investment vehicle at a higher rate. Commercial paper is a relatively secure, short-term investment.

Real Estate

In addition to its personal and financial values, real estate may also be extremely valuable as a tax shelter. At the time of this writing, couples over the age of fifty-five who are selling their home for the first time can retain up to $500,000 of the capital gain tax-free, individuals up to $250,000. (Capital gain is the profit the seller makes on the sale of the house.) Therefore, selling one's home is a potentially powerful strategy for creating an income-producing asset. But retaining one's home not only provides a place to live, it provides income tax relief in the form of deductions for either mortgage interest or real estate taxes paid. It may offer a rental income. The value of the home may also appreciate in the real estate market. The equity in real estate can be accessed through loans in the form of mortgages, equity loans, or reverse mortgages (For a discussion of reverse mortgages, see below).

A more aggressive strategy for putting the value of real estate to work is the capital transfer. In a capital transfer, money is borrowed against the value of the house, yielding a lump sum of cash as well as tax-deductible mortgage interest. The money is then invested with the intention of generating a capital gain. The client realizes up to a 40 percent tax deduction by paying mortgage interest, and only pays up to a 20 percent capital gains tax on the money that was invested. Even if they make the same amount on their investment as they pay in mortgage interest, because of the difference in tax payment and deduction rates, they make money. The money can then be used to pay for long-term care.

Mutual Funds

At the time of this writing there are eleven thousand different mutual funds. A mutual fund is a portfolio of investments managed by a mutual fund company. Investors can buy shares of the fund without paying large commissions on the purchase of individual stocks or bonds. For example, a stock mutual fund may hold over a million dollars of stock in each of a hundred different companies. The share value of the fund is calculated as the aggregate value of the fund's holdings divided by the number of shares the fund as a whole has sold. Mutual funds can be separated into the following subcategories.

Money Market Funds

These give the most liquidity for investors. Money Market Funds are similar to savings or checking accounts with one important exception–

they do not generally offer FDIC insurance against any failure of the investment. Large mutual fund companies offer money market funds that invest primarily in highly secure bonds, similar to those that FDIC-insured bank accounts may use for depositors' savings. When investors wish to purchase shares of another type of the company's mutual funds, or sell shares and turn them into immediate cash, money market funds can disburse or receive the asset transfers. Investors may opt to move money to and from money market funds within the company by telephone transfer rather than by mail.

Growth Funds

These funds are geared for long-term capital growth through both dividend payments and appreciation of stock value. Typically growth funds have higher risk and are comprised of newer, relatively small companies. So-called small cap (capitalization) stocks are issued by start-up companies seeking to establish themselves as big players in their respective markets. Their future is less "certain" than for their larger, blue chip cousins. The advantage of investing in small cap stocks is that their growth potential has not yet been realized due to their youth and relatively small capitalization or value. Buying small cap stocks gives investors more upside (capital gain) potential should the company grow at the higher rate.

Income Funds

These funds invest in preferred stocks, mortgages (Ginny Maes), bonds, and so forth, with the intention of producing higher dividends and/or interest payments to the mutual fund shareholders. Balanced funds, in which stocks and bonds are combined into one mutual fund, may fall into this category. Stocks issued by companies that pay dividends but generally do not share in the growth of the company may be part of an income fund's holdings.

Tax-Free Funds

Tax-Free funds are generally not for young investors. Typically, these funds help retirees generate fixed incomes with low risk to principal. These funds invest in many different types of bonds, paying particular attention to the tax advantages for the mutual fund shareholder. Thus, they favor instruments that are tax-free.

A word of caution is in order about the advertising associated with traditional mutual funds. The first and most obvious is the myth of annual growth. Quite often, mutual funds will select the period of time in which their fund grew the most and highlight this performance. Mutual fund companies are enamored of "mountain charts." These charts might show how $10,000 invested in 1965 would have grown to $10,000,000 today. The line on the graph ascends precipitously from left to right over the last thirty-five years. What they choose not to disclose is that some taxes were due along the way. The taxes are an expense that must be deducted from the earnings of the fund, and this deduction significantly reduces the ongoing growth potential of the fund.

Antiques and Collectibles

Typically, the sale of a collectible or an antique yields a 40 percent loss on the investment. Unless you are an expert you may find these to be bad investments. They are generally difficult to liquidate, and it is very difficult for a non-expert to get the full value of an item.

Certificates of Deposit (CDs)

CDs typically generate fairly low interest but offer liquidity and FDIC insurance on the principal up to $100,000. The money in a CD matures similarly to that invested in a bond. Early withdrawal incurs a "penalty" imposed by the bank holding the CD.

Annuities

Annuities are contracts, most often between an individual and an insurance company. Annuities can be powerful asset preservation vehicles, especially for those entering a nursing home. In some states (though not all), irrevocable, term-certain annuities may be considered exempt assets when determining Medicaid eligibility. Only the income they create is considered available. For this exemption to apply, however, they must be irrevocable, meaning that the annuity owner cannot cancel them and re-obtain the money invested in them. Also, the term (the length of time during which the investment is generating payments) must be certain (or fixed, based on the individual's life expectancy according to the state's actuarial tables), such that by the expiration of the term (should the investor live that long) the annuity would be spent down to zero. The states usually set life expectancy criteria based on insurance industry standards.

At the time of this writing, for example, a seventy-eight year old woman in Massachusetts is allowed to invest in an irrevocable, term-certain annuity that will be fully paid by the time she reaches age eighty-eight. If she dies prior to age eighty-eight, the payments may continue to go to the beneficiaries of her annuity. Some states may allow her to go on Medicaid despite the annuity (after all other criteria have been taken into account), but will put a lien on the annuity as an asset of her estate. This enables the state to recover Medicaid expenditures from her estate after her death. In this case, although the overall worth of a person's estate may be decreased after death by the state's recovery, the value of his or her personal assets are preserved in the annuity during his or her lifetime, generating monthly annuity payments that can be used to pay for long-term care.

Annuities are a way of deferring income through either fixed or variable interest rate agreements. A fixed rate of payment is generally guaranteed at the market rate at the time of the annuity's purchase. Variable annuities allow for fluctuations in interest rates or transfers between assets. For example, if either the annuity company or the annuity owner believe the annuity's investments are not going to work to their advantage, they can elect to move the annuity's assets out of a stock account into a money market fund to avoid an expected downturn in the stock market. This is done without paying any capital gain tax on the sale of that account at the time of the transfer. The disadvantage of an annuity is that the monthly payments are considered ordinary income when they begin. But monthly income from annuities may be an advantage if it puts an investor into a lower tax bracket than he or she would have been in prior to retirement. Transfers between accounts remain tax-free and the basis cost of the annuity also comes back tax-free.

Life Insurance

Life insurance may be one of the best kept secrets for financing long-term care. Most insurance companies allow policyholders to borrow against the policy's cash value or transform it into an annuity. This offers liquidity as well as tax deferral advantages. Additionally, many companies allow an "accelerated death benefit," allowing the policy owner to borrow up to half the death benefit if he or she becomes terminally ill. Life insurance policies also serve to guarantee that the surviving spouse will have a way of replenishing his or her assets if they have been spent to care for the dying spouse. Life insurance may ensure payment of reverse mortgage interest. Assets distributed to the surviving spouse from life insurance may also be used to replace government benefits lost by the death of a spouse. All of this information can help to reduce the anxiety of someone in need of long-term care, or one who is suffering from a terminal illness and may be concerned about the financial fate of a spouse once they die. The cost of life insurance is also predictable–a very important factor in retirement planning for those on fixed incomes. Policyholders can select how long the premiums will be guaranteed–ten years, twenty years, or for life–based on what they can afford.

One of the most interesting developments in insurance today is that the manufacturers of insurance products are buying back those products. Large insurers are willing now to buy back life insurance policies, albeit at a discount, ahead of the individual's death. Even healthy people are now selling their life insurance policies to a viatical company. Companies will buy back policies at a discount because they know the likelihood of a claim after age seventy is extremely high. Clients have even asked their agents to sell their life insurance policies for them. When manufacturers of life insurance products are willing to buy back their products, it's an important indication that they foresee many claims on their policies.

Viatical Settlements
Viatical settlements have gained popularity since the beginning of the AIDS epidemic. In viatical settlements, life insurance policies are bought by investors for less than face value. The policyholder may then use the cash settlement for long-term care prior to his or her death, and the investor makes a profit when the policyholder dies. Viatical settlements have become popular for other uses, as in the so-called "senior settlement." In such a settlement, those over a certain age can sell their life insurance policies and use the money for anything they like–a trip to Hawaii, for instance. Such options are excluded in certain states.

Viatical settlements offer a solution for many who lack capital assets to pay for long-term care. The accelerated death benefit mentioned above may be preferable for those who do not need as much cash prior to their death, or for those who have loved ones for whom they wish to provide following their death. The accelerated death benefit of most life insurance policies pays 50 percent of the benefit ahead of the policyholder's death and the remaining 50 percent when the policyholder dies. This guarantees 100 percent of the benefit will go to either the individual owner or the beneficiaries, as compared to 80 percent as is typical of viatical settlements.

Reverse Mortgages

Reverse mortgages can be a powerful income-generating tool, especially for the elderly, who may be perceived as too old to be a good risk for a long-term mortgage loan. In a reverse mortgage, the bank pays the borrower monthly payments in exchange for a lien on a property. Reverse mortgages may either require the sale of the home after a certain period of time or they may have a "life rights" feature, which precludes the bank from foreclosing on the home so long as the borrower either resides in it or intends to return to it (for example, from a nursing home). The bank calls the mortgage only when the borrower sells the home or dies. Borrowers may pay a premium for the life rights feature.

Q-Tip Trusts

Q-Tip trusts are established by attorneys to shelter assets and provide income to a surviving spouse. Because the money is in the name of the trust, the asset itself is protected in the same way that a term-certain annuity is protected. If the surviving spouse is placed in a nursing home, the assets are unavailable to him or her directly, and thus they are unavailable to the nursing home as well. Only the income in the surviving spouse's name is deemed available to the nursing home. This also ensures that money can pass to the next generation.

RETIREMENT PLANS

Retirement plans include 401(k) plans, IRAs, Money Purchase Plans, and other future financial plans approved by the IRS. These formal plans are generally marketed by mutual fund companies, banks, and insurance companies to individuals or to companies who purchase them for their employees. However, retirement plans can incorporate any of the assets above, with the exception of antiques and collectibles. Because of the federal and state tax liabilities attached to retirement plans, the face value of any plan stays intact only as long as the money remains untouched by the plan holder.

Retirement plans cannot be transferred without a cost. Because most retirement plans contain tax-deferred investments, they are subject to substantial taxes if they are transferred to a spouse or to another loved one prior to the death of the plan holder.

Capital asset protection strategies are part of both retirement and estate planning. Capital assets are those assets that a person could liquidate to obtain cash if needed. Capital assets are inherited estate tax free by spouses (for children and other beneficiaries the same holds true so long as the estate is valued at less than the allowable limit). Maintaining separate ownership of assets allows a surviving spouse to inherit a deceased spouse's assets free of income or estate tax. This should be considered when planning a financial strategy and considering long-term care resources.

Long Term Care Insurance

The last tool we will consider as part of a retirement plan for long-term care security is long-term care insurance (LTCI), which pays a daily benefit if one goes to a nursing home or if one needs home health care (as is also covered by many LTCI plans). Typically the beneficiary must be deficient in two or more activities of daily living (ADLs) to qualify for benefits. The ADLs include eating, bathing, using the toilet, dressing and ambulation.

Insurance companies, badly burned in the disability insurance market, are being conservative about long-term care insurance. Underwriting for long-term care insurance policies is getting stricter by the day. The applications denial rate for new policies in some agencies is as high as 35–40 percent. On the one hand, insurance companies recognize a potentially huge market that can benefit from this product and that can also be very profitable for them. On the other hand, it is getting more and more difficult to predict the amount of money that will be necessary to settle claims fifteen, twenty or even thirty years from now. It is possible to predict the likelihood of long-term disability for some, but certainly not for everyone.

The future costs of long-term care are also unpredictable. Today, the average cost of care in a nursing home is around $50,000 per year, but less than ten years ago the average was a little over $30,000 per year (costs vary regionally). As the costs of nursing home and home care rise, average LTCI benefits for nursing home and home health care will need to rise as well. Historically, rate increases for LTCI have been low, but premiums are rarely if ever guaranteed in LTCI policies.

Most LTCI policies do have a clause that informs policyholders that their policies are guaranteed renewable. This does not preclude the insurance company from raising premiums, however, only as allowed by the state's Department of Insurance. Given the history of both health and disability insurance premium increases, long-term care insurance premiums are almost sure to rise significantly over the years as both long-term care costs and long-term care claims increase.

LTCI insurers will insure only those who are healthy today, not those most likely to need long term care–the very elderly, the chronically ill, or the physically disabled. At the time of this writing, the odds that LTCI will be used to pay for nursing home care are relatively low, as can be seen from the following statistics:

- 9 percent of people over the age of sixty-five will spend five years or more in a nursing care facility.
- 25 percent will spend a year.
- 33 percent will spend three months or less.

Since those predictably in need of high levels of chronic care are uninsurable, we can conclude that for those who are insurable under LTCI, there is some question as to advantage of LTCI for nursing home coverage. But because LTCI policies also provide home health care, assisted living care, and respite care benefits, they can also be looked on as a way of *preventing* nursing home placement.

LTCI policy costs are determined by age and health, and generally cost about the same as a life insurance policy for a lifetime benefit with a similar cap. Premiums can run from several hundred dollars per year to as much as $20,000 per year. This is likely to be unaffordable for many Social Security recipients with an average income of around $800 per month.

LTCI has found favor with state and federal governments. A percentage of the cost of long-term care insurance premiums are tax deductible. Because LTCI can help defray the cost of nursing home or home care, certain states exempt either privately held assets or the homes of LTCI policyholders from consideration for Medicaid eligibility or from estate recovery.

For CLCP clients, weighing the advantages and disadvantages of purchasing LTCI can be very difficult. How can anyone accurately anticipate the probability of needing either nursing home placement or long-term care at home? In addition, one must also acknowledge the inherent conflict of interest when the professional advisor helping with the decision "to buy, or not to buy" may also stand to gain personally from the sale of a long-term care product.

There are legitimate arguments for and against the sale of LTCI by care managers. LTCI can be a very useful, even critical component of a long-term care plan. And who is better able to make this determination than a care manager who is familiar with all the lifecare planning alternatives, not just those subsidized by the insurance industry? On the other hand, care managers are as susceptible as any other professional to conflicts of interest. Care managers must sort out these issues on a case by case basis. For clients who can afford long-term care insurance, it can be a valuable component of estate and long-term care planning. For clients with little discretionary income, the purchase of LTCI must be considered very carefully, since if they ever have a need for nursing home or home health care, LTC insurance can prove invaluable.

Long-term care insurance is not the solution to all CLCP clients' long-term care needs. For the time being, only a few people are able to afford it, and those who will predictably need such insurance are generally not insurable. But those who cannot obtain long-term care insurance may be able to buy life insurance, or they may have even more useful resources available to them. Care managers need to be familiar with the many financial resources that may be used in constructing long-term care plans. They should be able to analyze each client's situation to help determine which options will work best and which advisor can best help the client.

SAMPLE RETIREMENT PLANNING LETTER

A retirement planning letter is presented here as an example of financial planning for long-term care. The letter was written by a financial planner to clarify some of the issues associated with financial decision making and the investment instruments available to meet one's long-term care needs.

$\mathfrak{Advanced}$ $\mathfrak{Retirement}$ $\mathfrak{Concepts}$, LLC

Masters of Science in Financial Services	***Enrique J. Alvarez***	463 South Main Street
Chartered Life Underwriter		P.O. Box 665
Chartered Financial Consultant		Suffield, CT 06078
Certified Insurance Consultant, State of CT		Phone: (860) 668-9700
Registered Health Underwriter		(800) 406-1595
Registered Employee Benefits Consultant		Fax: (860) 668-1182
Certified in Personal Financial Planning		
Certified in Estate Planning & Taxation		
Certified in Pensions & Executive Compensation		

May 17, 2000

Mr. and Mrs. Smith
100 College St.
Hudson, CT

Dear Jim and Mary:

After reviewing your finances and the best ways to finance your retirement and possible medical expenses, we should review your present financial situation. Let's start with your retirement assets:

1) Social Security currently pays Jim $1,150 per month, and Mary $1,100. You will continue to receive this money as long as you are alive. Based on your life expectancies, your Social Security benefits are worth in excess of $200,000 to your family.

2) Jim, your pension will pay $2,400 per month as long as you live. If you predecease Mary, then Mary would receive $1,600 per month.

3) Your 401(k) plans have approximately a $200,000 value. This would provide approximately $1,170 per month (adjusted for 3% inflation with a 7% rate of return during your normal life expectancy).

4) Your home could be sold and proceeds could be used to buy or lease a less expensive home and invest the difference for income.

5) You could take out a reverse mortgage and receive the income. When both of you die, the bank would sell the home and any equity in the home would go to your heirs.

6) Personal investments of $150,000 could be sold if additional income was required. The following is an example of your income stream under different scenarios:

1

	Jim and Mary Alive	Jim Dies	Mary Dies
Jim's Soc. Sec.	$1,150	0	$1,150
Mary's Soc. Sec.	$1,100	$1,150	0
Jim's Pension	$2,400	$1,600	$2,400
401(k)/IRA Income	$1,190	$1,190	$1,190
Total Income	**$5,840**	**$3,940**	**$4,740**

In the event that you, Jim, predecease Mary, Mary would have $1,900 less in income per month for the rest of her life. If you, Mary, predecease Jim, Jim would have $1,100 less per month to live on for the rest of his life. To offset this guaranteed loss of income you could spend down your assets to make up the difference, reduce your standard of living, or purchase life insurance. The proceeds could be used to offset the loss of income for the survivor.

The second concern we have—long-term care—is popularly financed in three ways:

	Pay As You Go	Long-Term Care Insurance	Life Insurance
Premium	None	Guaranteed renewable; Premiums may be increased by insurance company every time the insurance company typically hits a 60% loss ratio. Some companies have raised their rates.	Premiums are guaranteed
Amount of Benefits	Amount of Resources	Benefit you buy	Amount you purchase
When are Benefits Paid?	When You Choose	Typically, when you cannot perform two activities of daily living	Typically, when & if you become terminally ill
Frequency of Usage	As needed	25% either spouse	100% surviving spouse

% of people that will go into a nursing home for 5 years or longer – 9%
% of people that will die – 100%

When you die, what will happen to your policy?

Long-Term Care Insurance	Life Insurance
Premiums stop	Death benefit paid. Proceeds could be invested to offset the loss of Social Securiity benefits. Balance could be used to fund the survivor's long-term care needs.

I hope this information makes it easier for you to choose the method best suited to achieve your overall financial goals. I remain available to assist with your investment planning needs.

Sincerely,

Enrique J. Alvarez, CLU, ChFC, CIC, RHU, REBC
Master of Science in Financial Services

3

Suggested Readings

Bogle, John C. *Common Sense on Mutual Funds.* New York, NY: John Wiley & Sons, Inc., 1999.

Garner, Robert J., Charles L. Ratner, Barbara J. Raasch, and Martin Missenbaum. *Ernst & Young's Personal Financial Planning Guide*, 3rd ed. New York, NY: John Wiley & Sons, Inc., 1999.

Warner, Ralph. *Investing for Retirement: How to Make Good Choices Without Getting a Ph.D. in Finance.* Berkeley, CA: Nolo.com Publishers, 1999.

CHAPTER 10

The Community LifeCare Planning Alliance

Collaborative care planning is hardly new–lawyers, social workers, doctors, financial planners, insurance brokers, and families have been consulting with one another for years. What *is* new is the urgency with which collaborative care planning must now become more efficient and more effective.

More than ever before, the chronically ill and disabled need a coordinated response from the private sector. CLCP, and the care managers that practice it, will help long-term care planning clients meet their resource planning, emotional support, and health care needs more efficiently. They will help stave off the many assaults on their clients' independence once mitigated by liberally furnished health care and chronic-care benefits. If long-term care planning teams are to work, they will need what every team needs to win–a playbook. To be effective, new CLCP alliances should be organized around a few basic principles.

PRINCIPLES OF THE CLCP ALLIANCE

Principle #1 — Holism

Webster's defines the word "system" as "a set or arrangement of things so related or connected as to form a unity or organic whole." Whatever the system, various parts function in support of one another. If the parts are separated, the system disintegrates. Integration, however, yields a total effect that is greater than the sum of the individual parts. Holism is this "greater than" effect.

Holism is the most fundamental principle upon which truly effective CLCP is based. Achieving holism in CLCP can be extremely difficult. True synergy may become sabotaged by "domain poisoning."[1] The signature characteristic of domain poisoning is the usurpation of a CLCP

---

[1] Birmingham, J: Unpublished notes, Continuum Care Services, Suffield, CT April 21, 1997

task *from* the care planning professional most qualified to perform the task *by* a less qualified care-team member.

Domain poisoning can occur for any number of reasons. These may include the following:

- Inadequate understanding of roles within the Community LifeCare Planning alliance
- Lack of confidence between CLCP alliance members
- Care-team members' motivation for personal gain, i.e. financial gain, reputation, marketing, and so forth
- An individual team member's need to control the care planning process
- An individual team member's effort to satisfy their own need to be helpful

Whatever the cause, domain poisoning is the enemy of holism. It is the 7' 2" center insisting on dribbling the ball up the basketball court in a fast break, or the three hundred-pound tackle returning the kickoff. When domain poisoning sets in, the other team wins.

Domain poisoning decreases care-planning and care-management efficiency by increasing the time and cost of achieving the ultimate goal–client benefit. For efficiency's sake, CLCP tasks should be done by the least expensive care-team professional who is best suited to the task. The art of team care planning is the art of task sharing as well as the art of inter-professional communication, the second principle of Community LifeCare Planning.

Principle #2 — Communication: Talking
With One Another

Good communication can both prevent domain poisoning and act as an antidote for it. Candid, accurate, and honest communication is the second basic principle of interprofessional Community LifeCare Planning. Good communication enables effective action while poor communication is disintegrating.

Effective interprofessional communication requires that each member of the team talk *with* one another, not *at* one another. Each professional in the care-planning cluster must be willing to listen to one another, and each must be able to share opinions and recommendations and know that they will be heard. Effective communication requires mutual respect and an atmosphere of trust within the care plan alliance.

Although on the surface this seems obvious, in practice it is difficult to achieve. Effective communication must be intentionally nurtured and a facilitator may be needed to translate the goals of each discipline to the other CLCP alliance members in a meaningful way and keep the team from working at cross purposes. For several reasons, the care manager is often the most appropriate person to fill this facilitator role.

More than any of the other care-planning professionals, the care manager is free to ensure that good communication promotes the holism so favorable to the client's benefit. There are several reasons for this:

- The care manager is usually the least expensive member of the care-planning team. Families can often afford to pay the care manager to facilitate communication within the team.
- The care manager is likely to be the least specialized team member. He or she is therefore often useful in supporting the specialists when they cannot take the time from their specialized service to share information with the other team members, the client, or the client's family.
- Because of the care manager's professional background, he or she is probably most able to coordinate interdisciplinary team communication. This task has traditionally been within the purview of medical social work, discharge planning, and case management, from whose ranks care managers often come.

It is useful for someone to focus on identifying and eliminating obstacles that hinder the specialists' ability to perform tasks in a coordinated way. Poor communication is usually the primary obstacle, and facilitating communication becomes a specialty in itself. While the care manager may have been trained as a psychotherapist or nurse, he or she is more likely to serve as a care coordinator who helps the specialists serve as clinicians, estate planners, and financial managers.

It is also important to nurture the relationship the CLCP team develops with the client since the client's perspective is, after all, most important. The care-planning team needs to maintain a regular flow of information with the client. Once again, the least expensive and often best-suited interpreter for the client and the family is the care manager.

If the care manager is to facilitate effective communication, he or she must become the master of the two-minute conversation, the succinctly written memo, and the quickly returned e-mail. The care manager must understand the languages of medicine, law, psychotherapy, and insurance, and quickly and accurately translate each specialist's contributions for the others and the client.

Principle #3 — Shared Values

Common purpose is fueled by common values. Priorities must be negotiated and set by the members of the CLCP alliance to ensure effective action and to determine who will act and what will be done. There are certain values that must be shared by care-plan alliance members if the ultimate value–*client benefit*–is to be realized.

This book is the product of team collaboration. It grew out of a process that was a unique experience for each of the contributors and that produced a unique care-planning and care-management training resource–this book. All of the contributors are leaders in their fields. Each has a very sophisticated understanding of the basic tenets and principles upon which effective CLCP alliances are built. It was valuable to be a part of the process through which the group explored the complexities of task sharing, compromise, and values clarification.

There is a tale of blind men trying to describe an elephant to one another. One blind man was standing with his hand on an elephant's tail, describing the elephant to several other blind men. "An elephant is a creature similar to a whip with a tassel on the end of it," he proclaimed. Another blind man, with his hand on the elephant's tusk, responded, "Oh, but I beg to differ. The elephant is not a whip-like creature, but a sort of sword-like creature, long and hard with a point on the end." Another blind man, with his hand on the elephant's ear, objected further. "No, you are both wrong," he declared. "An elephant is flat and floppy with a hollow cavity in the middle." And so the debate continued with the leg, the head, et cetera, each blind man objecting to the other's characterization.

There were times when our group of care-planning specialists resembled these blind men. Each member had his or her perspective on what needed to be done first in each of the case examples we discussed. Without question, compromise and decision making were always enabled by the most commonly shared value–*dedication to client benefit.*

This value consistently promoted efficiency of effort and ensured the effectiveness of the outcomes.

Principle #4 — Dedication to Service

Alliances break apart when individual members serve themselves first and the client second. Inevitably, members of the CLCP alliance must make sacrifices if the benefits of holism are to be reliably achieved.

There are two rules that each member of the CLCP alliance can use to guarantee that the client receives the best possible service. First, each member of the care planning team should live by this motto: *Provide as much help as necessary and as little as possible.* Second, tasks should always be designated to the most qualified alliance member in the least expensive way possible. These two simple rules-of-thumb can check team members' selfish motivations and the domain poisoning that too often ensues.

Embracing the team-service approach is itself a value that each professional in the CLCP alliance must understand. The effort of the care *planning* professionals, including care manager, lawyer, financial planner, and so forth, creates the opportunity for care *giving* professionals, such as physicians and nurses, to keep the client healthy in the setting of his or her choice. Everyone in this formula must be dedicated to the same outcome. No single team member can facilitate that outcome without the help of the others.

Dedication to service compels each member of the team to compromise and sacrifice. It requires that team members serve one another no less intentionally than they serve the client or the client's family. The logic here is simple: "I help my client best by helping the person that can help my client best." Bickering within the team leads to wounded egos and obstructive behavior. This hardly serves the client's interests. The CLCP alliance members have a second motto: *The client's problems are our problems, not the reverse!*

Principle #5 — Institutional Diversion

Not all hospitalizations and nursing home placements can be avoided. For those that can, CLCP is a powerful model for preventing institutional placement. Care managers should seek to ensure that all members of the CLCP alliance are dedicated to preventing institutional placements whenever a competent client states this as his or her preference and whenever patient safety can be reasonably assured.

We may have arrived at the point in our developing health care crisis where many long-term care consumers are less safe in a nursing care facility than at home with part- or full-time personal care assistance. The one-to-one attention many chronic-care consumers need is less available in institutional settings every day. We have definitely arrived at the point where health care and long-term care, as currently financed through Medicare and Medicaid, are no longer affordable for the society that pays for them.

As compelling as these realities are, neither carries as much weight as the simple fact that, when given the choice, most long-term care planning clients adamantly prefer to remain in their homes rather than go to a hospital or nursing home. Thus, the primary reason that CLCP alliance members must be dedicated to the prevention of institutional placement is that nearly 100 percent of care-planning clients are unequivocally in favor of remaining independent—at home.

Whether or not to recommend hospitalization or nursing home placement is a decision that should be made by the most skilled medical treatment professional on the team. Most often this is the physician, the physician's assistant, or the nurse practitioner in charge of the client's primary medical care. But medical clinicians are not care planners in the broadest sense of the term. Their time is limited and their focus is usually on treatment, not resource management or resource development. They may need help seeing how additional resources or a different approach can create a community-care option that is safe and preferable to placement.

Many hospitalizations and nursing home placements for chronically and physically disabled patients are arranged for lack of personal care options. Placement recommendations are often made by the physician based on reports from the primary care nurse or the primary care therapist on the care management team. This may occur whether these clinicians are privately employed by the client or in the service of the home health care agency. In these cases, a care manager may be instrumental in helping medical practitioners understand how CLCP might be utilized to avoid an institutional admission. Most medical treatment professionals rarely assess resources from the CLCP perspective. They lack the training to do a thorough personal resource assessment. Among those who can do the assessment, few have the luxury of time to develop comprehensive resource management plans, in concert with a client's financial and legal advisors, that make community-based caregiving alternatives possible. Additionally, many health care and long-term care professionals—nurses, doctors, physical therapists, and medical social workers alike—regularly make the error of "permanency planning." An option that will not last "forever" is not pursued.

Why? Because most health care professionals operate from a third-party reimbursement mind-set. They may not yet consider health care from the private pay perspective. Consider the 75 year-old home care patient who suffers an exacerbation of her multiple sclerosis. She lives alone and has no close family relatives. She has a niece, with whom she talks regularly, and a husband, from whom she is separated, but both live over two hours away from her. During an extraordinary heat wave, she suddenly becomes incontinent and cannot transfer out of her bed and onto a commode or into a wheelchair. The home care nurse and physical therapist find her suddenly unsafe in a home care setting without twenty-four hour care.

While the health care professionals are accurate in their assessment of her safety risk, they are inaccurate in their belief that hospitalization and nursing home placement are necessary. The patient in question has $2,200 per month in income, $662,500 in liquid assets and stocks, and she owns a home worth $200,000. She is receptive to the idea of either live-in and/or long-shift personal care assistance from a home health aide.

The patient is placed in a nursing home because the nurse, the physical therapist, and the physician treating her make two flawed assumptions. First, they assume that since neither Medicare nor Medicaid will provide twenty-four hour care in the home, nursing home placement must be arranged. They do not see that a resource management intervention by a privately hired care manager may be sufficient to organize the patient and connect her with a home health aide or licensed practical nurse (LPN) who can live-in on a short-term basis until a more permanent solution can be found. Additionally, they mistakenly assume that since it is unlikely that this patient can pay for twenty-four hour care at home for the rest of her life, nursing home placement is automatically required. But what if the client, with a care manager's help, could find a live-in aide or sufficient long-shift personal care assistance, whether privately hired or agency-employed? Might this patient not spend several more months in a home care setting where she clearly wished to stay, rather than in a nursing home, during which another, more "permanent" option—moving to Virginia with her niece, perhaps—might be developed?

There is a paradox within the principle of institutional diversion. While institutional diversion is a fundamental goal and principle of the CLCP alliance, we recognize that hospitals, surgery centers, rehabilitation facilities, nursing homes and the health care professionals who staff them are, without question, indispensable and critically valuable. No one in the CLCP alliance should operate under the misapprehension that these institutions are not necessary. Indeed, without them, community lifecare options for most chronically-ill individuals disappear. Intensive care provided in state-of-the-art hospitals and rehabilitation facilities enables recovery from serious injury or illness and clears the way for chronic-care services to prevent subsequent injury or illness. Very few people with serious, debilitating, chronic conditions can forever avoid an episode of intensive medical treatment. Institutional care is a part of the community lifecare continuum.

However, CLCP can significantly alter the standards by which the need for institutional admissions is determined. It forces the institution-based, third party reimbursement model of health care to share the spotlight with a self reliance-based, self-pay, chronic-care model. The CLCP alliance creates opportunities for health care professionals to experiment with community-based, chronic-care options. At the same time, it provides protection for the institution-based health care professionals by developing safe discharge options. Without the support offered by the CLCP alliance, doctors, physician's assistants, and nurse practitioners may not be willing to accept the liability for authorizing "riskier" community-care arrangements when their at-risk patients might prefer such arrangements to nursing home placement.

At the very least, all members of the team should endorse the minimum standard of community-care planning. Following this standard, nursing home placement must be seen only as a last resort or respite option in cases where adequate custodial care services cannot be provided in the setting of the client's choice. We must remember that nursing homes are so named because of the availability of a registered nursing staff on a twenty-four hour basis. *Nursing* home implies *nursing* needs—services that can only be provided by a highly trained, experienced registered nurse (RN).

There are three main conditions that make long-term nursing home care a valid option:

- For sub-acute cases in which a patient's symptoms are volatile enough that twenty-four hour, on-site availability of a registered nurse is necessary to prevent hospitalization *and such services cannot be arranged in the client's preferred location*;
- For cases in which the patient's pain is too difficult to assess and manage without twenty-four hour skilled nursing services *and such services cannot be arranged in the client's preferred location*;
- And for cases in which custodial community-care resources *are* adequate but the chronic-care consumer's primary *caregiver* is not.

Billions of public dollars are wasted every year in nursing home placements that are elected as much to save physician labor (and liability) as to provide the most appropriate care. Physicians and other health care practitioners simply do not have the time to address the tasks necessary to develop alternatives that include family care coordination, home modification, locating private personal care assistance, and relocation to assisted living situations. But the CLCP alliance is skilled in developing alternatives to institutional placement, and dedicated to doing so. It helps clients maintain their independence and control; while at the same time protects the public coffers. It insulates medical treatment professionals from unacceptable liability and sustains the structural integrity of our acute-care institutions.

THE CLCP ALLIANCE'S SOCIAL SUPPORT MISSION

Every social institution is affected by our growing chronic-care problem. Health care and long-term care policy will soon become *the* hot political issues in America. Social, political, and economic stress associated with the rising numbers of chronically-ill and disabled people stem from two primary problems: the rising cost of health care and the demographic caregiving challenge we face.

These developments are having an impact upon families, communities, and businesses as never before. State budgets strain under the growing burden of Medicaid costs. Health care facilities are closing across the country as Medicare trims reimbursement for services. Employee absenteeism is on the rise as workers spend more time tending to the needs of elderly and/or disabled relatives.

These developments put the CLCP alliance at the center of the national health care and long-term care problem. The new (old) mission of all healthcare professionals is to empower their most vulnerable patients through prevention of illness and injury. The new mission of scores of budding care-plan alliances is to give these health care professionals the resources they need to do so. If physicians and nurses are to treat all the major and minor assaults on the health of our most vulnerable citizens, then lawyers, financial planners, accountants, brokers, and care managers must now serve as newly minted healthcare resource professionals. Their resource management is now directly responsible for health care and long-term care outcomes.

COMMUNICATION TECHNOLOGY

To communicate effectively, CLCP alliance members must utilize many new, hi-tech communication devices. They must be minimally competent with computers, and fluent with e-mail and Internet usage. It is important for them to be linked by cellular or digital phone, satellite pager, and easy-to-use message retrieval systems. For the care manager, perhaps more than any of the professionals in the care plan alliance, it is vital to be able to remain in communication, even when out on the road. Internet linkage is already available for automobile communication systems.

Communication is the transfer of information, and information is the *materiel* of decision making. Sharing information and making appropriate use of it is the primary task of the CLCP alliance. But hi-tech communication devices in no way assure effective communication. All members of the care-plan alliance must cultivate clear communication skills, particularly the care manager.

The two central communication challenges for the interdisciplinary care-planning team are *what* and *how*—*what* information is shared within the care-plan alliance, and *how* does this communication take place?

TECHNIQUES THAT FACILITATE COMMUNICATION AND HOLISM

Technique #1 — "How Can I Help?

As the saying goes, you catch more flies with honey than you do with vinegar. So it is with coordinating a care-planning team. At every possible opportunity the care manager should convey a clear message to the other members of the Community LifeCare Planning alliance that his or her job is to remove obstacles that are in the way of each team member; the care manager is there to provide support to the specialists within the alliance.

This message is conveyed by a simple technique. The care manager should ask one or all of the following questions of either the physician or the physician's nurse, the estate-planning attorney or the attorney's paralegal, the financial planner or the receptionist, every time the care manager calls.

- "What can I do to make your job easier?"
- "What does the client need to do to help *you*?"
- "What does another care-plan alliance member need to know from you?"
- "How can I interpret what you are doing to the client and his or her family?"

Approaching CLCP alliance members with a clear desire to help produces four results favorable to the care-planning outcome. First, it directs the CLCP alliance toward a more effective, holistic method of operation. Second, it establishes the care manager as both servant and leader at the same time. Third, it sets up the conditions for agreement about action steps between the care manager and an individual care-team member, while at the same time suggesting the team context. Fourth, it minimizes "me" and maximizes "we," the only effective antidote to domain poisoning.

Technique #2 — "I Don't Know."

Good Community Lifecare Planning often develops less from proclamations of knowledge and expertise than from acknowledgment of ignorance. All CLCP alliance members must seek out the questions that they can answer with a resounding– *"I don't know!"*

Care-team members afraid of their own ignorance serve poorly. No physician, lawyer, or accountant knows everything there is to know about medicine, law, and taxes. Consider then how much less the care manager can know about each of these professions. Suddenly, the value of learning becomes apparent. The care manager's ability to acknowledge what he or she doesn't know defines his or her usefulness to the client as well as to the CLCP alliance itself.

Acknowledgment of limitations forces the care manager to develop problem-solving and process-management skills. In many ways, how a care manager thinks is far more important than what he or she knows. In the face of a dilemma, the care manager's most creative response is, "The answers will be found, I just don't yet know where, how, or by whom!" This approach inevitably leads to collaborative problem solving and away from any one team member trying to take control.

Technique #3 — Use the Staff

Aside from care-plan alliance members' dedication to service, each must also be dedicated to a financial bottom line. It is inevitable, therefore, that frequently the physician, lawyer, broker, or accountant will not have time to talk. Sharing information with the care manager will not be his or her priority. So how do care managers acquire or share information without being pushy?

The answer is that they talk to the staff. Every lawyer relies on paralegals and clerical staff; every financial planner, stockbroker, and insurance agent relies on a secretary; every physician relies on a nurse. The staff knows all and sees all and can be relied upon to convey vital information to the specialist. The physician ready to recommend nursing home placement may not do so if he or she hears from the nurse that the patient has decided to search for a live-in home health aide. The lawyer's estate plan may change suddenly if he or she learns that the client has become hospitalized with risk of nursing home placement in the midst of the care-planning process.

Conversely, there are bits and pieces of care-planning information involving the specialist professionals that can be learned from their assistants. The secretary who sees the signed request for information in the patient's chart can apprise the care manager of the status of a Social Security Disability report. The paralegal can communicate whether or not a new power of attorney has been written. A financial planner's secretary can confirm that a CLCP client has made an appointment to purchase an annuity.

Technique #4 — Write it, Fax it, E-mail it!

Speaking is the fastest method of communication for the speaker, but reading is fastest for the listener. Writing also gets through more reliably. I have recently begun to receive telemarketing by fax. As little as I want to receive uninvited solicitations, I cannot hang up on what I've just read in the same way as I (politely) hang up on telemarketers before they have finished their first sentence.

If you have something important to communicate, do so in writing. The advantages of written communication are numerous. First, you will have evidence that the communication occurred. Nothing compensates for failed memories like the written word. Unless it was never received—because the fax broke down, the post office went on strike, or the secretary lost it—there is no disputing the nature of the information or that it was shared. For the care manager, this paper trail creates a record of service and perhaps evidence of due diligence (for the courts) if deposition or testimony is ever required. And, as mentioned above, this method of communication saves the reader time in the learning. Moreover, your message can be shared without having to be repeated—a considerable benefit when several lifecare professionals are coordinating a plan. In the long run, clear, succinct writing is a very efficient way for all care-plan alliance members to communicate. Admittedly, writing takes time, but voice recognition software is speeding up the process by enabling words to be spoken and typed simultaneously.

Technique #5 — Sweat the Details

It is not an overexaggeration to say that the life of a CLCP client, as well as the lives of his or her family, are in the hands of the care planning team. Members of the CLCP alliance must leave no margin for error. The physician's and the nurse's diagnosis, prognosis, and risk assessment must be as exact as possible; the lawyer's understanding of up-to-the-minute changes in Medicaid regulations must be accurate; the financial planner's calculations must be to the dollar. The care manager's contributions, including assessment of family-care capabilities, reports on a client's mental status, knowledge about community program service availability, and so forth, must be actual and realistic. Perfection may not be attainable, but that is no reason not to strive for it; there is too much at stake.

In health care and business development parlance, this approach has come to be known as Total Quality Improvement (TQI), Total Quality Management (TQM), or Continuous Quality Improvement (CQI). Whatever the acronym, the point is the same—only by striving for accuracy and a reduction in the margin of error can you achieve these goals. In other words, you hit what you aim for. In real estate, the adage is "location, location, location." In CLCP, it's "details, details, details."

Technique #6 — "I was In the Neighborhood."

We've all heard the saying "Out of sight, out of mind." Care managers must not forget the value of face-to-face contact. Recently I went to my doctor for a check-up. As it happens, my physician writes orders for many of the patients I care for as a medical social worker working for the visiting nurse agency. While I was legitimately in need his care, our contact and conversation will also have a favorable effect on the care we provide for both our VNA patients and, under my care-manager hat, our CLCP clients. On the one hand, he is my physician. On the other hand, he and I are colleagues. As of a few days ago, we met face-to-face, and professional-to-professional contact makes a difference.

While I don't suggest making a doctor's appointment every time you wish to discuss a client's care plan, there is no question but that meeting with someone, shaking hands, having eye contact—*being* with someone—sets up a relationship, and relationships pay dividends. This holds true for all CLCP alliance members. A good care manager visits the local Social Security office and makes a point of meeting the people behind the voices on the other end of the phone. Sooner or later, the meeting will pay dividends for a client. The Social Security worker is more likely to want to help the care manager he or she has met, however peripherally. People appreciate contact. The same holds true for the doctor, the lawyer, and the insurance broker.

VALUE

The basic premise of this chapter is that through collaboration, care-planning professionals increase their value and effectiveness. And again, professionals are also people. The solutions the CLCP alliance creates for a client are as much a reflection of who each team member is as a person, as they are a reflection of each person's professional competence. Humanness counts most. But it is not just the client that benefits from this collaboration. Team care planning promotes the personal growth and development of each member of the care-plan alliance as well.

This simple notion may present CLCP alliance members with the most difficult challenge of all. Each professional in the CLCP alliance must not only work to develop new skills, but must also make a commitment to self-scrutiny that challenges cherished notions of professional importance, leadership, and control. Thus, while a lawyer is learning to practice a different kind of law for the care-planning team, he or she is also challenged to become a different kind of lawyer. A physician must learn not just how to practice medicine differently, but also how to become a different kind of physician. The same is true for each care-team member.

In his book *The E-Myth* (or Entrepreneur's Myth), Michael E. Gerber explains why so many start-up businesses fail. His premise is simple. Many people are proficient in their chosen fields, but it takes more than technical proficiency to succeed in business. Too often, when good technicians start businesses they fall victim to the mistaken belief (or E-Myth) that because they are good at what they do, they will automatically be good at running the business that supports what they do. So the auto mechanic who repeatedly hears from his customers that he should leave his abusive boss and start his own shop does so. His business soon fails, however, because he neglected to learn the business management and entrepreneurial skills that must be mastered to run a business that fixes cars.

Here, for the benefit of all CLCP alliance members, we offer the *P-Myth* (or Professional Myth): *Proficiency in a specialized field of practice does not give any individual care-plan alliance member special status in the Community Lifecare Planning effort.* In fact, the opposite is most likely to be the case. An individual sense of "specialness", whether personal or professional, ensures the failure of a collaborative, holistic effort.

Overcoming the P-Myth requires that each member of the CLCP alliance embrace the notion that no single profession is *most* sacred– they *all* are. A good care plan evolves from collaboration, not specialization. The professions (or professionals) who resist this notion will find themselves falling behind as health care and long-term care services change. The evolution of CLCP alliances that promote prevention and better self-care management will occur *without* them.

CASE EXAMPLE

Readers are referred to Appendix E for an example of a coordinated long-term care and resource management plan developed by a care manager, an estate-planning attorney and a financial planner. Our example illustrates the sequence of tasks that often follows a care manager's initial assessment when professional resource management and estate-planning referrals are indicated.

Suggested Reading

Greenleaf, Robert K. *Servant Leadership: A Journey Into the Nature of Legitimate Power and Greatness.* New York, NY: Paulist Press, Publishers, 1991.

CHAPTER 11

The Private Market Response to Community LifeCare Planning

The ratio of working taxpayers to people over the age of sixty-five has dwindled from 17:1 in 1965 to less than 4:1 today. This means that there is less tax money available to Medicare, Medicaid and social services to pay for the chronic-care support that has been offered so liberally since the late sixties. As a consequence, community-based chronic-care programs have been cut at a time when they appear to be needed most. For example, between 1990 and 1999 Massachusetts reduced the number of clients served by its state-funded home care system from forty-six thousand to thirty-six thousand, despite the significant increase in those who are both eligible for and in need of this program's community-based services. While many long-term care professionals have opposed these and other drastic cutbacks in the funding of programs for frail and lower income elders, they can see the writing on the wall. These cuts will not simply be a temporary political trend that will eventually be reversed.

As budgets for many government subsidized services have been capped to control expenses, individuals needing chronic care have begun paying for these services privately in an effort to maintain their highest level of independence for as long as possible. Because of this we are likely to see considerable growth in demand for CLCP services in the private sector. There are likely to be several pay sources for these services that include chronic-care consumers themselves, their families and employers. To stay competitive in tight labor markets, businesses will pay for family-care benefits or risk losing employees who will leave or refuse to relocate due to elder caregiving responsibilities.

In the mid 1980s, the National Association of Professional Geriatric Care Managers (NAPGCM) was formed. Professionals from the geriatric services community, including hospital and home care social workers, mental health professionals, nurses, and other community service workers, accurately anticipated the advent of privately paid care-planning and care-management services. After watching their budgets shrink, the number of visits they could make dwindle, their

caseloads grow, and their reimbursement rates decline, these professionals saw the need for a non-governmental, fee-based alternative.

At the time of this writing, NAPGCM has grown to a network of
more than fifteen hundred nurses, social workers, and related long-term
care practitioners. The organization seeks to develop an alternative to
the rapidly deteriorating long-term care system. Geriatric care managers
(GCMs) have primarily marketed their services to affluent elders, their
affluent adult-children, and their legal, financial, and insurance advisors.

GCMs are growing in popularity. Private care managers throughout
the growing network of GCMs have learned that "adult-children" caregivers are *customers*. Their aging parents are the *consumers*, but it is typically their healthy family members who initially engage the services of
the care manager.

Even if they can only afford to pay for a few months of caregiving
services, more elderly or physically disabled citizens today are capable
of paying for these services than are willing to do so. But adult-children
may be able to persuade their parents to retain the services of private
care managers, or the children may pay for such help themselves if, for
example, they live a great distance from their aging parent and they
are in a better financial position to do so. The private pay alternative
is fast becoming the choice of first resort to maintain frail elders and
physically disabled individuals safely in community-care settings. The
adult-child serving as a long-distance caregiver wonders, "What good
does it do my chronically-ill, aging mother to receive Medicare subsidized personal care assistance in one-hour increments on Monday,
Wednesday and Friday, when she's no less at risk for a fall on Tuesday,
Thursday and the weekend? Whether Medicare will or will not authorize payment is irrelevant to her *chronic* care needs!"

CLCP must also take into account the needs and concerns of those
who offer support—involved family members, friends and neighbors
who are both care providers *and* customers. Serving the consumer
must always be the care manager's primary goal and focus, but meeting the consumer's needs invariably means caring for the caregivers.

COMMUNITY LIFECARE PLANNING "PRODUCTS"

Care managers perform a variety of tasks that can be priced and marketed. Their service is their product, as the services of auto mechanics,
lawyers, or architects are their products. CLCP products fall into three
main categories—the assessment, the care plan, and ongoing care man-

agement. These three services are highlighted below.

We emphasize that this is not an exhaustive list of the products and services care managers now provide or are likely to provide in the future. They may also perform training and education, consulting, employee assistance, guardianship, and other services. Many may remain employed within the health care system as part-time home-care nurses, medical social workers, in-patient facility discharge planners, and case managers while also practicing privately. However, many more of these professional care managers will move into full-time private practice as demand for their services grows.

The Assessment

The assessment is the first step in developing the care plan. An assessment performed by a care manager trained in CLCP is a comprehensive assessment of a client's continuing-care needs. It is not strictly a social service assessment, although social services are evaluated as potentially valuable resources for some clients. And it is not only an acute-care or chronic-care needs assessment, though a medical treatment plan may be part of it. A care manager's assessment also incorporates legal, financial and environmental considerations, yielding the broadest selection of caregiving options for the client.

The assessment itself is a considerable amount of work—*and not just for the care manager.* The assessment cannot be completed without a good deal of help from the client. The care manager asks the complicated questions, and the client and his or her family answers them. These questions and answers, and the dialogue that follows, pull the client's and the family's attention to long-term care issues. The assessment process focuses their minds on both the mechanical tasks that must be accomplished as well as the emotional adjustments necessary to make the care plan work.

The client becomes a partner in developing the care plan through the assessment process. The value for the client comes not only from the plan itself, but from having participated in its completion. The process *is* the product. Indeed, the assessment, which can vary in length from two to ten hours of the care manager's time, may ultimately be the only service provided. Often clients feel capable of continuing on their own after it has been completed.

As described in chapter 3, the care planning assessment yields a resource profile and a needs profile. Once these are understood, the care manager can begin the educational process that helps clients understand their long-term care options and, ultimately, decide upon the most beneficial plan.

The Care Plan

Rarely is there one best care plan for any one individual. There may be several possibilities—from home care to assisted living to family care to nursing home placement. For CLCP clients and their families, the challenge is to make the choice that appears to have the best odds of working. This often means balancing the wishes of the elderly or disabled person—such as remaining at home—with issues of affordability, practicality, and safety. Balancing these issues may require creative care planning and dogged determination. For example, in order to avoid a nursing home placement, it may be an option for a client to relocate to the home of an adult-child. But if this is unrealistic, then the care manager must consider the emotional support the client will need in order to adjust to his or her lost independence.

There is no guarantee that the best possible plan will be achieved. The ideal long-term plan may not be the most practical, but there is usually a best available plan to choose from among a selection of plans that are good enough. Neither the care manager, nor the client and his or her family should become obsessed with achieving the "perfect" plan. It's been said that the perfect is the enemy of the good.

Appendix F offers readers several examples of CarePlan Options Reports that illustrate how planning helps CLCP clients with the decision making process. Long-term care plans are often selected by process of elimination. It is useful to consider all the options from all angles, even if at first glance they appear to be unworkable. Indeed, there is no such thing as a "long-term" care plan. Most long-term care plans are a string of adaptations to constantly changing circumstances. But if all options have been considered, everyone concerned will be best prepared when the time comes to make changes. Long-term care clients and their families who have considered all the options are best informed to select the best plan for them.

Care Management

Care *planning* is a decision-making exercise. When the decisions are made, and the plan is established, the care *management* begins. As indicated previously, care management refers to oversight, coordination, and provision of care. While the following descriptions of tasks performed by care managers are by no means an all-inclusive list, they do convey the essence of the care management "product," which is ongoing support, advice and assistance.

An interdisciplinary team best performs care-management services. Here we describe care management as provided in the home care setting. Our focus on home care should not imply that independent care managers have no role when clients are hospitalized, placed in nursing homes, or elect alternatives to home health care such as assisted living or continuing-care retirement communities. And obviously, health care professionals in all caregiving venues are themselves also managing their patients' or residents' care.

Our home-care focus does reflect our bias toward the least restrictive care option, and the one that is most often preferred by the person in need of care. Our experience has shown that most Community Life-Care Planning clients want to stay at home. As care managers, our job is to help them do it and not to talk them out of it when home care management gets difficult. The exceptions to this philosophy would be those situations when the care manager's clinical judgement and that of the multidisciplinary team with whom he or she works is that it is truly not in the best interests of the person needing care to continue to remain at home.

Home health care is a specific kind of health care, and it is rarely appropriate for such care to be managed by a solo practitioner. Care managers with nursing backgrounds may create confusion for themselves and their clients when they offer client advocacy and planning services one day, and nursing services the next. The same applies to social workers trained as psychotherapists. They should not serve as care managers one day and mental health practitioners another.

Many of the strategies that facilitate team care planning (as highlighted in chapter 10) also apply to ongoing care management. The care-management team should share the same values. Communication and holism, for instance, are as important in care management as they are in establishing a care plan in the first place. And the care management team should understand the value of taking care of one another, as well as the client and his or her family.

Care management differs from care planning in its focus on clinical issues affecting the client's medical stability. These issues include medical management of chronic illness; psychological, emotional, social, and behavioral factors affecting the care management effort; and strategies to prevent illness and injury. Indeed, care management is often synonymous with medical treatment and medical management in a home care setting. Care managers must understand that they are part of a medical-treatment and chronic-illness management team.

In many ways, the term "care manager" is confusing. For a community-dwelling, frail-elderly or physically disabled adult, the physician is likely to be the *medical* care manager, the home health care or primary care nurse may be regarded as the manager of nursing care, and the home health care physical therapist is the manager of rehabilitation therapy. At first glance the care manager's role may appear at best redundant, at worst, presumptuous. Why does the client need a care manager when they are in the hands of so many competent caregivers?

While professional caregivers may provide essential medical treatment and medical-management services, they generally do not coordinate their services with other critically important members of the CLCP alliance such as attorneys, financial planners, insurance professionals, and trust officers. And with the exception of the physician, they generally do not cross the home care boundary to follow their clients into the hospital or the nursing home.

Care managers are useful whether the client is paying privately or receiving Medicare-subsidized home health care under a physician's order. Their value continues after the home health care agency discharges the patient/client from service, whether the patient has recovered or been re-hospitalized. In order to understand how necessary care managers can be, community health care practitioners must acknowledge that health care is not all medical. The Medicare home health care benefit operates within the constraints of "medical necessity," but many *necessary* continuing-care services cannot be justified as *medically* necessary. The patient/client may need private duty caregivers to do homemaking chores, and provide transportation and companion services. He or she may be interested in saving money by hiring someone from the community rather than from the home care agency.

A home care nurse is often not free to assist a client with remaining non-medical needs, but the care manager is. A physician may not have time or the expertise to provide assistance in this regard, but the care manager does. If the client needs live-in help that would cost $368 per day (at $17 per hour) for the home care agency to provide, but the client cannot afford this rate, and the care manager can locate someone to provide such care for \$100–\$200 per day, the care manager's status as a private, independent professional can both save the client money and improve his or her care. Fee-based care managers can also save family caregivers, especially adult-children, substantial travel costs and costs related to lost time at work.

The care manager's job is to provide the highest quality of support for the medical-management effort at the lowest cost for as long as possible. What may appear at first glance to be an additional or redundant service is, in fact, an integral part of the home health care continuum. Care managers help arrange and provide services for which the home care agency and the physician are not reimbursed and for which they have no time. They help create options that are privately paid or provided by the family and that compliment insurance-subsidized caregiving. And the private support services remain in place after the insurance company or Medicare/Medicaid terminates coverage.

Clearly, care managers must know how to work shoulder-to-shoulder with health care professionals. After a home care agency has discharged a client from service, it is likely that the client's care manager will remain teamed with his or her privately hired medical clinician in order to co-manage the client's in-home care. This clinician may be a nurse or nurse practitioner with home health care experience, practicing independently or through an agency. As mentioned above, it is rarely appropriate for a care manager to serve as both the administrative support person and as the nurse or mental health practitioner. It is definitely inappropriate for a care manager whose core discipline is non-medical to provide ongoing medical-management services.

As has been mentioned, many care management tasks are non-medical in nature. Relocation assistance, family care coordination, arranging for home modifications, and consultations with the resource management professionals who are advising the client—all fall into this category. And much of the ongoing care provided in a home care setting may be relatively simple and may entail nothing more than homemaking services (shopping, cleaning, laundry, and so on) or a few hours a week of personal care. But what appears to be simple today may get very complicated tomorrow. Sometimes the client's continuing-care needs are very sophisticated. Competent medical management offered by qualified medical managers is always indicated when caring for community-dwelling, chronically-ill individuals, no matter how simple some tasks may appear to be.

Care managers who lack agency-based home health care experience may not feel confident when co-managing complex cases. In this instance, it is appropriate to defer to agency-based medical management. Handing over the care-management reins may cut into the care manager's billable hours. He or she may lose the role of staffing the care team and coordinating care with privately hired staff, including the co-managing RN or adult nurse practitioner (ANP). He or she may also lose billable time for family care coordination. But it is better to lose all of this than to risk client injury or illness, let alone lose one's reputation or wind up in a lawsuit that holds one liable for negligence.

There is a fine line between care management and medical treatment. Care managers who engage in medical treatment must be licensed to do so and must know what they are doing. Reading this book does not automatically qualify a care manager to oversee the medical care of someone with serious, co-morbid chronic conditions who is also living in a community setting. For example, it does not prepare care managers to be the only care coordinator for a patient with amyotrophic lateral sclerosis (Lou Gherig's Disease) who wants desperately to stay home, has adequate financial resources to do so, but has no family caregiver to help with decisions. These and many other complicated home care cases require knowledge and experience that can only be gained by medical training and by working in health care settings.

Care managers can develop opportunities that are mutually beneficial for CLCP clients, home health care agencies, and care managers themselves. When done correctly, care planning helps clients adjust to the need for continuing care and helps them develop strategies to pay for it. As Medicare and Medicaid support for home health care diminishes, home care agencies will have no choice but to expand their non-certified, patient-pay business. Care managers will not only help home care patients organize their resources, but may enter into joint venture arrangements with home care agencies that are mutually beneficial to the providers involved. Such partnership arrangements can make it possible to provide seamless, professional care-planning and management services to the client.

However, many complicated home care cases *can* be well served by well-coordinated, experienced, private duty care teams. Private practitioners can operate without the burden of high administrative overhead costs and excessive regulatory oversight. It is difficult for agencies to match the care management potential of an adult nurse practitioner with years of home health care experience teamed with a similarly qualified medical social worker–both charging less per hour than often less experienced agency-based personnel. The same is true of physical therapists, live-in and hourly-rate home health aides, homemakers, and companions. Private care-management teams can operate in concert with physician care, but without constantly having to acquire physician orders for simple, medical-management services that the managing nurse or nurse practitioner deems necessary.

Admittedly, privately paid care management is unaffordable for many elderly and physically disabled individuals. Those chronically-ill and disabled individuals living on relatively low fixed incomes cannot pay the cost of private home care management services, which sometimes can exceed the cost of nursing home care. However, a combination of family resources and community support programs can sometimes pay these costs at levels high enough to provide twenty-four hour care. Care managers can connect people to community resources during the care-planning phase, enabling them to tap into sources offering as much as three to four thousand dollars per month in government subsidized home care services. As we discussed in chapter 7, many individuals are eligible for abundant community support services, but fail to acquire them for lack of a relatively low-cost assessment and referral opportunity.

Continuing-care management requires diligent adherence to predetermined prevention strategies and due caution against developing a false sense of security. The client that hasn't fallen in several weeks is still likely to fall again. Relationships between private duty caregivers and clients, between caregivers and client family members, spousal relationships, and relationships within the care management team must be nurtured. Relationship problems can have a negative effect on care-management outcomes equal to the more obvious medical or resource-management problems. Care management is more like tending a garden than constructing a building. It is not static; circumstances may change precipitously. Good care management therefore requires regular self-scrutiny and an awareness of risk especially when things have been going well.

"Success" in care management is hard to measure; many care management efforts result in hospitalization and nursing home placement. A client may fall less frequently at home than in a nursing home due to the increased supervision from 1:1 staffing the care manager has arranged. But are less frequent falls evidence of success or failure in the prevention effort? The care-management "cup" can be seen as half-full or half-empty depending upon one's frame of reference. While it is impossible to develop a system for perfectly managed care, care managers must be vigilant at all times, reducing margins for error and watching out for the accident-waiting-to-happen. Prevention planning doesn't stop when the aide is hired and all is well.

MARKETING CLCP

When people think of "health care" they think of doctors, hospitals, pharmaceuticals and health insurance. But health care also includes other vital services often brokered by care managers such as chronic care, wellness maintenance, supervised/supportive housing, care planning, and care management services. The problem for private care managers today is that their prospective customers—elders in need of chronic-care planning and care-management services, and their family members who may need guidance, advocacy and decision making assistance—probably don't know this service is available. And if they do, they may not understand the value of CLCP as a legitimate health care service. Care managers face a considerable marketing challenge. They must sell their service as part of a new health care paradigm to consumers who are mostly unaware of the value of CLCP for their own health care and long-term care security, as well as the security of their estates and the security of their family's future.

If marketing is an effort to generate demand for a product, the first marketing challenge for the care manager is to educate the public about the existence and value of the services listed above. Probably the single biggest reason why potential clients do not choose to hire care managers is that they do not understand that their chronic-care needs will not be met by Medicare or Medicaid. People at risk for hospitalization or long-term nursing home placement must first understand why it is necessary for them to pay for planning and management of their chronic, continuing-care needs. Care managers must find ways to educate care-planning consumers (elderly and physically or mentally disabled individuals), care-planning customers (consumers' adult children and spouses), and potential referral sources (health care professionals, lawyers, trust officers, and financial planners), about the limitations of Medicare, Medicaid, and private health insurance.

At the time of this writing, care managers are getting some help in overcoming the public's misunderstanding of the complexities and limitations of their health insurance. The federal government has begun a campaign to educate the public about the limits of Medicare and Medicaid, and there are now tax deductions available for long-term care insurance policy holders. Although the government's attention to these matters is helpful, it will still require marketing on the part of care managers to popularize CLCP. The utility of care planning and care management in helping people maintain their independence is a message care managers must emphasize to the media as often as possible. Developing and sustaining a high profile public awareness message will be necessary to build awareness of the value of Community LifeCare Planning.

As we have demonstrated in chapter 7 (Community Care Planning Resources) and chapter 8 (Estate Planning), CLCP can be critical for individuals with lower incomes and fewer assets. Unfortunately, both the government and the health care system that will authorize much of the CLCP needed by lower-income groups are coming slowly to recognize the value of prevention, much less pay for it. For the foreseeable future, the most fruitful sources of CLCP referrals are likely to be professionals who have influence in the lives of people in the middle- and upper-income and asset brackets. These professionals include attorneys, insurance professionals, financial planners, bank trust officers, and accountants. Health care professionals will also be fruitful referral sources. In the near term, those who can afford to pay for additional personal care assistance, home modification, relocation, and so forth, will be the most likely consumers of private care-planning and care-management services. And just as General Motors sells cars to the dealers and the dealers sell cars to the public, care managers will market their services not to consumers, but to those who can persuade clients to make use of their CLCP skills.

While it is true that those who have more assets may also have more to lose to catastrophic illness and nursing home placement, it is also true that wealthier individuals differ very little from lower- and middle-income people in their motivation to protect their resources. An individual who has $50,000 in the bank and a $70,000 home values what he or she has as dearly as someone with twenty times those assets, despite the notable difference in the amount of nursing home care each can afford. But there are significant differences in the asset protection strategies and home health care options each can consider

It may be a novel experience for a care manager who is used to working in the health care or social service systems to develop working relationships with lawyers, financial planners, and accountants. It may also be a novel experience to be regarded by such professionals as a referral source for them. Care managers must be careful to keep financial incentives for making referrals from compromising their services. To ensure objectivity, care managers should only accept payment from the client and his or her family. Marketing can cross the line to become a conflict of interest when payments are attached to referrals. It is one thing to develop collegial relationships to benefit the client; it is quite another to develop these relationships to benefit the care manager.

Private care managers must be mindful of the value of their reputation. Word travels when a care manager refers a client to another professional who performs a like service, but is either better at performing it and/or less costly. The satisfied client will tell a friend, "ElderCare Advisors, Inc. chose to save me money when they could have kept the work themselves. You should call them. You'll get a fair shake."

The greatest value of private care managers may be their personalized service and their commitment to customer satisfaction. Employee turnover in publicly-funded long-term care programs is staggeringly high. Some home care agencies and nursing homes lose as many as 50 percent of their employees each year. In contrast, independent, professional care managers offering Community LifeCare Planning at the local level are more likely to be there to follow through with the client. As small business owners, care managers are invested in the success of their business. As companies of care managers begin to flourish, as inevitably they will, individual care managers who have an investment in their parent corporation will drive the quality of service. People tend to invest themselves in what they own, and autonomy and personal investment are always advantages for the consumer.

The public perception that comprehensive CLCP services are provided by system-based professionals (such as hospital or nursing home discharge planners, health insurance case managers, or home care agency staff) is a considerable marketing challenge for care managers. Marketing efforts must accentuate three basic differences:

1) Community Lifecare Planning covers a lot of terrain, and includes financial and estate planning analysis, insurance brokerage, and many other professional services. These

services are normally not offered by either social service or health care system professionals.

2) Private care managers can follow the patient/client through-out the health care system–from hospital, to rehabilitation facility, to long-term care facility, to home health care agency and back to self-care.

3) Private care managers can spend more time serving individual clients than an employee of a health care facility because they have significantly smaller caseloads, much less paperwork, and considerably broader latitude and freedom of practice.

CASE EXAMPLE

We end this chapter with a true story that highlights several components of CLCP as practiced by an independent care manager. Readers are also referred to Appendix F at the end of the book for further examples of CarePlan Options Reports written by an independent CLCP practitioner.

Perhaps most noteworthy in the story that follows is the fact that the clients–Catherine and her daughter, Amy–are neither rich nor poor. They are from the proverbial middle class. As illustrated in chapter 7, CLCP can create care-plan options for a broad segment of the population and is not only for the very wealthy. Here we see how care managers can provide affordable CLCP services to those with moderate incomes and assets, yet who are keenly interested in remaining independent and preserving their life savings for their heirs, *and* who are willing to pay for the advise and help they need to do so. The value of CLCP, or any service for that matter, is in the difference it can make. Let's look at how Community LifeCare Planning was able to help one family achieve its long-term care goals.

A Family-Care Story — Catherine and Amy

Catherine is 83 years old, widowed and lives alone in her own home. She has approximately $82,000 in stock and cash equivalents. Her income from Social Security and an employee pension is approximately $1,300 per month. She has three children. Her daughter, Amy, is her primary caregiver.

Catherine's health is failing. She has recently suffered her fourth and by far most debilitating stroke. It has left her unable to walk or stand without assistance. She can no longer sign her name. Catherine also has osteoarthritis and osteoporosis. The treatment team at the rehabilitation facility, where Catherine has been recovering for almost two months, is telling Amy that Catherine needs 24-hour supervision and long term, custodial care—in other words, nursing home placement. Catherine does not want to go to a nursing home, but she knows she needs a lot of care. Amy works full-time. She cannot quit her job, leave her children and her husband, move in with Catherine and become her personal, full-time caregiver.

Catherine and Amy engage the services of a care manager to help them explore options for Catherine. Amy is the vital link to any option other than nursing home placement. The primary caregiver, in this case a supportive, committed, close relative, is the linch-pin connecting Catherine to alternatives.

The care manager helps Catherine and Amy understand the limits of Medicare, Medicaid, supplementary insurance, and the family's personal financial resources. The care manager familiarizes them with some of the estate-planning options available should Catherine wish to begin positioning for Medicaid eligibility in a nursing home or a community setting. Catherine's concession that she needs 24-hour custodial care, *and that she will have to spend her own money to obtain it*, makes community-based care planning a viable option. Creative deployment of resources always requires the client's support. For Catherine, this support follows her acknowledgement of the problems she faces.

For Catherine and Amy the decision to call in a care manager was the decision to explore an alternative to nursing home placement. Like most people, they were eager to avoid placement if possible. Catherine's means were limited. She had to acknowledge that any plan to care for her in the community, wherever she might live, might cost more than her monthly income and would, therefore, be time limited. Both Catherine and Amy agreed, however, that since Catherine preferred to remain either in her home or in another suitable community setting, even if it cost more than nursing home placement, it was worth it. The fact is that if she went to a nursing home as a privately paying resident, a good deal of the money would probably disappear rapidly anyway.

Since Catherine needed "only" 24-hour supervision and personal care assistance (and not an RN-level of skilled attention on a 24-hour basis), the care manager's recommendation was that Catherine and Amy try an experiment. They ran an ad in the local paper seeking live-in help, preferably from an experienced home health aide. Catherine's current caregiving needs were not too sophisticated, and training someone was a possibility as well.

Amy contracted with a friend, a nurse with home care experience, to supervise the live-in privately. They engaged the care manager to coordinate Catherine's private duty care plan with the nurse and MD. Amy and Catherine understood the importance of maintaining their emotional equilibrium. Both knew Amy would spend some weekends and some evenings with her mother when the aide was off duty. It was necessary for Amy to take care of herself as well.

Next, Catherine and Amy took a crash course from the care manager in being household employers. They then contacted Catherine's accountant and her insurance broker to learn about obtaining a household employer tax identification number and worker's compensation policy, and to check to see that Catherine had adequate homeowner's liability insurance. They then contacted a payroll service to handle their payroll and ensure they were making appropriate Social Security, Medicare, state and federal income tax deductions, and so on. Catherine's elder law attorney and her care manager worked together to resolve financial management, estate planning, and supplementary insurance questions. The care manager's home care expertise helped the elder law attorney maximize Catherine's community lifecare opportunities.

Catherine's income and assets precluded eligibility for *Community* (as opposed to *Institutional*) Medicaid without some planning. For Catherine, it was conceivable that she could qualify for Community Medicaid after her assets had been spent down or transferred. This would provide her a medication subsidy, transportation to and from her MD, and additional personal care assistance.

In Catherine's case it was advantageous both for her own well being, as well as for the state's fiscal health, that she plan for Community Medicaid eligibility. Acquiring Medicaid would expand her home care options, and, in the long run, might cost the state as little as $1,500 per month for medications, transportation and personal care assistance under a waiver. This compares favorably to the approximately $4000 per month the state might otherwise spend for her care in a nursing home (the total cost of a month's care in a nursing home minus her $1300 patient pay amount) after her own resources were exhausted.

Estate-planning activities included:

- Catherine assigned Amy general, durable power of attorney.
- Catherine funded an irrevocable burial trust and burial account.
- Catherine and Amy were advised of the possibility of funding an irrevocable, term-certain annuity with a ten-year payout as a way of creating an asset that would be immediately exempt from Medicaid recovery (only its income stream would be considered) should she continue to need nursing home placement. (NOTE: This is a provision of the State in which Catherine resides and may not pertain in other states.)
- Catherine and Amy met with a financial planner and insurance broker who counseled them on available annuity contracts should the annuity be selected.
- Family-gifting strategies were discussed that would both protect assets and position Catherine for eventual Medicaid eligibility.
- A decision concerning the status of Catherine's home was postponed to see how the live-in service worked out. Two possibilities were discussed, however. They were:

    1) Transferring the home to a life estate trust naming Catherine's children as beneficiaries while retaining life rights to the home for Catherine; or
    2) Selling the home and using the proceeds to put an addition onto Amy's home that would accommodate both Catherine and either a live-in or day/evening shift personal care attendant(s).

The upstairs of Catherine's home was readied for the live-in. Catherine was discharged to her home with a referral to a home health care agency that would care for her on a short term, intermittent basis under the Medicare "A" Home Health Care benefit. Her discharge took place almost 2 months after the care plan meeting at the rehabilitation facility. Catherine's nest egg was intact, minus the following expenses and transfers:

Catherine's Discharge Costs

- Care manager's fee (16 hours @ $60 p/hr) $960.00
- Attorney's fees (5 hours @ $175 p/hr) $875.00
- Home renovation costs (free labor from
  Catherine's son and son-in-law) $1450.00
- Irrevocable burial contract $5,000.00
- Gift to Amy $10,000.00
- Live-in advertisement and background check $350.00
- Accounting fees and worker's comp. insurance $300.00
- Barrier modifications with property lien $0.00
  (Barrier modifications to be paid through a
  residential rehab program or Dept. of
  Agriculture housing modification program)
- Purchase of lift chair (wheelchair and hospital
  bed covered by Medicare) $575.00
- Miscellaneous expenses $600.00

TOTAL $20,110.00

Catherine's discharge actually *cost* her $5110 ($22,110 minus $5000 burial contract and $10,000 gift to Amy, both of which assets remain for her use). For this fee she and Amy achieved the following:

- Obtained a new power of attorney and health care proxy
- Developed a preliminary estate plan that would both pro-tect assets and position Catherine for community supports should she need them to postpone nursing home placement
- Learned what they needed to know about long-term care options and community supports
- Found and hired a live-in caregiver (5 days per week) to care for her and offer respite to her daughter (with payroll set up and worker's comp. in place for a year)
- Installed a short ramp and widened the bathroom door
- Purchased needed durable medical equipment

The care manager served as the catalyst for Catherine's discharge by providing family care coordination services, resource management and decision-making advice, administrative help with staffing, and by coordinating the efforts of a quickly-formed CLCP alliance that included the estate-planning attorney, financial planner, insurance broker and home care nurse as medical manager.

Catherine's Estimated Monthly Home Care Budget

- Live-In Home Health Aide
  (5 days per week, $150 per day) $3150.00
- Extra shifts as needed $500.00
- RN supervision of HHAs $300.00
- Care Manager $300.00
- Cost of living (e.g. home maintenance,
  utilities, food, health insurance,et cetera) $1000.00

                     TOTAL   **$5250.00**

Catherine's ongoing community-care budget of $5250 per month means that she will spend down her own assets at the rate of almost $4000 per month ($5250 minus her monthly Social Security and Pension income), giving her 15 months to consider her alternatives before her liquid assets are gone. During that time, she and her daughter will consider a number of long-term alternatives with the care manager. These include modifying Amy's home and moving Catherine to live there, acquisition of community-supported chronic-care services once eligibility for Medicaid is established, and so on. While Catherine's future remains uncertain, for now, she is home—where she wants to be.

Suggested Readings

Kaplan, Mary, and Stephanie B. Hoffman. *Behaviors in Dementia: Best Practices for Successful Management.* Health Professions Press, 1998.

Kenney, James, et al. *Elder Care: Coping With Late-Life Crisis.* Golden Age Books: Perspectives on Aging, 1989.

Molloy, William. *Caring for Your Parents in Their Senior Years: A Guide for Grown-Up Children,* Firefly Books, 1998.

Tirrito, Terry, Nieli Langer, and Ilene L. Nathanson. *Elder Practice: A Multidisciplinary Approach to Working With Older Adults in the Community.* Univ. of South Carolina Press, 1996.

CHAPTER 12

Conclusion

When the United States of America was founded, health care was pretty basic. Most people did their own dental work, if you broke your leg you had a pretty good chance of dying, and childbirth was regularly fatal for the mother. At the beginning of this century, average life expectancy for men was not much over forty-five years of age and only .2 percent of our population was over the age of eighty-five. Prior to World War II, most paraplegics died from infections within a year of their paralysis.

A lot has changed in a few decades. Today, the chances of dying from complications of a fractured femur or the delivery of a child are extremely low. Most paraplegics now live normal life spans, and the percentage of people over the age of eighty-five is now 2 percent (ten times that a hundred years ago) and climbing fast. By the year 2050, 4 percent of the U.S. population will be over eighty-five years old—*twenty* times the percentage in 1900.

If life in the past was uncertain even for the young and healthy, it was exponentially more so for those with chronic health problems and physical disabilities. Many people died before they had the chance to experience old age and infirmity. But today, almost every once-fatal or disabling illness or injury now has an expensive treatment that didn't exist a few years ago. Our search for life-extending technologies has paid off with irresistible success.

The effort to care for the growing number of people with disabilities and chronic illnesses has never been as expansive or as expensive as it is now, thanks to these new treatment options. The question is, what consequence will these developments have for the future of our society?

No single issue will affect the future of our society more broadly than our health care crisis. Medicare and Medicaid together pay for most of the health care in America. But in the current political, economic, and social climate they are like the Titanic: as unsinkable as they once appeared to be, and as unthinkable as it is to abandon them, they are going down under the crushing cost of health care and the shear numbers of health care and long-term care consumers entitled to their benefit. Many believe these programs could sink our way of life and the social and economic systems we have created to protect it.

Again, consider the following facts:

1) Health care in the U.S. costs over a trillion dollars per year—more than 13 percent of GDP.

2) Seventy percent of all direct health care treatment is given to those with chronic health problems.

3) The most expensive people to treat are the thirteen-plus million U.S. citizens with one or more *disabling* chronic conditions—almost 5 percent of the total population.

4) Sixty percent of the disability is among those over age sixty-five.

5) By the year 2040, due primarily to the growth of the elderly population, 8.4 percent of the total population will be severely disabled.

6) At this rate, the cost of health care in 2040 will be far greater than today:

   - Of the total GDP, 23.5 percent will be devoted to health care for all.
   - Ten percent of the entire U.S. gross domestic product will be dedicated to providing health care for five percent of the population—those over sixty-five *and* disabled.

While the percentage of our population in need of care is growing, we face another equally vexing dilemma: the pool of able-bodied caregivers is shrinking. Today, half of the informal care needed by community-dwelling, frail-elderly, chronically-ill, or physically disabled citizens is provided by family caregivers between the ages of forty-five and sixty-five. Most of these caregivers are women. The ratio of caregivers in this age group to people over eighty-five years of age (those most in need of care) has dropped from twenty to one in 1970 to about eleven to one today. By the year 2030 it will be six to one. Lower birth rates and smaller families ensure its continued decline.

We face a demographic double whammy. The trend is clear—as the number of people with disabilities increases, able-bodied caregivers, in their most economically productive stage of life, will be forced to stop working to care for their sick, frail or disabled friends and relatives. Inevitably, we will face profound moral and ethical questions if we are to remain politically and economically viable. Something will have to change.

It is important to keep in mind that this shift in economic resources toward health care and away from other, arguably more productive purposes has not been brought on by the expansion of the aging population as such. Many of the circumstances driving this shift are amenable to change. The current rate of injury and exacerbation of chronic illnesses and disabilities can be reduced significantly through better self-care management and illness-prevention strategies. The increasing use of elective surgeries, expensive medications, and other medical treatments could be lessened through successful prevention and long-term care planning as well. The unnecessarily frequent placements of those with chronic conditions in hospitals and nursing homes, nearly all of which are paid for with federal and state tax dollars, could also be sharply reduced through creative community-based care planning.

Our health care crisis is manageable, but not without prevention-focused planning for those most likely to use expensive health care services. To keep our health care system from failing, we will need to face a few deeply disturbing questions. Can we or should we continue providing so much costly health care treatment for those in the end stages of life? Can we afford minimally life-extending surgeries for those who are predictably terminally ill? If so, how will we pay for them? If not, how do we go about instituting society-wide triage? How will we resolve difficult issues embedded in the politics of health care? At present, despite their numerical minority status, 40 percent of those who actually vote are over age sixty-five. Sometime in the next decade, despite the fact that they will still comprise a minority of the population (17 percent by 2030, 21 percent by 2050), they will likely become the voting majority. What sacrifices will they need to make to keep the health care system viable and the cost of health care from bankrupting the economy?

Economic insolvency is the enemy of our social and political systems. As Calvin Coolidge once so eloquently put it "The chief business of America is business." Health care is about life, healing, compassion and the relief of suffering, but it is also a business that must remain solvent, let alone thrive and grow. Health care must be paid for—by *all* of us. In health care, the cold reality is—no margin, no mission! CLCP can give form and direction to a less expensive, alternative health care approach based on self-reliance. It offers a way out of our addiction to an unaffordable approach to health care.

PREVENTION

Preventing illness and injury is the only way we will keep our health care institutions (not to mention the political and financial structures that support them) from being overwhelmed in the not-too-distant future. While prevention efforts may be supported by technological developments, for the most part prevention is low-tech, inexpensive and not very glamorous. There will not be a chronic-care mini-series competing with *ER* for Nielson ratings.

Prevention focuses on several key areas. These are:

- Engaging those most at risk for injury or exacerbation of a chronic illness in learning better self-care management;
- Supporting people as they work through the difficult emotions and changes in lifestyle associated with lost independence;
- Providing chronic-care services, in most cases recommended at levels higher than is apparently necessary, regardless of who pays the bill;
- Coordinating non-medical support services such as long-term care planning, individual and family counseling, housing modifications, estate planning, financial management, and links to community resources; and
- Organizing preventive medical services such as flu clinics, foot clinics, self-care management support groups, home visits by physicians, et cetera.

Unfortunately, our health care system focuses little on health maintenance. It is designed to provide treatment for illness and injury, whether or not they are preventable. It is also built around its billing processes, but it doesn't bill directly. Few of those who receive its services could afford them as individuals. In an arrangement enjoyed by no other segment of our economy, the health care system thrives on acute-care services provided to the chronically ill, elderly and disabled, that are all paid for by a third party. It is a trillion-dollar-a-year industry with no immediate incentive to prevent the consumption of acute-care services. Physicians' offices, hospitals, rehabilitation facilities and nursing homes can only bill when waiting rooms and beds are full, not empty.

Health care providers are in a double bind. They are dedicated to helping their patients stay well, and certainly do not maliciously seek to subsidize illness, but the system they must work in compensates them for healing and comforting patients only when they are ill, not for keeping them from getting sick to begin with. Here again, it is difficult to send a bill for prevention. The costs associated with making a sick person well are easy to identify and to charge for. But when a person remains healthy, how do we determine the value of the preventive care he or she has received? Prevention is, by definition, unmeasureable. When it is successful, nothing happens. How do we measure that which never occurred? Further, how do providers of health care charge insurance companies for it?

As we have seen, people with chronic conditions are the greatest consumers of direct health care services. Because exacerbation of illness or injury is most predictable among this population, preventive care is most effective for them. This need not be proven. It is reasonable to assume that planning promotes prevention and that preventive care reduces the costs that might have been incurred had a person's health declined. The question we must address is not whether prevention is worth it, but how is it done most effectively.

Our health care crisis is first a crisis of awareness. We are so focused on curing illness that we can't see the wellness-maintenance alternatives. In a treatment-only model, we cannot perceive the cost of illness or injury until it happens. When an illness or injury occurs we say, "Wow, this is so expensive! If only we could have prevented it." But when it comes right down to it, nowhere in our health care system is prevention a reality. Most health care professionals, and the patients they serve, are not really aware that prevention is a viable alternative. They can't see the forest (wellness and prevention opportunities) for the trees (so much illness and injury).

WHERE WE ARE

If you cut an apple in half, is it still an apple? The answer is yes—until you turn it around. The same question might be asked of public health insurance. Is Medicare still Medicare following the service cuts brought on by the Balanced Budget Act of 1997? Or, when we turn it around, has it not now become, more accurately, Medicare II? And when Medicare II becomes insolvent, will we simply create Medicare III (again, without changing the name) to maintain the illusion that "Medicare" is still there?

For nearly forty years Medicare and Medicaid have provided us with a financial safety net that has paid for most of the health care and long-term care needs of our most vulnerable citizens. However, these programs are not sustainable in their current forms for more than a few years. Indeed, Medicare has already become a very different program from what it was just a few short years ago. Many benefits have been cut by changing how providers are paid, rather than by changing the actual language describing the coverage. Medicare can remain solvent into the future only by reducing its scope. The same holds true for Medicaid.

Many solutions have been proposed to address our health care affordability problem. The imminent meltdown of our health care financing system is real, but we must also exercise caution and a healthy degree of skepticism as "studies" galore paint an unmanageable picture of the future of health care and long-term care. Too often these studies propose solutions that (coincidentally) depend on the mass purchase of their sponsor's products. Most over-emphasize long-term care financing schemes as our only salvation. However, even the most ardent supporters of managed care, long-term care insurance, and the entire panoply of system bail-out strategies must conclude that no funding mechanism will ever be developed by the private sector to replace Medicare and Medicaid. We are naive if we believe we can construct a financing scheme that will sustain our present health care and long-term care systems.

The recent economic boom notwithstanding, ours is a society no longer swimming in the post-World War II wealth upon which Medicare was built. The ratio between taxpayers and Social Security pensioners (by definition, also Medicare beneficiaries) is not forty to one (as it was in 1935), or twenty to one (as it was in 1965), but less than four to one and shrinking fast. Is it any wonder that hospitals are downsizing, home care agencies are closing, nursing homes are understaffed due to budget cuts and shortages of qualified staff, and health care sector stocks took a nosedive following the Medicare cuts in the Balanced Budget Act of 1997?

As important as inventing new insurance arrangements, tax incentive plans, and funding alternatives may be, these measures can also be seen as a last, desperate attempt to sustain health care approaches that can no longer work. But how do we actually make the transition from an institution-based system, to an approach based on self-reliance? How do we slow the juggernaut toward health care system collapse?

For health care to become manageable, the term "health care" must now be redefined to include "chronic care" as no less "medically necessary" than medical/surgical treatment and rehabilitation services. When chronic care and its precursor, prevention planning, become legitimate components of the health care equation, we will establish a health care system that includes patients as partners with health care providers and health care payers, sharing their part of the burden of health care responsibility and cost. By understanding that chronic care *is* health care, and by working from a model based on patient self-reliance, we can develop a creative response to the health care crisis we are facing. Here are a few suggestions that should make our transition easier.

THE THIRD PARTY IS OVER

We hold very dear the notion that we are entitled to third party reimbursement for health care. But the third-party mindset has become dangerous—it convinces us that there is such a thing as a free lunch. Now we are running out of sources for this reimbursement and soon enough, the party, as they say, will be over.

Visit any hospital, rehabilitation facility, or nursing home in the country. The majority of the occupants are receiving room, board, and expensive medical care for free. Consider the following:

- Over 60 percent of the occupants of most health care and long-term care institutions are Social Security beneficiaries whose care is paid for by Medicare or Medicaid.
- As indicated in chapter 3, many of these Social Security beneficiaries have long since consumed their personal contribution to the Social Security and Medicare systems.
- At the time of this writing, the Medicare "B" premium deducted from each Social Security beneficiary's check is a little less than $550 per year. However, the average Medicare beneficiary consumes over $4,000 worth of health care per year.

In other words, 60–70 percent of the health care we provide in this country is given to people who contribute only 10 percent toward the actual cost of the care. And that contribution comes from a pension benefit in large part supported by taxpayers who are not receiving that benefit. If we factor in the percentage of hospital residents covered by Medicaid, most of whom have made little or no financial contribution to their care, we must conclude that most direct treatment is provided to people who have paid nothing for it. Where does our sense of entitlement come from?

"Health care is a right!" is the battle cry of the more liberal faction in health care reform. This notion begs several questions:

- What *is* health care?
- What *is* a right?
- Can we afford to support everyone's "right" to health care?
- If so, how much are we willing to pay?

We can only add health care to the Constitution as a "right" if taxpayers are willing to finance it, and the cost will be different depending on how "health care" is defined. If health care is defined as medical treatment, then at the time of this writing health care in America costs over $1.2 trillion per year—one-seventh of the entire nation's gross domestic product. Are the American people willing to define such care as a right, in the same way that they define voting and free assembly as rights? Are we also ready to watch the cost and consumption of health care rise unchecked if we do define it as a right?

The right-to-health-care movement also touts national health insurance as the answer to all our woes. Socialized medicine, they say, will finally make health care affordable and available to everyone. They cite the fact that over forty-five million people in America currently lack health insurance. They ask how we can allow this to continue in the richest nation in the world.

The plight of the uninsured working poor and middle class is legitimate and should in no way be minimized. They certainly do need health insurance for access to primary care and medicines, and to cover the high cost of inpatient treatment. However, these uninsured are not the major consumers of health care, *and not only because they lack insurance*, nor will they become so if and when they are adequately covered. As has been demonstrated, the major consumers of health care are those people with chronic conditions, a relatively small percentage of the population. And virtually all of those with chronic illnesses and physical disabilities have the very best health insurance in the world—Medicare, plus either a private supplement, a public supplement, or Medicaid. Thus, the "health-care-is-a-right" battle cry, as noble and genuine a cause as it may be, does not acknowledge that the most expensive health care consumers are already covered. National health insurance does not solve the problem of affordability, nor does it reduce our sense of entitlement to expensive medical treatment that is in many ways at the heart of the affordability issue. National health insurance for still more acute care will not solve our primary health care challenge—caring for the chronically ill.

On the opposite end of the spectrum, the more conservative health care reformists wave the banner of managed care. They insist that market forces will solve the problem through HMOs (Health Maintenance Organizations) and other managed care arrangements that seek to engage patients (consumers) as partners in maintaining health. In this arrangement, they say, everybody wins. Health insurance consumers stay healthy. Doctors become teachers and teammates with their patients. And health insurers, by the way, make a little money.

But managed care doesn't work for the chronically ill. People with chronic illness need ongoing monitoring and regular access to care—exactly what managed care is designed *not* to offer. Managed care creates obstacles to care, not ready access. These obstacles come in the form of utilization reviews, treatment pre-authorization, and the various case management/gatekeeping services needed to slow the pace of treatment consumption. Managed care is very effective at cost containment, and it works for those of us who rarely get sick. It is a disaster for those of us who are sick all the time. The recent exodus of managed care companies from the Medicare+Choice program is evidence that even the inventors of managed care don't want to offer it to the elderly and disabled. For most health insurance companies, caring for such clients is a losing proposition.

To resolve our third party vendor dilemma, we need to begin by re-categorizing what we currently refer to as "health" care, but which is, more accurately, "sick" care. Our approach to health care is an allopathic one. By Webster's definition, allopathy is "Treatment of disease by remedies that produce effects different from or opposite to those produced by the disease." The criterion for admission to the health care system is *sickness*, not health. By any measure, therefore, ours is a sick-care system and not a health-care system at all. The system is perhaps better than any other at treating sickness and trauma, but its ability to care for and maintain our health is woefully inadequate.

If, as suggested above, we expand the definition of health care to include all of the self-directed action individuals can take to prevent illness, especially those individuals with chronic illness and physical disabilities, then suddenly health care is not just a right but also a responsibility. Suddenly we're asking the right questions: How many handrails can we install in the homes of persons with osteoporosis who are at risk for falling? How many people with insulin dependent diabetes can we help to better manage their diets? How many families can come together to help their relatives with chronic obstructive pulmonary disease feel less anxious and breathe just a little bit easier? How many physicians can we authorize to teach the chronically ill to better manage their illnesses? How many doctors can begin to visit patients with the greatest need and the least mobility in their homes? The irony is that once we expand the definition of health care, even if we decide that sick care is a right, we will probably be able to reduce the cost of sick care enough to make it available to all.

Common sense has become a casualty of health care's third party reimbursement system. Health care professionals consistently report that they believe most of the people under their care in hospitals and rehabilitation centers could have avoided being there by employing some reasonable preventive measures. They know that many of the chronic ailments that afflict their patients need not regularly become exacerbated to the point where hospitalization is needed. They know that their patients do not practice preventive planning or adequate self-care management. They know that the single most powerful health care reform will take place when patients themselves are disabused of the notion that it is the insurance company's job to maintain their health.

PHYSICIANS TO THE RESCUE

We cannot overemphasize the importance of maintaining a viable, acute-care, hospital-based, treatment component to our health care system. Ironically, sustaining the most important functions of our acute-care system requires movement away from institution-based health care delivery toward community-based alternatives. Institution-based health care has always accommodated the caregiver's interest in providing care in one location. Now, it's the patient's turn.

The trend toward community-based health care and chronic-care services is driven by several recent developments. First, in the face of health care subsidy cuts, "patients" are becoming "customers." They are paying for their own care and as a result they are demanding that the care be delivered in the venue of their choice—*their homes.* Second, recent technological advances in communication and diagnostic services have made health care far more portable. As described in chapter 6, health care has gained substantial high-tech support from tele-medicine, cellular and digital communication, laptop computing (especially for billing), miniaturized diagnostic equipment, the Internet, and so forth. Physicians, physician's assistants, and nurse practitioners have fewer excuses to remain in their offices or in the hospital. Third, the last great obstacle to home-delivered primary care—financial disincentives for physician home visits—is finally coming to an end. Medicare's recent pay rate increase for physician home visits has made home care services more financially feasible. And many physicians are finding that their distaste for managed care and steadily declining incomes under managed care arrangements have made home-delivered primary care a practice model that makes sense. In short, health care clinicians now have incentives to provide portable health care for the chronically ill and disabled. In the end, this development may be the most important contribution of the entire managed care movement.

While home-visiting physicians cannot see as many patients as their office-tethered colleagues, they will likely increase the chance that their community-dwelling, chronically-ill patients will stay out of the hospital. The simplest interventions made by a physician practicing from his or her car can prevent the most expensive form of crisis treatment—the emergency room visit—and the most expensive form of institution-based treatment—in-patient admissions. Physicians who are willing to sacrifice some income (although less of it than in the recent past) in exchange for increased patient contact and freedom of practice can create alternatives to much of the costly institution-based health care that is so inconsistent with the needs and the preferences of the chronically ill.

These three factors—patient demand, hi-tech support, and higher rates of compensation for traveling physicians—can forestall emergency room visits and hospital admissions for many who now regularly spend time in these institutions. Combine these developments with Community LifeCare Planning options, and we see that all of health care, including acute care, rehabilitation and chronic-care services, becomes an increasingly community-based service.

THE DYING RITUAL

It is impossible to say exactly how much money is spent on health care in America. We know we spend well over $1 trillion on measurable health care services. But this number comes from records kept by Medicare, Medicaid, private insurers and health care providers. A lot of care never gets recorded.

If we look more closely at that $1 trillion, we see some alarming trends. Perhaps most alarming is the amount we spend in hospitals and nursing homes caring for those who are certainly dying. End-of-life health care costs, defined as the cost of care provided within the last three weeks of life, have been estimated to be as much as 30 percent of all health care costs.

The exact figure is irrelevant. We know that billions are spent annually on surgeries and inpatient treatments that will only minimally extend the lives of those receiving them. In light of this, we may have only one choice—to *relearn* how to ritualize the dying process. Doing so will probably be the most difficult health care challenge we face.

In our culture, no individual or social priority supercedes longevity. But as the sheer volume of chronic illness and impairment overwhelms our health care and long-term care systems, we will lose the ability to aggressively treat both those who are dying slowly and those whose death is imminent. Extending life for everyone at all costs will no longer be an option. "Meaning" and "quality" at the end of life will need to be valued along with "longevity." Health care will be forced to embrace the withholding of treatment, and adopt a more spiritual aspect in doing so.

Sherwin Nuland's best seller, *How We Die*, may have set the stage for a yet-to-be-written sequel, *How We Live Just Before We Die*. In our health care system, we express our growing awareness of death's relationship to life through hospice. For the last twenty years the hospice movement has been growing in acceptability. Hospice provides a combined medical, spiritual and human touch when the end of life is a tangible certainty. It is the health care system's anteroom in which dying is authorized; it is our best effort when the system that wages war against death is about to lose the battle.

In order to qualify for hospice care, one must have an affliction that will take a patient's life and that modern medicine cannot forestall for more than six months. A patient's decision to "sign on" to hospice care is a resignation to this fact. With the help of physicians, hospice nurses, counselors and aides, hospice patients seek comfort and begin to consider the significance of their lives.

In fact, hospice care has been practiced since the beginning of time. When did we not comfort the dying? But hospice has acquired a special identity and status recently, perhaps in opposition to medical, pharmaceutical, and surgical treatments developed over the last fifty years or so. Hospice offers comfort, dignity, emotional support, and spiritual guidance when the modern medical cure is not yet available.

In hospice care, dying is not so much approved or embraced as it is surrendered to. Hospice care addresses not the causes of death but the symptoms of dying. It is the single most "non-medical" of Western medical disciplines. It incorporates pharmaceutical and medical/surgical science, to be sure. But it also readmits our emotions and our spirituality into the caregiving effort. For all our science, we remain intimidated in the face of death. When death is near, the non-scientific takes over.

But the hospice approach must also experiment with change. As enlightening as it can be for families and caregivers, and for the dying patients themselves, even hospice care remains fixed in the medical treatment model. Indeed, the hallmark of modern-day hospice care is pharmaceutical pain management. And today we use medications to relieve the physical pain of death as well as to buffer patients from the ultimate existential crisis of dying. But as well-meaning caregivers, we sometimes confuse our efforts, treating not our patients' discomfort, but our own. Prozac prescriptions have practically become a standing order in hospice care, as much to relieve patients of their sadness, fear, and apprehension as to relieve caregivers' fear of being ineffective. Yet there is a distinction between anesthetizing people to the grieving process with drugs, on the one hand, and mitigating their terror so that they can experience the grieving process on the other. Recognizing this difference requires an artful combination of bereavement counseling and pain management skills.

We pay a price when we equate physical pain with either the emotional pain or the spiritual crisis of dying. Even at the end of life, we should continue to have opportunities for emotional and spiritual growth. Grieving is a necessary part of this growth, and while it is painful, it is also a vital part of coping with death for the individual who is dying as well as for his or her family. Interrupting the grieving process with psychopharmacologic medications can rob the dying of death's meaning.

No one wants to die and everyone has to. We in the West are confused and terrified by death, and we will spare no expense to avoid it. Indeed, postponing death through medical treatment has become so seductive that we have become almost totally disconnected from the spiritual awareness that once aided us in the process of dying. Perhaps as a result we have also been disconnected from the significance of living.

All this is about to change. Our "damn-the-cost" search for any and all life-extending medical treatments is about to be short-circuited. Spending so much of our limited health care resources for patients in their often-predictable final weeks of life is no longer a viable option given current demographic trends. Death and dying will soon intrude on the public consciousness more immediately and more tangibly than they have in years. A century ago, 80 percent of us died at home. At the time of this writing, almost 80 percent of all deaths in America occur in hospitals. The pendulum is about to swing back.

In the near future, knowing our loved ones are dying and being with them as they die will be a far less sanitized *life* experience for most of us than it has been in the recent past. In response, we will need to look back into our cultural and religious heritage to learn, once again, to make of death a life ritual. This will have a far-reaching and unanticipated effect on the brewing health care and long-term care crisis.

How will this increased connectedness to death manifest itself? How will we modernize the community caregiving rituals that once helped us die in our beds? How will we move beyond the simplistic, medicinal focus on death? Will we see meditation groups to help us "leave" our bodies without physician assistance or euthanasia? Will comforting the dying finally make it's way into the medical school curriculum?

Few experiences in life affect us more profoundly than being with another human being as he or she dies. This experience is even more deeply moving when the dying person is a relative or a close friend. Life's impermanence becomes more tangible and spiritual connection becomes more immediate. Death alters us, and soon more of us will experience this profound change, holding our aging relatives in our arms as they die.

Increased proximity to death is likely to be the catalyst for far-reaching, unanticipated social change. Right now, the prepayment of funeral expenses, selection of a burial plot, and creation of a will are socially sanctioned death planning. Perhaps in the future we will supplement these protocols by designating in advance where we want to die. This brings up new questions—such as how would we know when it's time to go to that place? It is hard to say what the impact will be on calculations of health care and long-term care costs, and on such things as the cost of life insurance, but it is not difficult to imagine that it will be dramatic.

SUMMATION

Perhaps our health care and long-term care crisis will become the vehicle for broad, positive social change. Catastrophes have a way of creating opportunities. Our health care dilemma may be a catalyst for social development that we cannot yet see clearly.

In his book, *Illusions: The Confessions of a Reluctant Messiah*, Richard Bach (of *Jonathan Livingston Seagull* fame) writes from the perspective of a modern-day savior who decides he would rather dust crops than save mankind. He says, "Argue for your limitations and it's a surety they will be yours." The health care crisis we now face gives us pause, to consider which of our limitations are real and which are self-imposed.

Moving past limitations is the work of evolution. In that case, our long-term care challenge is likely to extend our evolutionary reach considerably. By the year 2050, one in five persons will be over age sixty-five. Chronic illness or impairment will disable one in ten persons. Nothing is certain about how we will manage so much disability except that the approaches we have been taking will not work much longer. What *is* certain is that we cannot spend our way to a solution—there isn't enough money.

We seem to have forgotten many things. Two stand out as we deal with the problems confronted by an aging society. First, what has happened to the time-honored ritual of respect for the elder generation? Since time immemorial, all societies have placed supreme value on the wisdom, the experience, and the counsel of their elders. Indeed, they have depended on this wisdom for survival. Has our obsession with ever-rising health care and long-term costs, and our fear of the consequences, robbed us of the perception of our elders as the valuable resource they have always been? With so many more elders alive today, should not all society be that much the wiser and more fortunate for it, both practically and spiritually? In our fear of a future demographic disaster, are we too quickly depreciating what soon will be a fifth of our people?

Second, where is the expression of sacrifice that has been an equally time-honored value held by elders in all societies throughout history as they move to the end of their life's journey? Indeed, is it not true that in many ways society needs the help of its elders now more than the elders need the help of society? Can we now ask that which no politician dares–Can our elders make sacrifices in health care entitlements, in income supports, and so on, to create opportunity for the able bodied workers and the young? Or has this become so politically infeasible that we must resign ourselves to exhausting the public coffers in service of their needs, but risk the creeping age-ism that is likely to follow?

We mustn't fear these questions. The young and able-bodied now depend on the consideration of the elderly, the disabled and the frail, no less than those who need care depend on the able-bodied to provide it. Those of us who are rearing children, developing careers, and shaping society's future understand that when we see our elders in nursing homes and hospitals, we see ourselves only a few years hence. We may not yet know with the same surety as they that "life is short," but we know we are all in this together.

We also know that history will measure us by how we care for the most vulnerable among us. And, in this, there is no "system" to bear the burden we must now share in our communities, in our homes and in our institutions. We *are* the system. This is the hard lesson we are learning as those who can no longer care for themselves grow in number.

Solving our health care and long-term care challenge requires that generations reconnect. By this path we can begin to move beyond an inadequate, utilitarian view of the value of human life. Economics needn't be all that is sacred. One thing is certain–this crisis will force us to take care of one another. And perhaps that isn't such a fearsome prospect after all. We hope this book will help everyone along.

Community LifeCare
Planning Forms

ELDERCARE ADVISORS, INC.
INITIAL CONSULTATION CHECKLIST

Husband _____ DOB _____

Social Security # _____

Wife _____ DOB _____

Social Security # _____

Telephone # _____ (h)   (w) _____

U.S. Citizens: ❑ Yes   ❑ No

Veteran: ❑ Yes   ❑ No (If yes, which spouse) _____

List of Children or Relatives:

Names	Address	Telephone # (h & w)

Contact Person	Address	Telephone # (h & w)

Health Care Proxy   ❑ Yes   ❑ No

Name/relationship #: _____

Power of Attorney: ❑ Yes   ❑ No

Name/relationship #: _____

Living Will: ❑ Yes   ❑ No

Copies given to/relationship:

_____

_____

_____

Real Property:
Primary Residence (if owned)

Approximate Value _____ Mortgage _____ Basis Cost _____

Ownership (names, sole, joint) _____

_____

Vacation Home/Investment Land

Approximate Value _____ Mortgage _____ Cost _____

Ownership (names, sole, joint) _____

_____

Bank Accounts/CD/Savings/Money Market/Checking/Etc.

Bank/Type Account	Names on Account	Approx. Value

Stocks/Bonds

No. Shares or Bonds/Type	Names on Shares/Bonds	Approx. Value

Other Asssets: (*Unlisted Stocks, Business or Partnership Interestss, Payable Notes,
Interest in Pension or Profit Sharing Plans, IRA, Keogh or Section 401(k) accounts, Annuities*)

Type	Owners	Value

Miscellaneous Personal Property: *(collectibles – furniture, cars, jewelry, antiques, etc.)*
Type   Approx. Value

Income: *(list monthly amounts)*	Husband	Wife
Earned	_____	_____
Social Security	_____	_____
Diability	_____	_____
Pension(s)	_____	_____
Investment *(split by ownership)*	_____	_____
	_____	_____
	_____	_____
	_____	_____
Annuity *(by ownership)*	_____	_____
	_____	_____
Other	_____	_____
Other	_____	_____
Total	_____	_____
Total	_____ (combined)	

Life Insurance Policies:

Company _____

Owner of policy _____

Insured _____

Beneficiary _____

Face Value _____

Cash Surrender Value (if any) _____

Company _____

Owner of policy _____

Insured _____

Beneficiary _____

Face Value _____

Cash Surrender Value (if any) _____

If you are unsure of the nature or specifics of the policy, bring a COPY with you.

Asset Transfers: *Have you (or either of you) made any transfer of any assets out of your name(s) in the past 36 months? If yes, please list names(s) on asset, date of transfer, value at date of transfer, and to whom it was transferred.*

Name   Date Transferred   Value at Transfer   Transferred to

_____

_____

_____

_____

Health Insurance/Long Term Care Insurance:

Company _____

Name of subscriber _____

Policy # _____

Group/Enrollment # _____

Phone # _____

Provider Phone _____

Claims Address _____

_____

Company _____

Name of subscriber _____

Policy # _____

Group/Enrollment # _____

Phone # _____

Provider Phone _____

Claims Address _____

_____

Physician Name/Address/Phone:

_____

_____

Questions you have for your care manager:

_____

_____

_____

_____

_____

_____

_____

ElderCare Advisors, Inc. – Initial Interview

Name _____ SS# _____ DOB _____ Date _____

Clinical Observations

Resources in Place:
Outside Agency(s)

❑ RN	❑ Health Care Proxy_____
❑ PT	❑ POA _____
❑ HHA	❑ DNR
❑ RN	❑ Living WIll
❑ Homemaker	❑ Will

Family Info/social supports:

Home Environment:

Medical HX (MD_____)

Employment/Education:

Finances (Income/Expenses, Assets, Supplementary Insurance)

Services Needs/Referrals

ELDERCARE ADVISORS, INC.
CONTINUING CARENEEDS ASSESSMENT

I. SOCIODEMOGRAPHICS

A. **Name** (Last, First, Middle Initial) B. **Address** _____ C. **Phone #**

_____   _____   _____

D. **Birthdate**   E. **Sex**   F. **Marital Status**   G. **Religion**   H. **Admission Date**

_____   ❑ M ❑ F   ❑ Married ❑ Single   ❑ Catholic ❑ Jewish   _____
                      ❑ Separated ❑ Divorced   ❑ Protestant ❑ Other
                      ❑ Widowed ❑ Unknown   ❑ Unknown

I. **Race**   J. **Education**   K. **Employment Status**

❑ American Indian/Alaskan Native   Highest Level Attained   ❑ Employed ❑ Unemployed
❑ African American ❑ Hispanic   _____   ❑ Retired ❑ Unknown
❑ White ❑ Other ❑ Unknown

L. **Health Care Coverage**   M. **Does Patient Speak English**

Medicare: ❑ Part A ❑ Part B ❑ Medicaid   ❑ Yes ❑ No
❑ Veteran ❑ Private Insurer (specify) _____   If no, primary language _____

II. HEALTH STATUS

A. **Reason for Referral** B. **Diagnosis(es)** (Principal & Secondary) C. **Surgical Procedure(s)**

_____   _____   _____

_____   _____   _____

Current or Recent Health Problems/Risk Factors that May Affect Care needs

❑ Heart Disease ❑ Head Injury   ❑ Arthritis   ❑ Falls/Unsteadiness
❑ Lung Disease ❑ Alzheimer's/Other Dementia's   ❑ Contractures   ❑ Impaired Vision
❑ Renal Disease ❑ Parkinson's   ❑ Amputations   ❑ Impaired Hearing
❑ Diabetes ❑ Neurodegenerative Disease   ❑ Pressure Ulcer   ❑ Substance Misuse
❑ Cancer ❑ Psychiatric Disorder   ❑ Obesity
❑ CVA ❑ Chronic Pain   ❑ Food/Fluid Intake Problem   ❑ Non-adherence
❑ PVD ❑ Toxin Exposure   ❑ Medication Interactions   with Therapeutic
❑ Other _____   Regimen

Level of Consciousness

❑ Alert (awake, responsive)   ❑ Semi-conscious (lethargic, drowsy, obtunded, stuporous)   ❑ Comatose (unresponsive)

Check Those Cognitive/Behavioral Factors that may affect Care Needs

❑ Impaired Orientation   ❑ Delusions and/or Hallucinations (perceives what does
(unaware of person, place or time)   does not exist, thoughts of persecution, paranoia or grandiosity)
❑ Impaired Memory   ❑ Wandering (Does not understand territorial constraints,
(forgetful to the point of being dysfunctional)   leading to unsafe situations)
❑ Impaired Comprehension   ❑ Agitation (Anxiety, restlessness)
(difficulty in understanding spoken or written directions)   ❑ Physically Assaultive
❑ Impaired Expression   (Strikes self or other, causing dangerous condition)
(difficulty in communicating needs verbally or in writing)   ❑ Suicidal (Hx attempts; verbalizes thoughts/plan)
❑ Depression   ❑ Unusual Behavior (Inappropriate verbalization,
(appears sad, helpless, hopeless; has difficulty   reclusivensess; hoarding
with concentration, sleep and/or appetite)   ❑ Other _____

III. FUNCTIONAL STATUS

A. Rate client's level of Independence
(Minimal assistance defined as including the need for supervision, verbal cueing or minimal physical assistance. Moderate assistance implies the need for physical assistance.)

Activities of Daily Living	Independent	Minimal Assistance	Moderate Assistance	Dependent	Assistive Device(s) Needed to Perform Activity	B. Additional Assistive Devices Currently in Use ❑ Glasses ❑ Dentures ❑ Hearing Aid ❑ Other (specify) _____
Eating						C. Instrumental Activities of Daily Living
Bathing						
Dressing						
Toilet Use						
Bowel Management						
Bladder Management						
Transfer						
Locomotion						

Check most frequent mode of locomotion: ❑ Walking ❑ Wheelchair		Independent	Minimal Assistance	Moderate Assistance
	Meal Preparation			
	Medication Administration			
	Telephone Use			
	Housekeeping			
	Shopping			
	Handling Finances			
	Transportation Use			

D. Communication

Comprehension
(Ability to understand auditory or visual communication)

❑ Able to understand directions
❑ Can follow directions with minimal prompting, repetition
❑ Has difficulty following directions, needs constant prompting
❑ Unable to follow simple directions

Expression
(Ability to communicate basic daily needs)

❑ Expresses needs clearly
❑ Expresses needs slowly or requires minimal prompting
❑ Expresses needs with difficulty, requiring much prompting
❑ Unable to express needs

Usual mode(s) of Communication

❑ Speech
❑ Writing
❑ Gestures/Sounds
❑ Sign Language
❑ Communication Device

E. List Restrictions that Would Affect Ability to Perform Above Functions:

F. Rehabilitation Potential:

IV. ENVIRONMENTAL FACTIORS AFFECTING CONTINUING CARE

A. Living Arrangements

❑ Own Home   ❑ Relative's home   ❑ Rental home/Apt.   ❑ Assisted Living
❑ Alone   ❑ With Spouse   ❑ With Others (specify) _____
❑ Other _____

B. Environmental Barriers	Yes	No	Comments
Are there barriers to building entry/exit?			
Are there internal barriers? (stairs, narrow doorway)			
Is the patient able to access emergency assistance?			
Other Barriers (specify)			

V. MEDICAL AND OTHER CARE REQUIREMENTS

A. Therapeutic Needs

1. Skin   ❑ Pressure Ulcer Care   ❑ Wound Care

2. Nutrition   ❑ Therapeutic Diet (specify) _____
     ❑ External Feeding   ❑ Nasogastric   ❑ Gastrostomy
     ❑ Parenteral Feeding

3. Hydration   ❑ Encourage Fluids   ❑ Restrict Fluids

4. Respiratory   ❑ Oxygen   ❑ Continuous   ❑ Intermittent
     ❑ Tracheostomy   ❑ Suctioning   ❑ Ventilation

5. Elimination   ❑ Urinary Catheter   ❑ Ostomy
     ❑ Dialysis: ___ Hemo ___ Peritoneal ___ CAPD   Treatment Frequency_____

6. Administration/Management of Medications:
     ❑ Oral   ❑ Subcutaneous/Intramuscular
     ❑ Intravenous: ___ Antibiotics ___ Chemotherapy ___ Blood Products
     ❑ Implanted Pump   ❑ Other_____

7. Skilled Services   ❑ RN   ❑ PT   ❑ OT   ❑ ST

8. Supervision/Evaluation _____

9. Other Care Needs _____

B. Patient/Family Educational Needs

❑ Self-Care Activities   ❑ Self-Management of Illness   ❑ Diet Instruction   ❑ Medication Administration
❑ Ostomy Care   ❑ Wound Care/Dressing Change   ❑ Tracheostomy Care/Suctioning
Other _____

C. List of Medications

_____
_____

VI. FAMILY AND COMMUNITY SUPPORT

A. Source(s) of Support

Primary Support	Relationship	Type of Support (physical, psychological, social and/or economic)	Availability	Limitation or Constraints	B. Community Services Utilized Prior to Admission
Name					Home Health Services ___
Address					Homemaker Services ___
Phone					Equipment/Supplies ___ Meals to Homebound ___
Other Caregiver:					Transportation ___ Adult Day Care ___
Name					Mental Health Services ___
Address					Hospice ___
Phone					Respite ___ Case Management ___
___ No Known Support					Other ___

C. Physician Responsible for Follow-up Care (Name/Phone #) _____

D. Other Individual Responsible for Coordinating Care (Name/Phone #) _____

VII. PATIENT/FAMILY GOALS AND PREFERENCES

A. Patient's Goals and Preferences for Continuing Care	B. Relgious or Ethnic Practices that May Affect Needs or for Continuing Care		
C. Family/Caregiver's Preferences for Continuing Care	D. Decision-Making Support:	Already Has	Desires/Requires
	DNR		
	Durable Power of Attorney		
	Health Care Proxy		
	Living Will		
	Guardian/Conservator		
E. Surrogate Decision-Maker (Name/Phone #)			

VIII. OPTIONS FOR CONTINUING CARE

A. Therapy/Service Needs:

❑ Nursing ❑ Respiratory Therapy ❑ Physical Therapy ❑ Social Work
❑ Occupational Therapy ❑ Mental Health ❑ Speech Therapy
Other _____

B. Durable Medical Equipment/Supply Needs

❑ Hospital Bed ❑ Siderails ❑ Trapeze ❑ Commode
❑ Walker ❑ Wheelchair ❑ Oxygen
Other _____
Disposable Supplies _____

C. The Following Options are Consistent with the Patient's Needs

❑ Home Care (no additional services necessary)
❑ Relative's Home _____
❑ Rehabilitation Facility
❑ Board & Care/Personal Care Facility/Retirement Home
❑ Nursing Facility
❑ Hospice
❑ Adult Day Care

❑ Other community services (specify type)
_____
❑ Home w/ Home Care Services (specify type)
_____
❑ Outpatient (specify type)
_____

D. Needs/Options Have Been Discussed with

❑ Patient ❑ Family/Representative ❑ Not Discussed

IX. CONTINUING CARE SERVICE NEEDS

A. The following actions are indicated to achieve service goals

❑ Obtain medical records
❑ Obtain psychiatric service records
❑ Review copies of: ___ POA
      ___ Living Will ___ Health Care Proxy
❑ Referral for legal services
❑ Application for community resources
❑ Acquisition of DME's:
❑ Referral to MD:
      ___ With recommendation of VNA services
      ___ With recommendation for nutrition services
      ___ Other recommendation _____
❑ Referral for other treatment/therapies (explain) _____

❑ Referral for mental health services/psych. evaluation
❑ Referral to support group
❑ Caregiver respite
❑ Financial planning
❑ Alcohol/Substance Abuse Treatment
❑ Long-term care insurance
❑ Alternative housing arranged:
      ___ Supported living arrangements
      ___ Move to family/friend's home
      ___ Nursing home placement

X. SERVICE GOALS / ASSESSMENT CONCLUSIONS

Care Manager's Signature _____ **Date** _____

Checklist of Suicide Risk Factors

ELDERCARE ADVISORS, INC.
CHECKLIST OF SUICIDE RISK FACTORS

Client _____ Date _____

The following ratings are based on my:
❑ Review of records *(specify)*

_____
_____

❑ Interview with staff, friends, relatives *(circle and name)*

_____

❑ Observations of this individual over the last: ❑ interview ❑ day ❑ week ❑ month
❑ Other *(specify)* _____

Historical Risk Factors
❑ A relative or close friend who died by suicide
❑ Criminal Behaviors
❑ Self-mutilating behaviors
❑ Substance abuse or dependence
❑ Checking off "suicide" on intake form or other assessments
❑ Suicidal behaviors ❑ multiple threats/attempts of:
    ❑ high lethality, ❑ high violence, ❑ clearly intended death.
    ❑ High pain tolerance ❑ Secretive attempts ❑ Anniversary attempts
    ❑ Chronic psychiatric problems ❑ Frequent accidents
❑ Other_____

Recent Specific Risk Factors
❑ In the last ❑ 24 hours ❑ few days ❑ week ❑ month ❑ few months ❑ year the client has:

❑ Had passive death wishes   ❑ Experienced fleeting ideation
❑ Experienced persistent ideation   ❑ Made threats
❑ Made gestures   ❑ Engaged in actions, rehearsals
❑ Made an attempt of ❑ high ❑ medium ❑ low lethality with:
    ❑ high ❑ medium ❑ low potential for rescue
❑ Seen recent/relevant media reports
❑ Talked with therapist or other staff about suicide intentions/plans
❑ Made a clear statement of intent to others
❑ Written a suicide note
❑ Described a practical/available method or plan
❑ Given away an important personal possession
❑ Made a will
❑ Made funeral arrangements
❑ Made suicide plans that involve a highly lethal method and a time without interruption
❑ Established access to means/methods
❑ Had a minimal social support system (no nearby friends, close relationships,
    therapeutic alliance; lives alone)
❑ Experienced significant stressors (major losses, irrevocable losses, failure in life roles,
    humiliation
❑ Other *(specify)* _____

Current Psychiatric Symptoms (*circle a number*)

- ❑ Psychological pain   Little   1   2   3   4   5   Intolerable
- ❑ Vegetative symptoms
  (sleep disturbances, restlessness)   Low   1   2   3   4   5   High
- ❑ Perceived external stressors   Low   1   2   3   4   5   High
- ❑ Agitation, irritability, rages, violence   Low   1   2   3   4   5   High
- ❑ Hopelessness   Hopeful   1   2   3   4   5   Hopeless
- ❑ Self-regard   Positive   1   2   3   4   5   Negative
- ❑ Implusivity
  (low self-control, distractibility)   Low   1   2   3   4   5   High
- ❑ Depression
  (blunted emotions, anhedonia, isolation)   Low   1   2   3   4   5   High
- ❑ Cognitive disorganization
  (organic brain syndrome, psychosis)   Low   1   2   3   4   5   High
- ❑ Other factors
  (homicidal intent with few/weak deterrents,
  motivated by revenge)   Low   1   2   3   4   5   High
- ❑ _____   Low   1   2   3   4   5   High
- ❑ _____   Low   1   2   3   4   5   High

Additional information on the items checked can be found in/at _____

Notes:

_____
_____
_____
_____
_____
_____
_____
_____
_____
_____
_____
_____
_____
_____
_____
_____
_____
_____
_____

Therapist _____ Date _____

APPENDIX C

Community Resources

Connecticut Home Care Program For Elders: Home Care Request Form

The State of Connecticut wants to give you an opportunity to stay home instead of going to a nursing home. That is the purpose of a home care program called the Connecticut Home Care Program for Elders. You can find out whether you may qualify for services from this program by completing this Request Form.

- We want to make sure that all elderly persons 65 years and over are informed about the program. We are asking that you complete, sign and return this form whether or not you qualify for services. Please refer to the back of this form for specific information regarding the income and asset level to determine if you may qualify for home care services.
- You will be expected to apply for Medicaid if you meet the financial criteria. If you do not meet the financial criteria for Medicaid, you may still be eligible for Home Care Services. Refer to the back of the form.
- If your income is below the program limit, but your counted assets currently exceed the applicable asset limit, you still may qualify to be screened for Home Care Program services when you reduce your assets to the limit. You are not required to spend your excess assets on health care. You may spend them on any goods or services for yourself or your spouse. However, you must receive fair market value in exchange for your excess assets and keep all of your receipts. When you have reduced your assets to the limit, you can submit another form like this one, which can be obtained by calling the toll-free number below.
- **Notice to Married Couples** – Under state and federal law, a married couple is allowed to protect assets for the person who is living in the community while his or her spouse is institutionalized or living at home and needing the kind of care that would otherwise be provided in a long term care institution. To obtain additional information or to request an Assessment of Spousal Assets, if you have not had one done already, and you are not applying for home care, please call toll-free 1-800-445-5394. If applying for home care services

please check appropriate box on the back of this form.

- Be advised that the Department may pursue legally liable relative contributions from spouses or recipients receiving services under the Connecticut Home Care Program for Elders.
- Be advised that the State has the right to recover monies from the estates of individuals who received services under the Connecticut Home Care Program for Elders.

INCOME AND ASSET INFORMATION

What Is Counted For Your Gross Monthly Income?

- Your total income before any deductions including any deductions for Medicare premiums.
- Count only your income and no one else's. (If married, do not count your spouse's income.)
- Count all income you get on a regular basis like your wages, pension, Social Security, Veterans benefits, and Supplemental Security Income.

What Are Your Countable Assets?

Do not count your house, furnishings, personal belongings (clothes, jewelry) or the motor vehicle that is your essential means of transportation. Also, do not count:

- **Burial Funds** – Irrevocable up to $5,400.00 for each person OR Revocable up to $1,200.00 for single person and $1,500.00 for each married individual under certain conditions.
- **Burial Plots** – For single individuals, one plot. For married individuals, one plot for each spouse and certain other family members under certain conditions.
- **Life Insurance Policies** – If the total face value of all policies does not exceed $1,500.00. (Otherwise count total cash surrender value of all policies.)

Count Assets Owned By You Or Your Spouse

All jointly held assets must be counted in full as yours unless you can show they are owned by someone else (not your spouse). This includes things like: real estate not used as your home, non-essential motor vehicles, campers, boats, bank/credit union accounts (savings, checking,

CD, IRA, Vacation or Christmas Club), stocks, revocable trust funds, bonds, U.S. Savings Bonds total cash surrender value of life insurance with a total face value that exceeds $1,500.00.

INCOME LIMITS – $1,500.00 per month or less

Asset Limits	Medicaid Waiver **	State Funded **
Individual –	$1,600.00	Individual – $16,392.00
Couple –	$3,200.00 (both receiving services)	Couple Combined Assets – $24,588.00 (one or both receiving services)
Couple –	$17,992.00* (One receiving services)	

*A higher amount may be allowed if you have a spousal assessment done (see Notice to Married Couples).

**Participation in program is based on availability of funds.

If your income and assets are within these amounts you may qualify for services.

Town of Hudson
Office of Community Development
Housing Rehabilitation Program Guidelines
For Single Family Owner-Occupied Properties

The Town of Hudson's Housing Rehabilitation Program is funded with federal and state monies made available through the Community Development Block Grant (CDBG) and Housing/Community Development (HCD) Program. The Rehab Program provides financial and technical assistance to eligible property owners for: 1) the correction of housing code violations, 2) the correction of fire code violations if applicable, 3) the implementation of cost-effective energy conservation measures, and 4) undertaking modifications to improve handicapped accessibility, as appropriate. Income restrictions apply to all residents of homes to be rehabilitated through this program.

HOUSING REHABILITATION PROGRAM POLICIES

Eligibility – In order to be eligible under the Town's Housing Rehabilitation Program, a property must: (a) be located in the Town of Hudson; (b) be in need of rehabilitation; and (c) be occupied by persons of low/moderate income (see Income Guidelines). In addition, all taxes must be current. The Town will not discriminate against any person because of race, creed, color, ancestry, religion, age, sex, marital status, lawful source of income, national origin, sexual orientation, familial status, learning disability or mental or physical disability.

Income Guidelines – The State Department of Housing utilizes Section 8 Program standards for qualifying participants in the Housing Rehabilitation Program. In most cases, income for the purposes of the Rehabilitation Program is defined in the following manner:

For all adult members of the household, income includes all: wages and salaries, interest, net business income, social security, pensions, and periodic payments including transfer payments, alimony, V.A. benefits, educational benefits, income from assets, etc. Income measure is gross income (except for business income) minus (a) $480 for each minor and $400 for each handicapped or disabled head of household; (b) medical expenses which exceed 3% of annual gross income (only deductible for elderly and handicapped); and (c) unusual expenses.

In order to be eligible for assistance under this program, each household income must be at or below 80% of the area median. Additional assistance may be available to you if you are an owner occupant and your household income is below 50% of median (see Financial Assistance, below). Median household income is based upon statistical data provided periodically by the U.S. Department of Housing and Urban Development (HUD). The income figures are adjusted for household size and are updated annually.

NUMBER IN HOUSEHOLD

	1	2	3	4	5	6	7	8
50% median:	$20,850	23,850	26,800	29,800	32,200	34,550	36,950	39,150
80% median:	$33,400	38,150	42,900	47,700	51,500	55,100	59,100	62,950

APPLICATION PROCESS

Applications will be handled on a first come first served basis based on the date the application is received in a completed form. If a waiting list for assistance exists at the time of your application, your project will then be added to the list. The OCD will inform you of your position on the waiting list. Please feel free to contact the OCD at any time to get an update on your current position. When it comes time for your application to be processed, if six (6) months have passed since your original application, you will be required to update any information that has changed.

FINANCIAL ASSISTANCE:
SINGLE FAMILY, OWNER OCCUPIED HOMES

Financial assistance is available to eligible property owners in the form of low interest (3%) and deferred payment (0% interest) loans. Low interest loans are available up to $25,000 for: 1) Owner occupants whose household income is between 50% and 80% of the area median. Deferred payment loans are available up to $25,000 for: 1) owner occupants whose income is below 50% of the area median, and/or 2) owner occupants in cases where the household income is at or below 80% of median and the head-of-household is either elderly (62+) or handicapped, or both.

Estate Planning For Long-Term Care: Sample Letter

PIERRO & ASSOCIATES, LLC

Attorneys at Law

21 Everett Road Extension, Albany, New York 12205   Telephone (518) 459-2100 • Telecopier (518) 459-2200

Louis W. Pierro
Edward V. Wilcenski
Douglas W. Stein*
Philip A. Di Giorgio

*Also admitted in
Massachusetts

Legal Assistants
Maura L. Clair
Jeanne D. Morris
Stefanie J. Zapach
Paul T. Copp
MSW, CSW-R

February 11, 2000

Mrs. Sally Smith
1675 Erie Boulevard
Albany, New York 12205

Dear Mrs. Smith:

It was a pleasure meeting with you and your financial advisor, Tom Buildweal, at my offices yesterday. I am writing as a follow-up to our meeting, in order to summarize for you several of the important points that we discussed regarding your estate planning, and the long-term care concerns that you expressed for your husband Harry.

You Are My Client

Preliminarily, I consider you my client at this time, and not your husband Harry. At some point Harry may need his own attorney, in particular if a guardianship becomes necessary for him. It would not be appropriate for me to represent Harry's interests at this juncture, and my recommendations will be based upon my representation of you.

Attorney-Client Privilege

As we also discussed, the communications that we had at our meeting are not "privileged" in the legal sense, due to the fact that the information was disclosed to Mr. Buildweal. I do not plan to volunteer the information to anyone absent your request, but you should be aware that communications shared with third parties are not protected by the attorney-client privilege. You indicated to me that Mr. Buildweal is a trusted friend and advisor to you, and you asked that I specifically share information with him with regard to your planning.

Your Husband

You have described your husband, Harry, age 74, as having advanced Alzheimer's disease. From your description, it does not appear that Harry currently has the ability to sign legal documents, although we may recommend an assessment to determine the precise level of

Sally Smith
February 11, 2000
Page 2

his mental abilities. The situation is such that Harry's condition may soon prevent him from continuing to live at home, and alternative placements should be considered. One option that is available is to seek out a facility which is designed for Alzheimer's and dementia patients, to provide a level of care called "Assisted Living". In our area, these facilities charge approximately $2,500.00 to $3,000.00 per month, which would have to be financed from your and Harry's income and resources. In light of Harry's violent behavior, however, it may be necessary to place him in a skilled nursing facility, which has a program for Alzheimer's patients. These types of facilities typically cost $5,500.00 to $6,500.00 per month, which can be paid for either by private resources and income, or by Medicaid.

Assets and Income

The assets and income that you have described to us may be summarized as follows:

House – owned as tenants by the entirety (no encumbrances)	$180,000
Brokerage account – jointly owned (highly appreciated stocks and mutual funds)	$200,000
IRA's: Yours (with Harry as beneficiary)	$ 50,000
Harry's (with you as beneficiary)	$200,000

Insurance: Harry has two policies (both with you as beneficiary):
  1) VA: $10,000 face value – $7,500 cash value
  2) Mass Mutual: $150,000 face value – $80,000 cash value (whole life policy)

You have one policy (with Harry as beneficiary):
  Mass Mutual: $100,000 face value – $22,000 cash value (whole life policy)

Bank Accounts:
  CD's – jointly owned $120,000
  Savings Account – Harry $35,000
  Savings Account – you $12,000
  Checking Account – joint $6,000

Harry's and your monthly income is as follows:

	Harry	Joint	You
Social Security	$1,100	0	$575
Pension (no survivor's benefit)	1,400	0	0
Dividends	0	$300	0
Interest	73	500	25
IRA required dist.	1,127	0	200
TOTAL	**$3,700**	**$800**	**$800**

Sally Smith
February 11, 2000
Page 3

Legal Documents

Harry currently has a Power of Attorney and a Will, but he does not have a Health Care Proxy. In addition, the Power of Attorney that Harry has signed does not include any gifting powers, or the ability to establish a trust on his behalf. In light of his questionable capacity, it may be impossible at this time to obtain new documents that would include health care decision-making and gifting powers.

You also have a Will and Power of Attorney, and after reviewing the documents, it is our recommendation that we execute on your behalf, at a minimum, a new Will, Power of Attorney and Health Care Proxy. In your Will, you should consider who will be the beneficiary of your estate, which you may want to leave directly to your children, with a portion of your estate passing into a "Supplemental Needs Trust" for Harry, which could be used to finance his care, without jeopardizing his eligibility in the future for Medicaid. You will also want to redesignate your Executor, perhaps using one or more of your children to fill that role. Your Power of Attorney should also name one or more of your children, and should include gifting and trust-making powers to accomplish your estate planning in the event that you lose the ability to do so yourself. The Health Care Proxy will appoint a health care decision-maker for you, and an alternate, and we will discuss further with you your intentions with regard to future health care decisions, including decisions with regard to life-sustaining measures. We will also discuss with you the structure of your assets, and possibly the establishment of a Trust, either revocable or irrevocable, which will be addressed in greater detail below.

Guardianship

If it is determined that Harry is unable to execute new legal documents, then consideration must be given to having a Guardian appointed to make health care decisions for him, including placement in a skilled nursing facility, and to do estate and long-term care planning on his behalf. In light of your substantial assets, and the potential long-term costs of Harry's catastrophic illness, it may become necessary to restructure assets, including the use of gifting or the establishment of trusts. The fact that Harry's Power of Attorney does not contain specific provisions to accomplish these tasks presents a potential problem, in that any such transfers by the current agent under the power of at-

Sally Smith
February 11, 2000
Page 4

torney are legally "voidable." That means they may be subject to challenge at a later date, for example when Medicaid is applied for. The need for a guardianship warrants further discussion, subsequent to the completion of Harry's psychological evaluation.

Tax Planning

The estate tax value of the assets currently owned by you and Harry is approximately $1,063,000.00. After reviewing your current wills and the structure of your assets, we determined that should Harry predecease you, he would have a "gross estate" for Federal estate tax purposes of $648,000.00. All of that property would pass to you, resulting in a full marital deduction of that same amount, and a "taxable estate" of $0.00. In that situation, your subsequent estate would then equal the full $1,063,000.00, resulting in a combined New York State and Federal estate tax of approximately $170,000.00. There would also be income tax generated by your IRA, and Harry's IRA, which would pass to you. In the event that you predeceased Harry, your "gross estate" would be approximately $415,000.00, which would all pass to Harry, leaving him with a taxable estate of $1,063,000.00. We discussed restructuring your assets, and your estate planning documents, to create a "Credit Shelter Trust", allowing you and Harry to maximize the use of each of your "exemption equivalents", which would allow you to completely shelter $1,300,000.00 ($650,000.00 for each of you) from estate tax in 1999.

Long-Term Care

Due to Harry's Alzheimer's disease, and given the fact that he is otherwise quite healthy, consideration must also be given to protecting your assets from Harry's potential prolonged long-term care stay. If Harry requires only assisted living, and not immediate nursing home placement, the $2,500.00 to $3,000.00 per month cost could be financed through existing income sources. Due to the progressive nature of his disease, however, and his long life expectancy, it is my recommendation that we prepare for his ultimate placement in a skilled nursing facility. We talked about applying for Medicaid on your husband's behalf, and the avenues that may be available to you to establish Medicaid eligibility.

Medicaid Planning

The fastest and most direct way for you to establish Medicaid eli-

Sally Smith
February 11, 2000
Page 5

gibility is to transfer all assets into your name, apply for Medicaid on your husband's behalf, and execute and file with the Medicaid application a "Spousal Refusal." As I advised you, spousal refusal is a technique that is employed quite frequently in New York, which provides immediate Medicaid eligibility. The risk in using spousal refusal is that the County may pursue a Family Court action, and seek contribution from you toward the cost of your husband's care. They may seek income and resources in this regard, and if successful you would be responsible for spending your assets down to the Community Spouse Resource Allowance (CSRA), approximately $80,000.00. Although spousal refusal lawsuits have not been common in the last few years, there has been recent activity reported from different areas of the state indicating that Counties are becoming more active and aggressive in seeking contribution from community spouses. If successful, remember that the County will only recover reimbursement for their cost, which is typically about two-thirds of the private pay nursing home rate. After discussing the use of a "Spousal Refusal" fully, you advised me that your sensitivities were such that you could not bring yourself to refuse to support your spouse. In addition, you advised that you would not be willing to undergo litigation, and therefore "Spousal Refusal" will no longer be considered as an option.

Without using your right to exercise a "Spousal Refusal", it will be necessary to reduce your total combined assets to approximately $80,000.00, plus your home, in order to obtain Medicaid for Harry. During our meeting we discussed the Medicaid "Look-Back" period, and "Penalty"period, which pertain to transfers of assets prior to a Medicaid application. If assets are gifted outright, the "look-back" period is 36 months, whereas if assets are gifted to an irrevocable trust, the "look-back" period is 60 months. The penalty period in our region is calculated by identifying transfers within the appropriate "look-back" period, and dividing the value of those transfers by $5,058.00, the "Average Monthly Cost" of nursing home care in this area. The transfer of your assets must be done with an eye toward tax planning, as several of your assets have separate and distinct treatment under the tax law. In addition, we must remain conscious of your need for income and security that your standard of living will not deteriorate in light of your husband's catastrophic illness.

Sally Smith
February 11, 2000
Page 6

Planning Recommendations

The plan that we explored at our meeting consists of a series of transfers, and the establishment of an Irrevocable Trust in your name. Again, one overriding concern in carrying out any such plan is Harry's inability to sign documents transferring his assets, and the questionable authority that exists under the current power of attorney for the agent to carry out such transfers. Provided the issue of legal authority to make transfers is resolved (which may necessitate a guardianship), we believe that a detailed plan can be established to create Medicaid eligibility for Harry in three (3) years, preserving sufficient assets to pay privately for his care during that time period, while minimizing the tax impact to you and your heirs from income, capital gains, gift and estate taxes.

One recommendation is for you to create an irrevocable trust, and fund the trust with your $200,000.00 of highly appreciated stocks and mutual funds. You will remain the income beneficiary of the trust, although access to principal will be limited to allowing your trustees to make gifts to your children and grandchildren. You indicated that you would like to have your daughter Jennifer as the Trustee of your trust, with Jonathan as the alternate, and that you would like to have all three of your children as beneficiaries equally. We also discussed potentially using an additional trust for Roger, to protect his assets from creditors, which you can establish at a later date through the exercise of your "Power of Appointment", which retains for you the right to change beneficiaries through your will. You also have the right to change Trustees under terms of the trust. Upon your death, if Harry survives you, the will can be used to create a "Supplemental Needs Trust" for him, which will allow the Trustee to use both principal and income for him, without jeopardizing his eligibility for Medicaid. If he does not survive you, the $200,000.00, plus any appreciated value, will pass directly to your children, and they will receive a "step-up" in basis, thereby avoiding capital gains tax on the sale of their securities.

We also recommend transfers of your and Harry's life insurance policies, which will have the dual effect of reducing your estate for Medicaid purposes, while at the same time eliminating the face value of the policies from your taxable estate (this will occur after 3 years—the tax "inclusion period"). With regard to Harry's life insurance, we

Sally Smith
February 11, 2000
Page 7

recommend that you consider transferring ownership of his two policies to your three children as joint owners with right of survivorship, and naming as beneficiary an irrevocable trust for your benefit, which will go unfunded at the present time, but upon Harry's death will receive the proceeds from the children's life insurance. That amount, or $160,000.00, can be held in a "Supplemental Needs Trust" for you, which would allow your trustees to use both income and principal from the trust while preserving your right to Medicaid in the future. The transfer of ownership of the policy is subject to a 36-month "look-back" period, and therefore would not be considered as a penalized transfer in month 37. Your life insurance policy can be transferred to the three children as well, naming them as the beneficiaries. You indicated that the cooperation of the children, and their willingness to hold assets, is not an issue, but I do recommend that prior to executing any transfers the children be educated as to their roles in your planning.

With regard to your home, we recommend that you transfer a remainder interest to your three children, and retain for yourself (but not Harry) a legal life estate in the premises. Again, such a transfer is subject to a 36-month "look-back" period, and your retained life estate will not be a countable asset under the Medicaid rules. With regard to tax implications of this transaction, you will retain your Star exemption, and you will continue to be able to deduct your real property tax payments. During your lifetime, you will be responsible for all carrying charges on the property, and upon your death your children will receive the property with a full step-up in basis. If Harry should require Medicaid after the expiration of the 36-month "look-back" period, and you predecease him, the house will transfer to the children with no impact on Harry's Medicaid eligibility.

With regard to your IRA valued at $50,000.00, and the bank accounts which you and Harry own, a portion of these assets will be retained by you as your CSRA of $80,000.00, and the balance will be gifted to your children, to be held by them in a joint bank account. Federal regulations provide that your IRA is "exempt" with regard to Harry's Medicaid eligibility. New York State, however, has treated the IRA of a "community spouse," in this case you, as part of the CSRA calculation. Therefore, it is likely that when Harry applies for Medicaid, your $50,000.00 will be considered a part of your $80,000.00 exempt

Sally Smith
February 11, 2000
Page 8

amount. As such, you will be able to retain only $30,000.00 of cash at the time Harry applies for Medicaid. Finally, the beneficiary of the IRA should be changed to your children.

With regard to Harry's IRA, it is recommended that you withdraw sufficient amounts on an annual basis from his IRA to pay the private costs of either assisted living or nursing home care. A budget will have to be developed to insure that adequate funds are available to private pay for three years, which will depend upon Harry's placement in either an assisted living or nursing facility. By utilizing the IRA funds, which are fully taxable as income, and matching withdrawals from the IRA to payment of nursing home expenses, it is possible to obtain an income tax deduction for the nursing home payments which will off-set the tax consequences of withdrawing the IRA funds. Nursing home expenses are deductible as a medical expense, and subject to a 7.5% floor.

We will also need to establish a budget for you during the three-year "look-back" period, and set aside sufficient assets to pay for any expenses you may incur during that time. We recommend that you prepay your burial and funeral account, make necessary repairs to your home and pay for other "spend-down" items during the three-year period, to achieve the goal of Medicaid eligibility.

At the expiration of a 36 month period, your plan will be designed so that the penalty period for the transfer of assets to your trust ($200,000.00) will expire, based upon the current average monthly cost of nursing home care of $5,058.00, and projected increases in that average. The 3 year "look-back" period on all other transfers will also expire simultaneously, resulting in Medicaid eligibility in month 37. With regard to your estate tax planning, your remaining taxable estate after Harry's and your gifting and three (3) years of "spending-down" will be approximately $460,000.00, based on current asset values. Harry's taxable estate will be $3,550.00, and he will have made prior taxable gifts of approximately $120,000.00 to transfer the remaining assets (including life insurance) to your children, which will be sheltered using Harry's unified credit. The income tax consequences of Harry's IRA will also have been off-set utilizing the nursing home deduction. Consequently, we anticipate the total cost to your estate, for both long-term care costs and estate and gift taxes, to be the net cost

Sally Smith
February 11, 2000
Page 9

of spending the $200,000.00 IRA on Harry's care during the three (3) year period.

If Harry does begin to receive Medicaid at the end of the three- (3) year spend-down period, your income will be at least $2,049.00 per month, which you indicated would be sufficient to maintain your standard of living in your home.

Once you have had an opportunity to review this letter, please call me at your convenience so that we can discuss the recommended planning, and the costs of carrying out the plan.

Very truly yours,
PIERRO & ASSOCIATES, LLC

Louis W. Pierro

LWP/kls

The CLCP/Estate Planning/ Financial Planning Alliance

A Case Example

In our example we start by presenting an investment portfolio for an elderly couple. The story of the portfolio's organization bears repeating. The wife of a nursing home resident who was about to lose his coverage under the Medicare benefit came to a care manager on referral from the nursing home social worker. Mrs. Dana Underhill was worried that the couple's assets were at risk for the cost of Mr. Francis Underhill's nursing home care. When the care manager met with Dana Underhill, she reported that the couple had approximately $150,000 in liquid assets, plus a home worth approximately $125,000. After three meetings between the care manager, Dana Underhill and her daughter-in-law at the couple's home, an additional $300,000 in liquid assets were found. *Until the care manager's financial resource analysis, the existence of these assets was unknown to Mrs. Underhill!* The daughter-in-law found one stock certificate worth over $38,000 in a shoebox under the bed. The portfolio assets that were discovered by the care manager and the daughter-in-law are indicated in bold in the following portfolio.

Obviously, these revelations had significant consequences for the couple's long-term care, financial planning, and estate-planning options. Unfortunately, this scenario is repeatedly encountered by care managers who find clients unprepared to deal with the cost of long term care, not to mention overwhelmed and confused by the medical problems they encounter.

A care manager must be able to help clients begin the work of sorting out their financial resources under the most stressful circumstances. The Underhill's estate plan could only be created accurately following the care manager's resource assessment and the portfolio organization effort the family engaged in to complete it. The care manager referred them to an elder law/estate-planning attorney for assistance. Planning was complicated by the fact that the nursing home in which Francis Underhill was placed was in Massachusetts, but his and his wife's residence was in New York. A copy of the elder law attorney's preliminary estate-planning recommendations is attached for readers to study as an example of how the care manager/estate-planning attorney alliance served the client's best interests. Note the letter's reference to a second attorney's recommendations. Attorney Wilcenski, the author of the attached letter, sought advice from a Massachusetts attorney in developing these estate-planning recommendations.

Subsequent to the estate-planning referral, the care manager also referred Dana Underhill to a financial planner to improve the quality of the couple's holdings. The financial planner's recommendations, offered following his consultation with both the care manager and estate-planning attorney, completed the initial work of the care-plan alliance. Reader's should note that the financial planner was able to establish basis costs for the stocks described in the portfolio, a key ingredient in the development of any estate planning/financial planning effort.

This coordinated planning effort served the family's asset preservation goals as they appropriately anticipated both Dana *and* Francis Underhill's possible long-term care needs. It also helped the couple to prepare for Mr. Underhill's continued residence in the nursing care facility, as well as for his possible return home were that to become an option at some future date.

Again, the following investment portfolio was organized by a care manager during three meetings over approximately six weeks time. The assets in bold text were unknown to Mrs. Underhill until the care manager and Mrs. Underhill's daughter-in-law assisted her in organizing her affairs. The question marks indicate where the financial planner needed to investigate further.

DANA & FRANCIS UNDERHILL INVESTMENT PORTFOLIO

Total Countable Assets (excluding residence): $613,079.35

I. CASH, CD'S AND BANK BALANCES

Bank Name/Acct. #	Type	Title	Current Value
Carson City Savings			
75-256784	CD	Dana/Francis	27,603.00
75-224562	CD	Dana	12,045.00
74-499075	CD	Dana	14,111.00
75-20449027	CD	Dana	11,310.00
75-23309057	CD	Dana	20,200.00
Mason Bank			
6064330980	Checking	Francis & Dana	7,816.00
9384450638	Money Market	Both	36,000.00
9320997066	Money Market	Dana (Trust–Heather)	12,052.00
6060000494	CD	Dana	6,569.00
8026784106	CD	Dana	18,520.00
8093756486	CD	Dana	26,034.00
TOTAL			**$192,260.00**

II. SECURITIES (BONDS, MARKETABLE SECURITIES, ETC.)

Company/Bond Type	Shares	Title	Cost	Current Value
Carson Cty. Muni (Water) **CUSIP – 228946H54**	50000	**Both**	?	27,603.00
Town of Morgan Muni (Airport)	50000	**Both**	?	50,763.00
Mason Financial Group (Stock)	936	**Dana**	?	38,493.00
Mason Financial Group (Stock)	710	Dana	?	29,198.75
Gibson Securities	204	Francis	?	3,151.80
TOTAL				**$173,192.55**

III. IRA, 401(k), KEOGH AND/OR OTHER RETIREMENT ACCOUNTS

Institution No.	Owner	Beneficiary	Current Value
Mohawk Bank & Trust Certif. No. 33672056	Dana	?	1,831.84
TOTAL			**$1,831.84**

IV. LIFE AND ACCIDENT INSURANCE/ANNUITIES

Company/Policy Type & No.	Owner	Beneficiary	Current Value
AETNA (Annuity) **Contract No. N044893200**	**Dana**	**All children**	55,624.96
AETNA (Annuity	**Dana**	**All children**	50,670.00
TOTAL			**$106,294.96**

V. REAL ESTATE

Description/Location	Title	Cost/Basis	Outstanding	Current Value
Smithville Family Home Smithville, NY	Dana	$120,000	00.00	125,000.00
TOTAL				**$106,294.96**

VI. BUSINESS INTERESTS

If the individual(s) needing long-term care has any current business interests, please provide a short description giving the name, location, percentage owned, names and relationship of co-owners, and the form of ownership (i.e. sole proprietorship, closely held corporation, partnership, etc.) of the business.

Please bring a copy of any agreements, financial statements, etc.

N/A

Rights or Interests in Trusts, Estates, or Prospective Inheritance:

Briefly describe or give the name of the trust in which the individual(s) needing long-term care has an interest, or the person who is the source of the inheritance. Please provide a copy of the instrument, which creates the interest, if available. If not, please advise how we may obtain a copy.

N/A

VII. MISCELLANEOUS

Asset Type	Owner	Date Purchased	Current Value
Promissory Note* (approx.)	Dana	9/94	45,000.00
Mortgage+ (approx.)	Dana	7/94	94,500.00
Mortgage (paid 6/99)++	Dana	1984	(approx) 50,000.00
TOTAL			**$139,500.00**

Remarks:

*The above Promissory note is to a family member. Note is 7% annual interest rate. Monthly payments: $291.67 (no principal curtailment provision). In my opinion, asset is not sellable. Monthly payments are interest-only payments and income only. See attached.

+The above mortgage is to a non-family member. 7% annual interest rate. Monthly payments: $699.22. Amortization schedule and note available.

++The above-paid mortagage was issued to a family member. All relevant affidavits are available.

PIERRO & ASSOCIATES, LLC

Attorneys at Law

21 Everett Road Extension, Albany, New York 12205   Telephone (518) 459-2100 • Telecopier (518) 459-2200

Louis W. Pierro
Edward V. Wilcenski
Douglas W. Stein*
Philip A. Di Giorgio

*Also admitted in
Massachusetts

Legal Assistants
Maura L. Clair
Jeanne D. Morris
Stefanie J. Zapach
Paul T. Copp
MSW, CSW-R

July 15, 1999

Dear Mrs. Underhill:

I am enclosing a copy of Attorney Warren Atley's response to my June 23rd correspondence. The letter is somewhat technical, but should be sufficient to provide you with an idea of some of the difficulties in planning for Medicaid across state lines. On page 3 of his letter, Attorney Atley highlights three possible strategies for establishing eligibility for Medicaid for Mr. Underhill in the State of Massachusetts:

- An immediate transfer of approximately $117,000, either to your children or to an irrevocable trust established for your benefit;
- Converting the excess resource amount (approximately $234,000) into annuity contracts. An annuity contract would involve an irrevocable transfer of that sum to an insurance company, which would guarantee you a stream of income for either a term of years or the rest of your life, based on your age and current interest rate.
- The use of a "caretaker agreement," which would be drawn somewhat differently in the State of Massachusetts than they are in the State of New York. According to Mr. Jones, they usually involve an up-front transfer of assets to your proposed caretaker, who agrees to provide services for the rest of your life, with the agreement reduced to writing in the form of a "caretaker agreement." This technique would not, in my opinion, be appropriate to protect a substantial amount of money.

All of these techniques present some very viable planning opportunities. However, in order to establish immediate eligibility for Medicaid for your husband, the use of the annuity presents the only alter-

1

native. I must confess, however, that I do not favor this technique for such a large sum of money, especially considering that your and your husband's care needs are in such a state of flux.

Another item that is clear on reading Attorney Atley's letter is that the estate and long-term care planning techniques that we would use in establishing your husband's Medicaid in the state of Massachusetts may adversely impact our planning for your long-term care needs. In other words, by focusing all of your planning on establishing eligibility for your husband in the short term, we may be jeopardizing your own planning needs over the long term.

In summary, after reading Attorney Atley's letter and after speaking with your care manager, I believe that what you need most at this point is time to monitor your husband's health, and time to discuss your own long term needs with your family. Thus, it is my recommendation that you continue to private pay for your husband's care for the next six months or so. I recall that during our last meeting, you were considering using some of your funds to build an addition onto your daughter-in-law's home in anticipation of an eventual move out of your current residence. If you were still seriously considering this option, now would be the time to make your final decision so that you can budget accordingly.

During this "wait and see" period, I would recommend the preparation of the following documents:

1) The six-month waiting period would be generated by establishing an irrevocable trust for your benefit, into which you would transfer approximately $31,000.00. This transfer would generate a penalty period of approximately six months before you could apply for Medicaid on your husband's behalf. The trust would hold those funds for your benefit, and any income or dividends earned on those funds would be paid directly to you. Upon your passing, the balance of the trust fund would be distributed to your children in equal shares;

2) The balance of your property, including your real property, would be transferred into a revocable or "living" trust. These trusts are asset management tools, not asset protection tools; all of the assets held in such a trust would be fully available to you upon demand, and can be the source of additional gifts to your irrevocable trust in connection with your spend down plan. This trust would be used to centralize management of your as-

2

sets and, more importantly, to avoid the need to probate your estate upon your death. Upon your death, the balance would be distributed to your children in equal shares. As we discussed, if you use this technique, there is a possibility that in the event you were to predecease your husband while he was receiving Medicaid, there is a risk that the County Department of Social Services might seek to exercise your husband's "elective share" rights against your estate, and on his behalf. In order to do so, however, the County would have to initiate a Petition in Surrogate's Court, and I am not aware of any circumstances in this area of the state where such a proceeding has been initiated by a Social Services agency;

3) A new will would be drafted as a precaution in the event any of your assets were not successfully transferred into your revocable (or living) trust prior to your death. The will would be designed to sweep any of those assets into your revocable trust, to be held and distributed according to that trust's terms;

4) We would prepare an expanded durable power of attorney granting your agent explicit authority to engage in long-term care planning on your behalf, including the power to create trusts and make transfers of your assets.

5) A deed transferring your residence into your revocable trust would be prepared and filed with the County Clerk..

You currently have a health care proxy and living will in place. They are sufficient, although somewhat less detailed than the documents that we use for our clients. I would be happy to provide you with a draft of our form and leave the decision as to whether you would want to execute a new Health Care Proxy up to you.

I believe that the caretaker agreement discussed in Mr. Atley's letter should be put on hold for now, as it is currently unclear whether that agreement would be submitted to a New York or Massachusetts Medicaid agency. This issue should be a topic of discussion with your care manager.

Executing these documents will accomplish a number of equally important objectives: in the short term you will continue to have full control over the majority of your assets, which will be in the revocable trust. As your needs change, you will have the flexibility to address them. At the same time, by creating the irrevocable trust, you will have established the mechanism for making future gifts that will be protected

3

from having to be spent on your and your husband's long-term care. Finally, these documents will streamline the management of your assets in the event you become unable to actively participate in investment and spending decisions, and will streamline the costs and minimize the risks of transitioning the property to your children at death.

Once we receive your approval to proceed with this plan of action, we would prepare the documents referenced above within the next few weeks, and then arrange to have them executed as soon as you have reviewed and approved them in their final form. The trusts would then need to be "funded," which is the process of transferring title of your current holdings into the name of either the revocable or irrevocable trust, upon our recommendation. You can complete much of this work with the assistance of your family. If you would like our office to supervise the funding, we would be happy to do so, although trust funding is a service for which we would bill separately, based on time spent.

Finally, as we approach the end of the month of July, I would recommend that you make an additional transfer of $5,010.00 to one of your children (preferably one who has not received any of the prior gifts, if possible) to continue the Medicaid transfer penalty period running. This transfer should be completed before the end of the month of July. Because your care manager and I have discussed your case at length, I have taken the liberty of forwarding a copy of this letter to him. I look forward to hearing from you.

Very truly yours,
PIERRO & ASSOCIATES, LLC

Edward V. Wilcenski

EVW/prd
cc: Joseph A. Jackson, LICSW, CCM
Agreed and Accepted:

_____
Client

Dated: _____, 1999

APPELBAUM *FINANCIAL* SERVICES

ORE BED ROAD – P.O. BOX 1493
LANESBORO, MA 01237
KENNETH N. APPELBAUM

17 EAST HOUSATONIC ST.
PITTSFIELD, MA 01201
(413) 442-5858
FAX (413) 499-6180

July 25, 1999

Mrs. Dana Underhill
87 Cross Hill Rd.
Stephentown, NY

Dear Mrs. Underhill,

I have analyzed your current investments in light of your husband's recent nursing home placement and Attorney Wilcenski's estate planning recommendations. The attached repositioning strategy illustrates how you might better prepare for meeting your and your husband's long-term care needs. Should you wish to pursue my recommendations, either before or after the creation of any trusts, I would be happy to meet with you at your home to begin setting up your new accounts. Please note that there are still a few issues to address. As indicated at the bottom of page 2, they include Medicaid planning for yourself, inclusion of your home's equity in your long-term care financing plans, the possible purchase of long term care insurance for you, and the status of the promissory notes you currently hold.

Please feel free to contact me with any questions you may have concerning these recommendations. I also remain available to consult with your attorney and your care manager at any convenient time.

Thank you for the opportunity to assist you and your family.

Sincerely,

Kenneth N. Appelbaum

KNG/khg
Enclosures
cc: Attorney Edward Wilcenski
    Joseph A. Jackson, LICSW, CCM

1

APPELBAUM FINANCIAL SERVICES

ORE BED ROAD – P.O. BOX 1493
LANESBORO, MA 01237
KENNETH N. APPELBAUM

17 EAST HOUSATONIC ST.
PITTSFIELD, MA 01201
(413) 442-5858
FAX (413) 499-6180

INVESTMENT REPOSITIONING STRATEGY: DANA AND FRANCIS UNDERHILL

CURRENT ASSETS: $613,080

Current Asset Registration:	Dana	Francis	Jointly Held
Local Banks	120,841.00	0.00	71,419.00
Bonds	102,349.00		
Stocks	67,692.00	3,152.00	
IRA	1,832.00		
Annuities	106,295.00		
Promissory Notes	139,500.00		

Recommendations from Attorney Wilcneski:

- $31,000 transfer to Irrevocable Trust for the benefit of Dana
- $117,000 transfer to Living Trust or gifted to Dana's children
- $234,000 transfer to an immediate annuity for Dana

Action Plan:

Funding mechanism for above recommendations:

$31,000 Irrevocable Trust
- $3,152 sale of Stock registered to Francis
- $27,603 Carson City CD #75-256784 registered to Dana & Francis

$117,000 Living Trust or Gift
- $102,349 sale of the two Municipal Bonds registered to Dana & Francis
- $14,651 from the sale of Mason Financial Group Stock registered to Dana

$234,000 Annuity
- $106,295 transfer by way of 1035 exchange from Aetna Annuities
- $53,041 balance of sale from Mason Financial & Mason Financial, both registered to Dana
- $36,000 Joint Money Market Account Mason Bank #9384450638
- $14,111 Carson City CD #74-499075 registered to Dana
- $20,200 Carson City CD #75-23309057 registered to Dana
- $3,908 half of joint checking account Mason Bank #6064330980.

Result: With the addition of reregistering the balance of the jointly held checking account ($3,908) to Dana, no assets will be registered to Francis.

1

TAX CONSEQUENCES FOR ABOVE

$23,871 Long Term Capital Gain (LTCG)

- $3,152 sale of stock registered to Francis (204 shares Gilson Securities)
  - purchased @ $10.00 p/sh = $2,040 Basis
  - sale   @ $15.45 p/sh = $3,152

               LTCG = $1,112

- $102,349 Sale of the two Muni Bonds
  - 51,586 Carson City purchased @ $50,000   LTCG = $1,586
  - 50,763 Town of Morgan purchased @ $50,000   LTCG = $ 763
- $106,295 Annuity 1035 exchanges – NON TAXABLE
- $67,692 Sale of the two financial stocks

       $38,493 = 936 shares Mason Financial
  - purchased   @ $27.00 p/sh = $25,272 Basis
  - sale   @ $41.125 p/sh = $38,493

               LTCG = $13,221

       $29,199 = 710 shares Mason Financial
  - purchased   @ $31.00 p/sh = $22,010 Basis
  - sale   @ $41.125 p/sh = $29,199

               LTCG = $ 7,189

         Total   LTCG = $23,871

- Bank Account transfers will have no tax consequence.
- The LTCG total of $23,871 will be offset by the self pay portion of Francis's nursing home cost.

INVESTMENT RECOMMENDATIONS FOR ACTION PLAN:

$31,000: Irrevocable Trust

+$117,000: (if added to Living Trust)

$148,000: Total Invested in Trusts

- 50% in Balanced Mutual Fund (12.48% avg. return of all Balanced Funds*)
- 25% in Growth & Income Mutual Fund (12.74% avg. return all G&I Funds*)
- 25% in Long Term Growth Mutual Fund (17.60% avg. return all LTG Funds*)
  *10 year average returns going back from 4/28/00

$234,000: Immediate Annuity

- Dana is the owner and annuitant, her children are the beneficiaries
- Monthly Income: $2,496.50 per month for 126 months
- Yearly Income: $29,958
- Taxable Yearly Income: $7,625.00
- Nontaxable Yearly Income: $22,333.00

REMAINING ISSUES TO BE ADDRESSED:

- Medicaid Planning for Dana
- Residence
- Long Term Care Insurance for Dana
- Promissory Notes

2

Three CarePlan Options Reports

CarePlan Options Reports

In Community Lifecare Planning, whenever possible, the "team captain" role is reserved for the primary decision-maker and beneficiary of the plan—the client. Here are some real-life examples of how clients have benefited from the services of a care manager dedicated to their priorities and not the priorities as set by either the health care or long-term care systems.

As one can see from these examples, an assessment may indicate an assortment of care plan options, any of which are realistic, but only one of which will be selected. As the saying goes, "There is more than one way to skin a cat." So it is with care planning. The care plan that is selected by the decision-makers—the client and his or her family—may ultimately be formed by a compromise between a list of priorities and the limited resources available to achieve them. The best plan is nearly always the one most acceptable to and supported by the client. Hopefully, the plan the client settles on will most closely match the resources available with the goods and services that can best address his or her continuing-care needs. These goods and services include, but are not limited to, the following:

- Personal care assistance
- Housing alternatives/modification
- Emotional support/mental health services
- Medical care/Medication assistance
- Assistive devices/durable medical equipment
- Transportation
- Socialization
- Vocational rehabilitation
- Caregiver support
- Long-term care financing
- Estate plans
- Family care coordination
- Homemaking
- Insurance analysis/advocacy

The following CarePlan Options Reports will further familiarize you with how the care manager describes the long-term care opportunities and helps clients understand their choices.

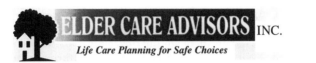

ELDER CARE ADVISORS INC.
Life Care Planning for Safe Choices

CarePlan Options Report

Clients: Bob and Loraine Soden
Care Planner: Joseph A. Jackson, LICSW, CCM
Submitted To: Lisa and Frank Damon; Patricia Olsen
Date: 10/26/99

CLIENT STATUS

Loraine Soden is an 81 y/o married white female. She is currently a resident of Stoville Health Care Center in Fitchburg, MA. Loraine has been a nursing home resident at Stoville since 8/31/99. She has had several hospitalizations in 1999 that have been precipitated by injuries she has received from falls and that also have been complicated by her seizure disorder.

Loraine's functioning is compromised in all spheres. She is wheelchair bound, dependent for transfers, dependent for toileting and bathing. Loraine's speech is impaired. Upper extremities are tremulous. According to Lisa Damon, her niece, Parkinson's Disease has not been ruled out, however, her speech and motor impairments are undoubtedly related to her left-side subdural hematoma as well. Loraine needs 24-hour supervision, personal care assistance on a custodial care basis, and regular RN assessment.

Bob Soden is an 81 y/o married white male. Bob currently lives in his own home and is eager for his wife to return there. Bob is an insulin dependent diabetic. Family members report that his physician suspects he is in early stages of Alzheimer's Disease. Bob is ambulatory and independent to all ADLs. Family reports that he can be belligerent and oppositional at times. Bob's short-term memory is impaired, however, family reports that he is currently safe in a home care setting while alone. They report no incidents of wandering, nor other unsafe behaviors such as unsafe cooking, smoking, et cetera.

RESOURCES

Health Insurance

Both Bob and Loraine have excellent health insurance. Bob is enrolled in Managed Care/Medicare through Wellcare Health Plan. His

1

daughter, Patricia Olsen, has maintained his Blue Cross/Blue Shield carve-out policy through Soden Manufacturing Co., the company that Bob founded. He has adequate pharmaceutical assistance. Loraine is covered by Medicare and a Medigap policy through her Massachusetts State employment. Her Medicare rehabilitation coverage was exhausted on 9/29/99. She has been a private pay nursing home resident at $210 per day since that time.

Income/Assets

Bob and Loraine have a joint fixed income of approximately $3,000 per month. Investments have generated additional income of up to $5000 per month. They have two joint checking accounts, one individually owned checking account (Loraine's), and one savings account in trust for Bob that totals approximately $197,000. They have revocable trusts funded in 1996, each worth approximately $200,000. Their home is unencumbered by loans and worth approximately $150,000. Joint available assets, including the home equal $747,000.

Community Resources

Bob and Loraine have received services from a home health care agency in the past. Bill receives Meals on Wheels. Due to excess income and assets, community resources do not play into their long-term care planning options to any significant degree at this time.

Living Environment

Bob and Loraine own a modest 2-3-bedroom home with one full bath. The home is small and has one floor only. The first floor is 4-5 steps above ground level. Rooms and corridors are small and narrow. Bathroom is inaccessible.

Social and Family Supports

Bob and Loraine were married late in life and had no children together. Loraine has a niece, Lisa Damon. Lisa and her husband, Frank visit Bob and Loraine often. They are are retired themselves and live approximately 45 minutes from Bob and Loraine's home. Bob has two daughters from his first marriage, Patricia Olsen and Jane Soden. Patricia lives in Fitchburg and is very attentive. She brings Bob to her home for evening meals and stops by his home every morning to make sure he takes his insulin. Jane Soden lives in Portland, Oregon and, while keenly interested in assisting in any way she can, is obviously limited by geographic distance. Patricia Olsen is joint power of attorney for Bob Soden. Bob Soden is solo power of attorney for Loraine Soden.

2

At the time of this writing Frank and Lisa Damon are planning to live-in with Bob and Loraine to enable Loraine's discharge from the nursing care facility. They intend to provide 24-hour care and supervision for a limited period of time. Lisa is a retired RN with long-term care experience.

Loraine has one surviving brother and one surviving sister, both of whom are mentioned in her will as minor beneficiaries. Lisa Damon is the primary beneficiary of Loraine's will at this time. Bob Soden's will leaves his estate to Jane and Patricia, his daughters.

Patient Self Efficacy

It is this care manager's opinion that neither Bob nor Loraine are adequate self-care managers. Both have chronic, progressive illnesses that will continue to negatively impact cognitive capacity. Neither is reliable with medication compliance or clinical status reporting. As mentioned above, Loraine is dependent for toileting, bathing, mobility, and dressing. It is not clear whether or not she can feed herself adequately. Loraine's speech impairment further reduces her ability to contribute to her own care.

CARE PLAN OPTIONS

Home Care

Loraine and Bob would both like to see Loraine return home from the nursing care facility. There are several obstacles to overcome in creating a safe, long-term home care plan for them. Should these obstacles be overcome, and under even the best of circumstances, Loraine's medical instability will continue to put her at significant risk for hospitalization.

In my opinion, it is likely that with 24-hour supervision and personal care assistance, Loraine would be safer in a home care setting than she currently is at a nursing home. Loraine has fallen in the nursing home and injured herself severely on at least three occasions. With 24-hour live-in or long-shift home health aide services, Loraine would receive 1:1 or 1:2 attention throughout the course of the day. This represents a significant increase in care and supervision than she currently receives in the nursing home and should greatly decrease her risk for falls.

There are two primary obstacles to developing a safe plan of care for Loraine Soden at home. They are accessibility and staffing.

Accessibility

The Soden's may choose to modify their home as follows:

3

1) Installing a ramp
2) Widening key doorways
3) Installing an accessible bath
4) Repositioning furniture to accommodate durable medical equipment (hospital bed, lift chair, walker, commode)
5) Constructing an additional room onto the back of the house for live-in and/or long-shift personal care attendants

Loraine and Bob's home is inaccessible to a wheelchair. It has no ramp, however, there is sufficient space on the property to install one. Any ramp would need to be over 24-feet long (or longer) due to the first floor elevation. Standard building code for wheelchair ramps is usually one foot of ramp length for every one inch of rise. If the ramp issued from the front porch, it would need to run the length of the side of the home, toward the rear along the driveway. If it issued from the back of the house it would probably need to be longer given the greater number of steps in the back of the house. The back entrance of the home also requires considerable modification for wheelchair accessibility.

The only full bathroom in this home is also inaccessible. We discussed the installation of a roll-in shower in the back room of the house during our 11/2/99 meeting.

Staffing

Frank and Lisa Damon cannot offer 24-hour supervision and personal care assistance indefinitely, nor would it be appropriate for them to do so, if only for safety reasons associated with Loraine Soden's need for assistance with transfers. Loraine will need a minimum of 8 to 10 transfers per day, some days probably more. Nursing home staff reports that she is difficult to transfer. Her ability to assist with transfers by bearing her own weight may also continue to decline. To be safe in a home care setting, Loraine will need 24-hour custodial care offered by a highly skilled home health aide serving under the supervision of an RN providing medical management services.

Aside from the caregiving needs—close supervision to prevent falls, skilled assessment to prevent skin breakdown, assistance with transfers, personal care assistance, homemaking, and so on—there are two staffing obstacles to overcome. They are:

1) If a live-in home health aide were to be sought, the home environment, as small as it is, would present any live-in attendant with a considerable psychological challenge. The home

4

has very few rooms. This would practically eliminate the
possibility of any privacy or separation time for the live-in.

2) Living-in is difficult enough with one patient. There may be
times when a live-in assistant would have two patients to
care for, however, given Bob Soden's current and imminent
decline. Moreover, if Bob does have Alzheimer's Disease,
we must anticipate typical personality changes associated
with his illness. Mr. Soden will likely become more difficult
to live with, not less. Anticipating these stressors, we must
acknowledge that in a home this small, there would be little respite or privacy for the caregivers. Staffing schedules
should therefore be spread among several different people,
rather than relying on one live-in aide.

HOME CARE RECOMMENDATIONS

I recommend the following action steps to create an adequate plan
of care for Loraine and Bob Soden's medical management and caregiver support needs:

1) **Installation of a roll-in shower** – In our 11/2/99 meeting we
discussed the design and installation of an accessible
shower. It appears that the back room of the home is both
close enough to plumbing and large enough for this installation.

2) **Ramp installation** – We also discussed the simple design for
a ramp that proceeds from the front porch along the driveway side of the house down to ground level. This would significantly improve access and egress for Loraine and her
home health aide.

3) **Staffing** – There are six care management tasks that will
need to be performed for Bob and Loraine to remain safe
in their home. These are:

- Homemaking
- Personal care assistance
- Medical management
- Transportation
- Care coordination
- Crisis intervention

While all of these tasks are important, none is more important than
personal care assistance. Good personal care will compensate for the
two biggest risks to Loraine's long-term stability–falls and skin break-

down. Given the above-cited concerns associated with the lack of privacy in this relatively small home, I recommend that personal care assistance and supervision be provided on a custodial care basis, 24-hours per day, by combination of family caregivers, long-shift private-duty home health aide services, and brief, two-day live-in arrangements.

As was discussed during the 11/2/99 care-planning visit, I believe the following schedule would suffice to expedite Loraine's safe discharge from the nursing home. This arrangement would increase Loraine's safety and stability, and at the same time will enable considerable savings over the current $6,700 per month nursing home costs. It will also provide adequate respite for family caregivers.

I therefore recommend that the following caregiver schedule be discussed with Loretta's physician:

- 8 AM – 6 PM home health aide shifts, 5 days per week, provided by private duty home health aide. (approximate cost: $2520/mo)
- 2 – 2½ days per week and three overnights covered by a private duty, live-in home health aide. (Approximate cost: $1575/mo)
- 4 – 5 evenings/nights per week family caregiver

The above staffing would cost approximately $4,000 per month, assuming a $12 per hour rate for shift work and a $150 per day rate for live-in services, calculated at 4.2 weeks per month. Home health aide and live-in help would be expected to perform supervision, personal care, homemaking, and meal prep services. Meals should be provided for the staff by the employer(s), in this case Bob or Loraine. The aides should expect to receive two weeks notice and/or severance pay should Loraine become hospitalized for an extended period of time. For brief, in-patient or respite admissions, they should be retained on salary. Conversely, private-duty staff would be expected to give a minimum of two weeks' notice before leaving Bob and Loraine's employ.

Unless the family can find qualified candidates through personal connections, locating experienced staff may require running an ad in the local paper, interviewing prospective employees, and performing criminal background checks and reference checks on them. All household employer arrangements should be made, including acquisition of a federal tax ID number for Robert and Loraine Soden, workers compensation policy, adequate homeowner's liability, payroll deductions, issuance of 1099's, et cetera.

6

Loraine's physician should be consulted prior to the initiation of this staffing effort. Dr. Levin will be signing for Loraine's discharge and any subsequent Medicare-subsidized home health aide services. He will need assurance that medications will be appropriately dispensed and that private-duty caregivers will be adequately supervised for him to discharge Loraine with orders. It is my recommendation that an experienced RN or nurse practitioner also be retained to provide medical management on behalf of and in concert with Dr. Levin following discharge from Medicare home health care services. I recommend finding an RN or ANP with home health care experience willing to work privately. Nurses that practice independently can exercise a broad degree of latitude in terms of both their services and availability that is not usually offered by agency-based RN's. Skilled professionals, either RN's or physical therapists, practicing privately need not become employees. They can serve as independent practitioners responsible for their own malpractice, workers comp., and tax deductions.

ElderCare Advisors, Inc. can assist in locating the above-cited home health aides and professional caregivers. Because Lisa Damon is an RN with long-term care experience, she is capable of performing some medical management and staffing functions in the interim. It is hoped that an experienced RN can be located to provide her with assistance in this regard. ElderCare Advisors, Inc. will provide the following affidavits to assist in locating appropriate staff:

- employment application
- home health aide job description
- household employer information
- sample home health aide interview questions
- referral for assistance with background check
- consultation throughout hiring process as needed

CARE MANAGEMENT

As mentioned above, Lisa Damon intends to perform both a care giving and care-management role in facilitating Loraine's discharge to her home. Lisa states that her ability to do so is time limited, however. It is appropriate, therefore, for Bob and Loraine Soden to expect increased involvement from a private care manager as Lisa's availability decreases. ElderCare Advisors, Inc. has provided care planning and decision making assistance throughout the assessment and submission of this report. We will continue to provide care-management assistance in collaboration with the medical management staff following Loraine's

7

discharge from the nursing care facility.

TAX CONSIDERATIONS

All of the above barrier modifications, as well as the medically necessary and medically remedial services may be tax deductible. An accountant should be consulted regarding this issue.

SUMMARY

It is clear that both Bob and Loraine Soden wish for Loraine to return home. For this reason and because they have the resources to arrange for Loraine's care and Bob's ongoing support in a home care setting, it is appropriate to consider the home care alternative at this time. Loraine's home care services are not likely to exceed the cost of nursing home care. More importantly, Loraine and Bob are likely to be happier living in their own home than in either a nursing home or in an assisted living or independent living facility.

Thank you for the opportunity to submit this report and to assist in the care planning and care management for Bob and Loraine.

8

ELDER CARE ADVISORS INC.
Life Care Planning for Safe Choices

CarePlan Options Report

Client Name: Caroline West
Submitted to: Sean Atwood and John West
Submitted by: Joseph A. Jackson, LICSW, CCM
Date: 4/12/00

CLIENT STATUS

Caroline West is an 80 y/o widowed African-American female. She currently lives with her daughter and son-in-law, Sean and Ellis Atwood, in their home in Guilford, NY. Mrs. West has been diagnosed with early stage Alzheimer's Disease. The diagnosis was made at Southwestern Vermont Medical Center's Memory Disorders Clinic.

On 3/18/00 I met with Sean and Ellis Atwood and Caroline West at their home. Mrs. West was pleasant and responsive. She was intermittently disoriented to place and time, however, she knew that she was in her daughter's home, which she considers her home as well. Mrs. West lives in a very pleasant "mother-in-law" apartment that has been meticulously designed to enable family caregiving and supervision. She states that she finds her accommodations satisfactory. Her physical level of functioning appears to be quite high. She is ambulatory and able to feed and dress herself. According to Sean she needs minimal prompting and supervision for toileting and bathing. She is quite agile for anyone who is 80 years old, let alone an Alzheimer's patient. (She eagerly demonstrated her physical prowess by standing up and touching her toes during the interview.)

Mrs. West's short-term memory is impaired. Long-term memory appears intact. She was able to identify historical sequences involving her childhood (e.g. relocation from Newark, NJ to Cleveland, OH as a young girl), high school years, birth of children, marriages and career milestones. She denied any emotional or behavioral disturbances, stating that she was happy to live where she lived and enjoyed spending time alone. She does not wish to expand her socialization opportunities, but indicated she enjoys her role as a board member for an unspecified "organization" that she stated she works for locally.

1

Mrs. West was able to communicate effectively and to answer questions in sequence relevantly. Her attention wandered at times and she displayed some tangentiality in ideation. Her responses were regularly interrupted as she had difficulty with word-finding and pronunciation. Mrs. West was smiling and engaging throughout the interview. She denied any sleep or appetite disturbance. Neither she nor her daughter reported any recent falls or problems with ongoing disequilibrium.

At the present time Caroline West is being supervised by her daughter Sean, who takes her to work with her daily. Sean owns a private bookkeeping and payroll service. Until recently the family had employed a personal care attendant for Mrs. West, however, the PCA resigned after an incident in which Mrs. West bit her. No serious injury was sustained by the PCA. Mrs. West resisted being restrained from taking a walk outside during inclement weather without adequate clothing. Sean Atwood reports other incidents where Mrs. West has bitten her also, usually following minor confrontations. Obviously, Mrs. West is now demonstrating both aggressive behaviors and problems with impulse control. Should Sean decide to continue caring for her in a home care setting, she will need to find personal care assistants who are capable of managing aggressive behaviors correctly.

CAREPLAN OPTIONS

Caroline West is in the early stages of Alzheimer's Disease. Thus, her family should prepare for an extended caregiving effort. Sean Atwood and Caroline West's son, John West, have initiated important resource management tasks by engaging the services of an estate planning attorney to help them develop an estate plan that will ensure access to community support services while protecting private pay options. The following areas should be investigated over the next few months to ensure preparedness for all eventualities:

- Respite Services
- Placement Options
- Adult Day Health
- Geriatric Psychiatry
- Family Education
- Care Management
- Community Resource Access

Respite Services

While Sean is willing to continue taking her mother to work with her, she knows this cannot continue much longer. Sean will need respite.

2

There are two primary obstacles to overcome in finding a day-shift home health aide. First, Mrs. West can become aggressive and inflict injury. It may be difficult to find someone who is willing and able to manage this behavior effectively. The possibility of aggressive behavior *should be disclosed* to any candidates as a precautionary measure prior to the home health aide's employment. A worker's compensation policy should also be in effect. Second, the pool of caregivers from which the home health aide can be drawn is relatively small to begin with given the rural location of the Atwood home. If after a preliminary search, such an individual cannot be located, the Atwood's may need to expand their search into nearby urban areas including the capital district to the north, and possibly even as far south as New York City, should they choose to seek live-in help. Qualified candidates should be certified as either a certified nurse's aide or home health aide—at minimum—if not a licensed practical nurse (LPN) or RN, preferably with home health care experience.

There are considerable risks to hiring a day-shift or live-in personal care attendant. Many of these risks can be reduced by doing a criminal and employment background check, checking references and additionally providing supervision for the aide (see the Care Management Section below). The Atwood's have compensated for some of this risk by installing video monitoring devices in the home that can monitor both the caregiver and the client and verify the cause of any injury to either Mrs. West or her caregiver that may occur while family members are away from the home. It should be emphasized that this monitoring can serve as protection both for Mrs. West (from potentially abusive caregivers) and for the caregivers (from potentially aggressive or manipulative behavior from Mrs. West).

The greatest risk to caregiver and client alike is Mrs. West's lack of impulse control. The caregiver may need to restrain Mrs. West to protect her from herself, let alone for the caregiver to protect him or herself from harm. Any home health aide whom the Atwood's hire should be trained in the proper way to restrain combative/assaultive individuals. He or she should also have an emergency response communication capability (such as a life-call pendant) to ensure that if circumstances get out of his or her control, trained personnel from either First Aide or the police department can respond immediately. At the same time, every effort should be made to keep the home environment as restraint-free as possible. If Mrs. West show signs of wandering, the

3

family should consider obtaining a CareTrak system that could ensure she would be easily located.

Placement Options

At this time, it is reasonable for Sean and Ellis to begin touring nursing care facilities that specialize in caring for people with Alzheimer's Disease and other dementing illnesses. While I am not recommending placement now, it may become necessary at some point in the future. Should placement become necessary the family is well advised to have done their research ahead of any urgent need. I have recommended that Sean Atwood visit the following four facilities:

1) Woodside Place, Oakmont, PA
2) Marjorie Doyle Rockwell Center, Troy, NY
3) Hearthstone (a specialized dementia unit) at Laurel Lake Nursing Care and Assisted Living Facility, Lee, MA
4) The "Bridges" Program at Melbourne Place, Pittsfield, MA

These facilities are appropriate placement options for Mrs. West should she need residential, custodial care. Visiting them will also initiate the family into the process of planning for all eventualities in a realistic and tangible way. There may also be other potential placements nearer to Guilford, NY. I encourage the family to do their own investigations through the Alzheimer's Foundation. I will also continue my investigations in this regard to see if other appropriate placement options are available nearby.

Adult Day Health

I am not recommending that the family investigate adult day health programs at this time. Mrs. West has indicated that she is not interested in taking part in social or group recreational activities, nor does it appear that an adequate program currently exists in the Catskill/Hudson area. There are indications that a local home care agency will be opening an adult day program for people with Alzheimer's Disease in Hudson, NY sometime this year. The family should stay apprised of this and visit the program when it does open.

Geriatric Psychiatry

It is not too soon for Mrs. West to begin developing a relationship with a geriatric psychiatrist with specialized training and experience in behavioral management for people with dementing illnesses. I have indicated to Sean that I have a connection with such a psychiatrist in the Berkshires who also has an office in Valatia, NY. As part of the overall plan I am recommending that the family begin interviewing psychia-

4

trists in the Catskill/Hudson region in anticipation of Mrs. West's fur-ther cognitive decline and potential need for psychopharmacologic in-tervention. It should be noted that a psychiatrist's intervention for people with dementing illnesses is justified for precisely the same rea-son as for people with other emotional disorders. The purpose is to im-prove the client's/patient's subjective experience rather than to accommodate the caregiver by administering pharmaceutical restraints to the patient. Conversely, medication is appropriately utilized to miti-gate behavioral disturbances that can put both the client and caregivers at risk, as well as to manage sleep disturbance, for example.

Family Education

Alzheimer's Disease is a chronic, progressive illness. As with all chronic illnesses, health management is affected as much by caregiver and patient knowledge about the illness as by the disease process itself. It is entirely appropriate for Mrs. West's family to educate themselves as much as possible about current Alzheimer's research, treatment op-tions, behavioral management techniques, and so on. Attached to this report is an article, "Clinical Stages of Alzheimer's Disease," by Barry Reisberg and Emile H. Franssen, as well as the most recent assessment tools for determining the stages of the illness. The Memory Disorders Clinic at the Southwestern Vermont Medical Center is an excellent re-source for additional information. From time to time as I come upon relevant information I will share it with the family as well.

Care Management

Mrs. West's long-term care plan must be adaptable given the like-lihood that her care needs will change over time. Her family will likely be confronted with an ongoing decision-making challenge to address behavioral management, placement, respite, staffing, and resource management issues. Aside from the actual caregiving arrangements, it is appropriate to consider the cost of care both now and into the fu-ture. Mrs. West's resources are not unlimited and the pace at which she will decline is unpredictable. It is therefore appropriate for the family to engage the services of a care management team skilled at providing ongoing care planning, medical management and crisis intervention services.

It is useful to anticipate three phases of care for Mrs. West. This will help the family to understand the care manager's role in ensuring that Mrs. West's care is of the highest quality and that cost considerations are appropriately addressed. We can identify these phases based on the realistic expectation that at some point during the progression of her illness Mrs. West will need a temporary placement in a supervised setting that specializes in caring for people with Alzheimer's Disease. The care management team would provide different services during pre-placement (current phase), placement, and post-placement phases.

Pre-Placement

Mrs. West's family has decided to care for her in a home care setting for as long as possible, but only so long as it is manageable for the family and, most importantly, clinically indicated for Mrs. West's care. The care manager's role during this phase is to help the family make home care arrangements, provide ongoing supervision and assessment, and offer objective, decision-making assistance and crisis intervention services as needed. The care manager can help address administrative issues, behavioral management issues, staffing and long-term care planning concerns. Medical management is not seen as critical at this point in time, however, it is appropriate to begin looking for a home health care clinician at the RN or adult nurse practitioner (ANP) level who can begin to develop a relationship with the family and Mrs. West, and who can provide appropriate supervision of privately-hired home health aide staff. Developing a relationship now with an RN or ANP willing to work privately for the family as a medical manager will also prepare the family for the post-placement phase during which medical management may be the primary focus of Mrs. West's care. For the pre-placement phase, the RN or ANP would need to be willing to make home visits and would focus on minor medical-management issues, medication monitoring, and home health aide supervision for any personal care that will be provided in the home.

Placement

If placement becomes necessary, the care manager would provide an important decision-making support and advocacy service for the family. At the very least the care manager will again be able to offer an objective opinion as to whether or not placement is best for all concerned. Following placement, the care manager can also offer advocacy services as warranted and can follow Mrs. West's course to help the family with discharge planning should they wish to bring Mrs. West home for custodial care during the end-stage of her illness.

Placement is likely to happen following one of three developments—either Mrs. West will become hospitalized for a medical reason and subsequently placed in a nursing care facility, she will become un-

6

manageable in the home in a crisis with an ensuing hospitalization, or she will be directly placed in a residential facility of the family's choice. If Mrs. West is hospitalized for either behavioral or medical/surgical reasons, placement in the family's residential facility-of-choice may follow an interim placement at a post-acute facility that cannot be determined at this time. Hospitals are always under pressure to discharge patients quickly from the acute-care setting to either rehabilitation or nursing care facilities. Patients and their families may not be able to exercise the latitude of choice when the acute-care bed is no longer covered by insurance, but the preferred placement option does not have a bed available at that time.

Under this circumstance the family may wish to employ the care manager to assist with both the discharge planning and transition to the placement-of-choice. The care manager's familiarity with how the system works (and sometimes doesn't work) may enable a smoother, faster transition.

Post-Placement

In my experience, people with Alzheimer's Disease whose illness has progressed to the point where they have lost mobility are considerably less difficult to care for in a home care setting than those in the earlier stages of the illness. Bed-bound and wheelchair-bound home care patients are, by definition, less able to wander, less able to resist caregiving, and less capable of inflicting injury on their caregivers. Those with Alzheimer's Disease are also less communicative and may need more immediately responsive personal care. A 1:1 staffing ratio can provide care in a home care setting by hiring long-shift or live-in home health aides who care for the patient under the supervision of an RN or ANP, and often for less money than the cost of nursing home care. In most instances, such a care management approach is actually safer than the nursing care facility which may have a ratio of 12 patients to one aide, or higher.

Should the family decide to bring Mrs. West home following her decline, the care manager would assist by working in concert with a medical manager to ensure the patient's medical stability is maintained in a well-coordinated, home care team effort. Such an effort need not be agency-based. Privately hired caregivers, including nurses and nurse practitioners, may offer services equal in quality to those of home care agencies and often at less cost. They also can practice independently, giving the family and client a more responsive, consistent service.

7

COMMUNITY RESOURCE ACCESS

Your estate-planning attorney has also advised me that upon full execution of his estate plan, Mrs. West will be eligible for community Medicaid in New York. This adds a significant resource to her personal and family long-term care resources.

I have had a great deal of experience supplementing both Medicare home care benefits and personal resources with Medicaid waiver programs in community settings. It is possible that if Mrs. West is approved for community Medicaid (as opposed to institutional Medicaid) she could qualify for significant home care supports in the form of both homemaking services (shopping, cleaning and laundry), personal care assistance from an agency-based home health aide, medication assistance, transportation assistance, skilled services (nursing, physical therapy), and so on. Mrs. West and her family may realize significant benefit (and savings) from New York's long-term home care waiver program if/when Mrs. West's level of functioning declines to within eligibility limits and if/when she becomes income and asset eligible. It should be noted that as liberal as the home care benefit may be under this program, home care agencies may not be able to fill staffing needs regardless of how much care Mrs. West is authorized to receive. Here again the family may face obstacles to meeting home care needs because of the home's rural location. These problems notwithstanding, it is entirely appropriate to acquire information about the benefits of New York State Medicaid home care waivers at this time.

SUMMARY

It is not possible to anticipate the exact course of Mrs. West's illness. It *is* possible to prepare for any number of eventualities. Mrs. West has excellent resources in all the major resource categories—health insurance, financial resources, community resources, the home's accessibility and design, her family, and her own relatively good health. None of these resources are more important than the commitment of her family. The key to the success of Mrs. West's long-term care is for the family to use their financial, community and personal resources wisely and to take care of themselves as supportively as they take care of Mrs. West. I hope this report is useful in this regard.

8

Community Resource Access and Estate Planning

The following report illustrates the often-complex planning challenge facing those who have financial resources, but who must also plan for the long-term care of both an aging parent and a disabled adult-child. This report, written by a care manager, called upon the care manager's community resource access and estate planning expertise in addressing the care planning needs of a mother and daughter. Each client had different disabilities and different life expectancies, but shared the same interwoven financial resources. Such plans may begin by addressing asset allocation issues first, and care planning considerations second. They always involve the family as a whole in the difficult process of budgeting limited resources for unpredictable long-term care needs.

The report is complicated in parts, but a detailed reading will further your knowledge of how resource management, estate planning and long-term care planning dovetail to create long-term care options for CLCP clients.

9

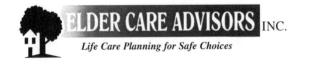

ELDER CARE ADVISORS INC.
Life Care Planning for Safe Choices

CarePlan Options Report

Submitted to: Daniel McCallum
Re: Long-term Care Planning for Jill R. and Maureen P. McCallum
Submitted by: Joseph A. Jackson, LICSW, CCM
Date: 3/16/00

CASE DESCRIPTION

Jill McCallum is an 85-year-old widow who lives in her own home with her 50-year-old daughter, Maureen. Maureen has epilepsy and is mentally retarded. At the time of this writing, Jill is recovering from valve replacement surgery in a rehabilitation facility. Her son, Daniel, also reports that she has congestive heart failure. Her current care needs are unknown to ElderCare Advisors, Inc. Jill currently owns her own home in Woburn, MA individually.

Jill McCallum has Social Security Retirement income of $585 per month. Her approximately $300,000 investment portfolio yields an additional $1000 per month. Maureen has approximately $666 per month from her state pension. She has $80,000 in assets, currently held individually in her own mutual fund. Jill has a Medex Gold health insurance policy (carrier unknown). Maureen has health insurance as a retired state employee (carrier unknown).

Jill has created two unfunded trusts for Maureen's benefit–a "supplemental" trust and a "special needs" trust. The supplemental trust is fundable only at Jill's death. The special needs trust can be funded at any time prior to Jill's death. The trusts qualify as "Medicaid trusts" or "payback" trusts. They will not preclude Medicaid eligibility for Maureen in either a community or long-term care setting. They are irrevocable, and any money left in them following Maureen's death will be paid back to the state for any care it may have subsidized during her lifetime.

Jill has two sons, Daniel and James, both of whom are actively involved and committed to helping with Jill and their sister Maureen's short-term and long-term care planning. At the time of this writing, preliminary discharge plans for Jill include retaining personal care as-

1

sistance for her on a private duty basis to provide for her needs in a home care setting. Daniel reports that a qualified individual is already in Jill's employ for 4–5 hours per day. This individual has been providing companionship and supervision for Maureen for quite some time; however, she is now willing to focus on Jill's care. Daniel also reports that Jill is considering selling her home and purchasing a smaller home nearer to James, enabling closer supervision of her care by him. Daniel has begun investigating alternative housing arrangements for Maureen. He has inquired as to whether Maureen can move nearer to his home in Cape Cod to live at The Tides, an independent living facility that houses primarily elderly individuals.

OPTION 1: AGGRESSIVE ASSET TRANSFERS

Should Jill and her family decide to transfer assets out of Jill's name (whether to protect those assets for Maureen's future care needs or to position Jill immediately for either community or institutional Medicaid eligibility) a few options might be considered. As with all options described below, the McCallum's are advised to consult with their attorney prior to initiating any estate-planning actions. The following options are described to familiarize the family with the possible benefits to Jill and Maureen's long-term care, and should not be interpreted as recommendations. The family should also consult their accountant regarding the tax consequences of any estate-planning activities involving the sale or transfer of assets.

Medicaid Eligibility

Jill can qualify for Medicaid immediately by transferring assets to the special needs trust she has created for her daughter. There is an obvious negative consequence to doing this–the assets she transfers to the trust would subsequently be unavailable for her own care should she need them. However, by creating the supplemental and special needs trusts for her daughter Maureen, Jill has clearly signaled her intention to provide for her daughter's long-term care needs both during and after her (Jill's) death.

Both of these trusts are set up to provide for Maureen's special needs–above and beyond housing, clothing, food, and medical care. Their existence provides a failsafe asset-transfer strategy should Jill suddenly become so disabled that she needs nursing home care and wishes to qualify for Medicaid (the supplemental needs trust would not qualify in this strategy, however, as it is fundable only in the event of Jill's death). They could also be used as an advance-planning option

2

ahead of nursing home placement to qualify Jill for community Medicaid. According to Rebecca Ohlander, Esq., Jill's estate-planning attorney who drafted the trusts, Maureen's special needs trust is fundable at any time and asset transfers into it do not impose a period of ineligibility for Medicaid on the grantor (Jill).

Should Jill elect to transfer all of her assets into the special needs trust at any time, whether proactively during a period of wellness, or reactively in response to a nursing home placement, she could become immediately eligible for Medicaid in the State of Massachusetts in a home care or assisted living setting as her fixed income from Social Security is below the $696 per month eligibility limit for seniors in the community. This would qualify her for certain state-subsidized chronic care benefits in the community (see discussion below). She would also become immediately financially eligible for long-term care Medicaid in an institutional setting, however, applicants for institutional Medicaid at any age must also meet the state's standard of need for care as determined by their physical disability.

Jill's home is an exempt asset under Medicaid eligibility rules so long as she lives in it as her primary residence or intends to return to it (e.g. from a nursing home). It, too, could be sold to fund Maureen's trust at any time, or may be transferable to Maureen without imposition of a period of ineligibility for Medicaid for Jill (see below).

The obvious consequence of transferring assets into Maureen's special needs trust in advance of Jill's death is that these assets become unavailable to pay privately for Jill's continuing-care needs in either her home or an independent- or assisted-living setting. Her chronic-care needs would therefore need to be met by a community support program or by family subsidy. Conversely, leaving Jill's assets intact as currently owned makes her ineligible for community Medicaid. Aside from the above-cited income eligibility limits, individuals over age 65 cannot have more than $2000 in available cash or cash equivalents. They may have up to $8000 in an irrevocable funeral contract, $1500 in a burial fund, and up to $2000 in savings. Community Medicaid eligibility may be the most significant consideration in deciding whether or not to leave assets in Jill's name at this time.

Community Medicaid

Medicaid is the state-/federally-subsidized health insurance for low-income and special-needs populations. It is available in institutional and community settings. In the State of Massachusetts, acquisition of community Medicaid for community-dwelling, frail-elderly, chronically-ill or physically disabled individuals offers not just health insurance but also enables access to several long-term care supports, four of which are vital. These are pharmaceutical assistance, transportation assistance, the Personal Care Attendant program, and the Home Health Initiative.

Medical Transportation

Community Medicaid beneficiaries may enroll in the medical transportation program which provides transportation by cab, wheelchair-accessible vans, or by ambulance to and from outpatient medical appointments. This program also subsidizes home health aide accompaniment to and from appointments.

Pharmaceutical Assistance

Medicaid currently pays for medications without limit and with low co-pays.

Personal Care Attendant Program

The Personal Care Attendant Program (PCA) is available to community-dwelling Medicaid beneficiaries who are at risk for nursing home placement by virtue of their disability. The program was started over a decade ago to empower people with disabilities by creating personal care options to prevent nursing home placement as well as to put consumers more directly in charge of their own care. The PCA Program may authorize up to 56 hours per week of personal care assistance paid for by the state at the current rate of $9.75 per hour. Program participants may hire and train anyone they choose to be their personal care attendant. The state gives the subsidy directly to the program beneficiary ("employer") who then pays his or her personal care attendant ("employee"). The state does not pay either the personal care attendant or a home care agency directly. The state also provides a fiscal intermediary to those program participants that want assistance with payroll deductions, workers compensation, et cetera.

Home Health Initiative

Community-dwelling, frail-elderly individuals who are also on Medicaid may also qualify for the Home Health Initiative administered by Area Access Agencies in contract with the state Division of Medical Assistance. This is a chronic-care program that provides a limited monthly amount of skilled home care services offered by certified agency personnel.

Transfer of Home

Another asset transfer option might be to move Jill's investments into the special needs trust, but give her home directly to Maureen, characterizing the transfer as eligible for the caregiver-child exception. Under Medicaid eligibility transfer rules, if an adult-child has been living in the home of a homeowner for more than two years and one day, and has been providing either medically necessary or medically remedial services to the homeowner (as verified by a competent medical authority), the homeowner may transfer the home into the name of the adult-child as an exempt transfer that does not otherwise impose a period of ineligibility for Medicaid on the homeowner. Such a transfer of the home from Jill to Maureen may be a plausible way of protecting Maureen's long-term housing options after Jill has died. If Maureen owns the home she can subsequently sell it and buy into a living situation she would not otherwise have been able to acquire had everything been put into the trust. There could be capital gain tax implications if following the transfer of the home to Maureen she did not live in it for two years and one day. Of course, the same disadvantages associated with other transfers also pertain here, namely, that Jill would no longer be able to either borrow money against the home or sell it and utilize the money for her care after moving to a less expensive living situation.

Qualified Term-Certain Annuity

An additional option might be to transfer some or all of Jill's assets into a qualified term-certain annuity that immediately exempts the principle in the annuity from long-term care Medicaid eligibility consideration. The state considers only the income from a qualified annuity as available to the long-term care or institutional Medicaid applicant.

At the time of this writing, Massachusetts residents are allowed to transfer assets into an annuity that is irrevocable and that will spend down to zero during their term-certain life expectancy (as set by state actuarial rules). The annuitant can designate family members as beneficiaries of the annuity. Should the annuitant die before the annuity is exhausted of funds, the proceeds can go to the beneficiaries as a lump sum payment or as monthly payments, depending on the terms of the annuity. For example, for a woman at age 85, the State of Massachusetts will authorize a term-certain annuity for a period of seven and a half years. If Jill were to purchase such an annuity today for $100,000, she would receive approximately $1500 per month for the next 7.5 years. If Jill purchased such an annuity now and other assets were transferred either to Maureen's name (such as the home) or into Maureen's special needs trust, and Jill required nursing home placement, her patient-pay amount in the nursing home would be approximately $2035 per month ($1500 from her annuity plus her $585 Social Security, minus a $60 per month personal needs allowance). The State of Massachusetts would pay the difference between her patient-pay amount and her assigned per-diem Medicaid rate. If she regained functioning to where her now $2085 per month fixed income was sufficient to privately pay for some community-based care, she could retain a discharge option that would not otherwise have been available to her had she transferred all of her assets into Maureen's special needs trust.

It should be noted that this plan would make community Medicaid very difficult to acquire, as the annuity disbursements would be regarded as income, placing Jill well over the $696 per month income limit. It would be *possible* for her to qualify for community Medicaid but not without an aggressive "spend-down" strategy–she would need to spend six times the difference between her fixed income and the federal poverty level for a senior in the community on medically necessary or medically remedial expenses to be eligible for community Medicaid for the balance of the six-month period. It is this care manager's opinion that this spend-down strategy is too complicated for the purposes of this writing and would require more advanced consideration than is warranted at this time

If assets were transferred through any combination of the above-cited strategies and Jill needed incrementally greater amounts of personal care assistance in a home care setting this could be paid for in combination by the proceeds from her annuity and family contributions. Additionally, as cited above, the existence of the annuity would not preclude Medicaid eligibility in a long-term care facility but it would create a discharge option that might not have otherwise been available. If Jill were to need nursing home care, and she had also funded her own special needs trust by incremental transfers (see discussion under Option 2 below) her own special needs trust could provide additional resources rather than those of her family while at the same time she would be Medicaid eligible.

OPTION 2: ADDITIONAL ESTATE PLANNING

At the time of this writing, Jill's estate plan is geared toward protecting assets for Maureen by transferring assets to qualified Medicaid trusts, either while Jill is alive or after her death. As mentioned above, the special needs trust is the only vehicle currently set up to protect assets for Maureen ahead of Jill's death. Other estate-planning options exist that might enable Jill to protect assets for her own care while moving assets out of her name to position her for eventual Medicaid eligibility. They are worth considering if for no other reason than that Jill's life span is unpredictable–she could live to 95 or 100. If all of her assets were transferred to a special needs trust for her daughter following her own nursing home placement, Daniel and James could be called upon to offer substantial resources to meet her special needs.

Family Gifts and Trusts

If Jill and her family are interested in preserving assets for her care while positioning her for Medicaid eligibility, assets can be moved gradually into a living trust for Jill or gifted outright. Such gifts have been made to children with the expectation that the money would be retained for the long-term care of the donor (but with no legal attachment or agreement to that effect) as this would disqualify the transfer as a bonafide gift. The advantage of this strategy is that once the wait period associated with the asset transfer is over, the donor becomes eligible for Medicaid. The money that has been gifted to a family member may be used at the family member's discretion, should he or she choose to do so, to pay for extra care for the disabled family member. Whether Jill funded her own Medicaid-qualified trust or gave money to her family, these asset transfers would impose a period of ineligibility for Medicaid of approximately one month for every \$5010 transferred counting from the date of the transfer.

The disadvantage of outright gifting is that the donor is separated from her money and has no guarantees that the receiver of the gift will make the money available. Nor is there any assurance that the money won't be spent or consumed in, for example, either a divorce or a lawsuit against the receiver of the gift. There are also tax consequences to the receivers as the money begins to generate income, dividends, capital gains, and so forth. For the McCallum's, family gifting will not be pursued as Daniel has unequivocally stated his disinterest in it. Therefore, creating an irrevocable special needs or irrevocable living trust for Jill is probably the only way to preserve assets for her needs should she wish to qualify for Medicaid over time.

Funding her own trust may be useful for Jill and Daniel given

7

Daniel's willingness to pay for some of Jill's long-term care himself. If Jill recovers from her most recent medical treatment episode and begins transferring money to a qualified trust of her own at the rate of $5010 per month, she continues to retain control over most of her assets while protecting incremental amounts of them for her own special needs (and waiting out the wait period associated with each transfer, month by month). She also moves toward Medicaid eligibility.

One Scenario

To achieve her asset protection and eventual Medicaid eligibility goals, and to preserve assets for Maureen's long-term care needs, Jill could follow an incremental asset transfer strategy, say, for a year. If her care needs in her home remained relatively constant while making these monthly transfers, she could pay privately for her care out of her own savings, with or without supplements from Daniel. Continuing with this hypothetical example, if her care needs did not exceed five hours per day for the first year ($1800 per month at $12 per hour), by the time the year would be over, she would have spent $21,600 on her care, transferred $60,000 to her own qualified Medicaid trust, leaving approximately $220,000 in her name. Her "unprotected" $220,000 could be utilized to continue paying privately or could be transferred entirely to Maureen's special needs trust if/when immediate Medicaid eligibility was advantageous. Going forward, should Jill need long-term nursing home care, her $60,000 trust could be utilized to improve the quality of her life in the nursing care facility.

A word of caution is in order concerning the virtues of Medicaid eligibility. While it is true that Medicaid-eligible individuals in institutional settings receive considerable support from their state of residence in paying for their care, their placement options may become more limited than for those capable of paying privately. All licensed nursing homes in all states must agree to accept a certain minimum percentage of Medicaid residents. It is a condition of licensure. However, once the nursing home has met its minimum Medicaid percentage quota it can exercise discretion in its admissions strategies. Nearly all nursing homes receive a higher rate of compensation from privately paying residents. Competition for beds at the "better" nursing homes can become very keen and Medicaid admissions may be refused in preference for those who can pay privately. It is possible that a Medicaid-subsidized nursing home resident could become hospitalized, remain in the hospital longer than his or her "bed hold" authorization, and lose the opportunity to return to the nursing home of his or her choice—even if it has beds available. It is important that the McCallum family understand that this remote possibility is part of the chance that Jill takes in transferring assets into irrevocable trusts. Gradual asset transfers may protect Jill's private pay options.

It should also be noted that once admitted to a nursing care facility, Medicaid beneficiaries receive the same level of care as privately paying residents. Nursing home staff members do not discriminate in the quality of the attention they offer. Nor can a nursing home decide on room changes or discharges based on the pay source.

It is also this care manager's opinion that because nursing homes are stretched to their limits, it is always beneficial for Medicaid-qualified and privately paying residents to be able to pay for extra private duty care *when they are in the nursing home!* A few hours a week of special attention can go a long way in improving the quality of life and the safety of any nursing home resident.

OPTION 3: NO ESTATE-PLANNING CHANGES / NO ASSET TRANSFERS

Should Jill elect to make no changes in her estate plan or in how her assets are held, and should she need either nursing home care or ongoing home care, she would have to pay privately for her care in both caregiving venues. She would not qualify for even the minimum state-subsidized care through the Home Care Program for Elders let alone higher levels of care through the PCA Program, the Home Health Initiative, or Medicaid.

By electing Option 3, Jill would rely on the estate plan as currently constructed and on her own and her family's resources. If she died suddenly, all of her remaining assets would be transferred into the supplemental needs trust for Maureen. As a result, none of these assets would be available to pay for Maureen's "non-special" needs such as personal care, food, clothing, or shelter needs. Maureen would be reliant on her own pension as well as family contributions to meet these needs. It is unclear to this care manager if Maureen would qualify for Social Security Survivor's benefits as a disabled, dependent child of Jill's (see discussion below). The supplemental trust could be used to pay for incidentals, recreational activities, et cetera.

Keeping Jill's estate intact will enable her to remain in the community for a longer period of time should she and her family choose to utilize the assets to pay privately for progressively higher levels of care. Obviously, if Jill were to remain in a community setting and spend her assets on her own care, less of her assets would be available to fund Maureen's supplemental or special needs trusts. It is entirely possible that Jill could need live-in services and the assistance of a care management team in a home care setting. Her care, combined with housing, utilities, food, and medical costs, could easily reach $6000-7000 per month. Her assets could be entirely depleted after four years. Should Option 3 be selected, and should Jill need incrementally higher levels of personal care assistance or nursing home care, she and her family will inevitably have to confront the difficult question—Do we transfer assets to protect Maureen's long-term care options at the expense of Jill's home care option?

SUMMARY

Clearly, Jill's intention is to provide for her daughter's long-term care security. This intention may be well served at this time through community resource planning for Maureen. Per Daniel McCallum's report, Maureen has an Intelligence Quotient below 70, qualifying her as disabled by mental retardation. With an income of $666 per month from her state employee's pension and $80,000 in the bank, if Maureen were to be formally certified as disabled, whether through a Medicaid application or through the Division of Mental Retardation (DMR) sponsorship process, Maureen would be eligible for Medicaid now. No asset transfers would be necessary as Maureen is under age 65. DMR sponsorship could also qualify her for subsidized placement in a group home, vocational rehabilitation, and expose her to appropriate recreational and socialization opportunities.

Maureen is 50 years old. Any additional resources she is able to acquire at this time will likely extend the life of her special needs and supplemental trusts considerably into the future. Acquisition of DMR sponsorship may also lay the groundwork for Daniel's and James' guardianship of their sister. Her acquisition of Medicaid may also enable her to develop a relationship with her own personal care attendant outside the DMR system. This, too, could prove to be a valuable resource for the family as Maureen has already been privately paying for personal care assistance and supervision in Woburn, MA.

Finally, one additional long-term care option for Jill bears mentioning. Jill's income from Social Security is relatively low. If she was to enter an assisted living facility and transferred all of her assets to her

10

daughter's special needs trust she may qualify for SSI-G benefits. (SSI transfer rules changed in December 1999. This transfer may be exempt from Medicaid look back, but SSI may be different.)

SSI-G is an income and medical support program for Social Security beneficiaries with incomes below $966 per month, who are physically disabled (dependent in two or more activities of daily living-bathing, feeding, dressing, toileting, and mobility), and who reside in an intermediate care facility or assisted living facility that has qualified as a Group Adult Foster Care home (GAFC). For these SSI-G eligible residents, the federal government provides additional income up to the $966 per month SSI-G limit, and the state provides Medicaid benefits as well as a medical support subsidy of $1000 per month. The SSI-G income and state medical stipend is paid directly to the assisted living facility or intermediate care facility. Some facilities offer shared living quarters to SSI-G residents, such as two bedroom suites with a common bath, that allow these GAFC program beneficiaries to reside in the shared apartment without need for additional family subsidy. (The assisted living facility receives $3800 per month from the two residents combined, approximately that which they would otherwise have received had they rented the two-bedroom suite to a privately paying individual.) Those SSI-G/GAFC program beneficiaries wishing to live in single-occupancy apartments, but for which their $1900 per month stipend is insufficient for the assisted living facility, may be able to have the cost of their residency offset by family members supplementing the SSI-G and medical stipend.

Thank you for the opportunity to submit this report. I hope it has helped you and your family in your long-term care planning efforts.

11

REFERENCES

1984–90 The Longitudinal Study of Aging. U.S. Department of Health and Human Services, Centers for Disease Control and Prevention, National Center for Health Statistics. CD-Rom LSOA, No. 1. Issued September 1993.

1994 National Health Interview Survey on Disability, Phase 1. U.S. Department of Health and Human Services, Centers for Disease Control and Prevention, National Center for Health Statistics. CD-Rom Series 10, No. 8. Reissued September 1996.

1*994 Summary: The National Home and Hospice Care Survey.* U.S. Department of Health and Human Services, Centers for Disease Control and Prevention, National Center for Health Statistics. A Vital and Health Statistics Publication. Issued February 1997.

1995 Accident and Health Direct Written Premiums: Property/Casualty, Life/ Health, Fraternal, HMDI Insurers. National Association of Insurance Commissioners. Kansas City, MO. 1996.

1995 Medicare Supplement Insurance Experience Summary: Country-Wide. National Association of Insurance Commissioners. Kansas City, MO. 1996.

1995 National Nursing Home Survey. U.S. Department of Health and Human Services, Centers for Disease Control and Prevention, National Center for Health Statistics. CD-Rom Series 13, No. 9. Issued June 1997.

Aging Parents and Common Sense: A Practical Guide for You and Your Parents. New York, NY: Equitable Foundation and Children of Aging Parents, Inc., 1996.

Ascher, Barbara Lazear. *Landscape Without Gravity.* New York, NY: Delphinium Books, 1992.

Bogle, John C. *Common Sense on Mutual Funds.* New York, NY: John Wiley & Sons, Inc., 1999.

Blythe, R. *The View in Winter.* New York, NY: Harcourt Brace Jovanovich, 1979. Boland, P. Making Managed Healthcare Work. Aspen Publishers, 1993.

Cancer Facts and Figures. American Cancer Society. Atlanta, GA. 1997

Clifford, Dennis and Cora Jordan. *Plan Your Estate: Absolutely Everything You Need to Know to Protect Your Loved Ones.* 4th ed. Berkeley, CA: Nolo.com, Publishers, 1998.

Cowan, C., and B. Braden. *Business, Household and Government: Health Care Spending.* Health Care Financing Review. Vol. 18, No. 3. U.S. Department of Health and Human Services, Health Care Finance Administration. Washington, D.C., Spring 1997.

Diagnostic and Statistical Manual of Mental Disorders, 4th ed. Washington, D.C.: American Psychiatric Association, Publishers, 1994.

Doka, K. *Disenfranchising Grief.* Lexington, MA: Lexington Books, 1989.

Duffy, Michael. *Handbook of Counseling and Psychotherapy with Older Adults.* New York, NY: John Wiley & Sons, Inc., Publishers, 1999.

Freedman, Donald N., and Emily S. Starr. *Estate Planning for the Aging or Incapacitated Client in Massachusetts.* Boston, MA: Massachusetts Continuing Legal Education, Inc., 1999 Revised Edition.

Fries, J. and C. E. Koop, et al. "Reducing Health Care Costs by Reducing the Need and Demand for Medical Services." *New England Journal of Medicine* 329:321-325 (July 29, 1993).

Garner, Robert J., Charles L. Ratner, Barbara J. Raasch, and Martin Missenbaum. *Ernst & Young's Personal Financial Planning Guide,* Third ed. New York, NY: John Wiley & Sons, Inc., 1999.

Gladwell, M. "The Alzheimer's Strain: The Next Health Care Crisis." *The New Yorker,* 20 and 27 October 1997, 124-139.

Greenleaf, Robert K. *Servant Leadership: A Journey Into the Nature of Legitimate Power and Greatness.* New York, NY: Paulist Press, Publishers, 1991.

Grosel, Charles, Melinda Hamilton, Julie Koyano, and Susan Eastwood. *Health & Health Care 2010: The Forecast, the Challenge.* Prepared by The Institute for the Future. San Francisco, CA: Jossey-Bass, Publishers, 2000.

Haupt, B. *Characteristics of Hospice Care Discharges: United States, 1993–94.* U.S. Department of Health and Human Services, Centers for Disease Control and Prevention, National Center for Health Statistics. Advance Data, No. 287. April, 1997.

Hoffman, C., Rice D., et al. *Chronic Care in America: A 21st Century Challenge.* San Francisco, CA: The Institute for Health and Aging. Princeton: The Robert Wood Johnson Foundation. August 1996.

Holloway, Nancy. *Medical Surgical Care Planning-Second Edition.* Spring House, PA: Spring House Corporation, 1993.

Kaplan, Mary, and Stephanie B. Hoffman. *Behaviors in Dementia: Best Practices for Successful Management.* Health Professions Press, 1998.

Kasle, Annette Levinson. *New York Elder Law Handbook.* New York, NY: Practicing Law Institute, 1999.

Kenney, James, et al. *Elder Care: Coping With Late-Life Crisis.* Golden Age Books: Perspectives on Aging, 1989.

Levit, K., Lazenby, H., et al. *National Health Expenditures, 1995.* Health Care Financing Review. Vol. 18, No. 1 U.S. Department of Health and Human Services, Health Care Finance Administration, Washington, D.C., Fall, 1996.

Lorig, K., et al. *Living a Healthy Life With Chronic Conditions.* Palo Alto, CA: Bull Publishing Company, 1994.

The Merck Manual, 16th ed. Rahway, NJ: Merck Research Laboratories, 1992.

The Merck Manual of Geriatrics, 2nd ed. Rahway, NJ: Merck Research Laboratories, 1995.

Molloy, William. *Caring for Your Parents in Their Senior Years: A Guide for Grown-Up Children*, Firefly Books, 1998.

Moses, Ken, and Robert Kearney. *Transition Therapy: An Existential Approach to Facilitating Growth in the Light of Loss.* Evanston, IL: Resource Networks, Inc., 1995.

Orodenker, S. *Family Caregiving in a Changing Society: The Effects of Employment on Caregivers Stress.* Garland. Studies on Elderly in America, 1991.

Pastan, Linda. *The Five Stages of Grief.* New York, NY: W.W. Norton & Co., Inc., 1978.

Phillips, S., and P. Benner. *The Crisis of Care: Affirming and Restoring Caring Practices in the Helping Professions.* Washington, D.C.: Georgetown University Press, 1994.

Pick, T. Pickering, Robert Howden, and Henry Gray. *Gray's Anatomy.* New York, NY: Gramercy Books, 1977.

Regan, John J, J.S.D. *Tax, Estate & Financial Planning for the Elderly.* Albany, NY: Matthew Bender, 1998.

Reuben, David B., George T. Grossbert, Lorraine C. Mion, James T. Pacala, Jane F. Potter, Todd P. Semla, *Geriatrics At Your Fingertips.* 1998/99 edition. Belle Mead, NJ: Excerpta Medica, Inc.

Stern, E. Mark. *Psychotherapy and the Grieving Patient.* New York , NY: Hadworth Press, Inc., 1985.

Strauss, Peter J., and Nancy M. Lederman. *The Elder Law Handbook.* New York, NY: Facts On File, Inc., 1996.

Tatelbaum, Judy. *The Courage to Grieve.* New York, NY: Harper and Row.

Thomas, Clayton, L. *Taber's Cyclopedic Medical Dictionary*, 18th ed. Philadelphia, PA: F. A. Davis Company, Publishers, 1997.

Tirrito, Terry, Nieli Langer, and Ilene L. Nathanson. *Elder Practice: A Multidisciplinary Approach to Working With Older Adults in the Community.* Univ. of South Carolina Press, 1996.

Warner, Ralph. *Investing for Retirement: How to Make Good Choices Without Getting a Ph. D. in Finance.* Berkeley, CA: Nolo.com Publishers, 1999.

Worden, J. William. *Grief Counseling & Grief Therapy: A Handbook for the Mental Health Practitioner.* New York, NY: Springer Co., Inc., 1992.

Wright, Beatrice. *Physical Disability: A Psychological Approach.* New York, NY: Harper & Row, 1960.

INDEX

ABOUT THE CONTRIBUTORS

Jackie Birmingham, RN, MS, CMAC is the Director of Network Integration for Integrated Healthcare Networks, Inc. of Newton, MA. Nationally and internationally recognized as a leader in continuity of care reform, Jackie provides expertise in discharge planning and case management. Jackie was director of Discharge Planning at Hartford Hospital from 1983–1993, has worked in high-tech home care, and has provided services to both acute-care and provider-based case managers. She has authored several books and journal articles focusing on clinical issues related to continuity of care. In 2000, the Case Management Society of America honored Jackie as "Distinguished Case Manager of the Year."

David N. Hornick, MD, MPH is board certified in emergency medicine and board prepared in internal medicine, geriatrics and public health. Dr. Hornick's research interests center around developing optimized systems for the delivery of non-institutional, community-based, long-term care. He has directed demonstration projects in home tele-healthcare and redesign of apartments for the elderly utilizing universal design technology. He is recent past president of the Capital Area Consortium on Aging and Disability in Albany, NY and former member of the board of directors of the American Academy of Home Care Physicians. He is currently developing a medical practice limited to home medical care in Schenectady, N.Y.

Roberta Miller, MD is board certified in Internal Medicine and certified in Hospice and Palliative Care. Dr. Miller is an Assistant Professor of Medicine at Albany Medical College and the Medical Director of the Home Based Primary Care Program at the Upstate Veterans Affairs Medical Center New York At Albany. She has received a grant for The Expansion of Home Care into Academic Medicine from the John A. Hartford Foundation and the Director of the Home Care Training Institute. Dr. Miller is an active member of the American Academy of Home Care Physicians and is currently involved in telemedicine applications in home health care.

Louis W. Pierro, Esq. is a practicing attorney who for the past 16 years has focused on representing individuals, families and small business owners in Estate and Long-Term Care Planning, Elder Law, Estate and Trust Administration, and Business Succession Planning. Mr. Pierro is Chair-Elect of the New York State Bar Association Elder Law Section, Vice-Chair of the Trusts and Estates Law Section Estate Planning Committee, and serves as a member of both Sections' Executive Committees. He is a member of the National Academy of Elder Law Attorneys and the American Bar Association Probate and Property Section. His law firm, Pierro & Associates, LLC, is located in Albany, NY.

Robert E. O'Toole, LICSW, BCD is a founding member of the National Association of Professional Geriatric Care Managers. He is a former editor of Geriatric Care Management Journal and is adjunct Professor of Gerontology at Stonehill College. His articles on elder care issues have appeared in several publications. Mr. O'Toole is also an independent broker specializing in Long Term Care insurance, viatical settlements and other approaches to paying the costs of long-term care. He owns and operates Informed Decisions, Inc., based in Dedham, MA.

Enrique J. Alvarez, MSFS, CLU, ChFC owns and operates Professional Insurance Brokerage, Inc. and Advanced Retirement Concepts, LLC in Suffield, CT. Enrique is a Chartered Life Underwriter, Chartered Financial Consultant, Registered Health Underwriter, Registered Employee Benefits Consultant and Master of Science in Financial Services. He is on the advisory board of The American College and is a member of The Society of Financial Professionals as well as Suffield Chamber of Commerce.

Debra A. Jarck, RN, ACNP is an Acute Care Nurse Practitioner currently providing outpatient primary care services in Pittsfield, MA. Debra is an experienced ICU and IV therapy nurse and has a decade-long career in home health care. Debra has been a consultant and author for numerous nursing publications, including *The Nurse Practitioner Drug Book* and *The IV Therapy Handbook* (Springhouse Publications). She is also developing an independent private practice offering medical management and chronic care for homebound long-term care consumers in western Massachusetts.

Paul T. Copp, MSW, CSW-R is Executive Director of the National Alliance for the Mentally Ill–New York. His 20-year professional and academic career has included health and human service administration, health economics education, institutional medical, case management, preventive health care, medical social work, long-term care and end-of-life care. Mr. Copp is an authority in geriatrics and gerontology. He is a licensed therapist specializing in family therapy and helping individuals challenged by chronic disease.